Pharmaceutics-I

[*Revised Sixth Edition*]

R. M. Mehta

B. Sc., M. Pharm., A.I.C.

VALLABH PRAKASHAN®

ISBN 978-93-85529-00-9
VPBN 26

First Edition 1994
Second Edition 1996
Third Edition 2002
Fourth Edition 2007
Fifth Edition 2010
Sixth Edition 2015
7th Reprint 2023

Published by
M K Jain for VALLABH PRAKASHAN®
C-5, SMA Cooperative Industrial Estate
GT Karnal Road, DELHI-110033
phone : 9868678074
e-mail : mail@vallabhprakashan.in

₹ **200** (local)
₹ **210** (outstation)
₹ **600** (overseas)

Printed at
Deepak Pustak Bandhnalaya, UP

Preface to the Sixth Edition

It is a great pleasure for me to place the Sixth (Revised) Edition 2015. The subject matter particularly the chapters on 'Introduction to dosage forms', Introduction to pharmacopoeias, metrology, packing of pharmaceuticals, extraction processes have been revised and updated for the benefit of students.

I hope the present edition will prove to be more useful to the faculty and students. The suggestions for further improvement will be thankfully acknowledged.

ROHTAK
28 May, 2015

– R.M. Mehta

Preface to the First Edition

Since writing my earlier book on Pharmaceutics II, the curriculum for Diploma in Pharmacy has been considerably revised by the Pharmacy Council of India by its new Education Regulations 1991.

The present book has been written strictly in accordance with the revised syllabus of Pharmaceutics I. The subject-matter is presented in simple, concise and easily understandable language. I have tried to incorporate the latest information available on various subjects to enable the students to accurately prepare various dosage form. The other salient features of the book are as under:

(*i*) The illustrations and diagrams have been included to help the student in comprehending the various processes discussed easily.

(*ii*) The diagrams are neatly drawn and adequately labelled.

(*iii*) As an aid to the student to test his own comprehension of the subject matter discussed, several types of exhaustive Revision Questions have been given at the end of each chapter.

(*iv*) To enhance the utility of the Revision Questions, these have been given in the form of multiple choice questions, fill in the blanks type, match the columns, very short answer questions, short answer questions and long answer questions.

(*v*) The useful terms are given at the end of the book.

I have tried to make the book as informative and exhaustive as possible within the constraints of time allotted to the subject.

Thanks are due to my wife Mrs. Madhu Mehta for her inspiration and cooperation and valuable suggestions from time to time in preparing this book.

I also express my gratitude to Mr. Manish K. Jain of M/s Vallabh Prakashan for his keen interest and painstaking efforts in the publication of this book and for its fine get-up.

Suggestion and comments from teachers and students are welcome and will be gratefully acknowledged.

ROHTAK
10 October, 1993

– R.M. Mehta

Syllabus of Pharmaceutics-I

(as per Education Regulations 1991)

Theory (75 hours)

1. Introduction of different dosage forms. Their classification with examples—their relative applications. Familiarisation with new drug delivery systems.

2. Introduction to Pharmacopœias with special reference to the Indian Pharmacopoeia.

3. Metrology—Systems of weights and measures. Calculations including conversion from one to another system, Percentage calculations and adjustment of products. Use of alligation method in calculations. Isotonic solutions.

4. Packaging of Pharmaceuticals-Desirable features of a container-types of containers. Study of glass and plastics as materials for containers and rubber as a material for closures-their merits and demerits. Introduction to aerosol packaging.

5. Size reduction—Objectives, and factors affecting size reduction, methods of size reduction—Study of Hammer Mill, Ball Mill, Fluid Energy Mill and Disintegrator.

6. Size separation-Size separation by sifting. Official standards for powders. Sedimentation methods of size separation. Construction and working of Cyclone Separator.

7. Mixing and Homogenisation-Liquid mixing and powder mixing, Mixing of semisolids. Study of Silverson Mixer-Homogeniser, Planetary Mixer, Agitated powder mixer; Triple Roller Mill; Propeller Mixer, Colloidal Mill and Hand Homogeniser, Double Cone Mixer.

8. Clarification and Filtration—Theory of filtration, Filter media; Filter aids and selection of filters. Study of the following filtration equipment-Filter Press, Sintered Filters, Filter Candles, Metafilter.

9. Extraction and Galenicals—(*a*) Study of percolation and maceration and their modifications, continuous hot extraction-Applications in the preparation of tinctures and extracts. (*b*) Introduction to Ayurvedic dosage forms.

10. Heat processes—Evaporation-Definition Factors affecting evaporation-Study of Evaporating Still and Evaporating Pan.

11. Distillation—Simple distillation and Fractional distillation; Steam distillation and Vacuum distillation. Study of Vacuum still, preparation of Purified Water I.P. and Water for Injection I.P. Construction and working of the still used for the same.

12. Introduction to drying processes—Study of Tray Dryers: Fluidized Bed Dryer, Vacuum Dryer and Freeze Dryer.

13. Sterilization—Concept of sterilization and its difference from disinfection-Thermal resistance of microorganisms. Detailed study of the following sterilisation processes.

(*i*) Sterilization with moist heat,

(*ii*) Dry heat sterilization,

(*iii*) Sterilization by radiation,

(*iv*) Sterilization filtration and

(*v*) Gaseous sterilization.

Aseptic techniques—Application of sterilization processes in hospitals particularly with reference to surgical dressings and intravenous fluids. Precautions for safe and effective handling of sterilization equipment.

14. Processing of Tablets-Definition; Different types of compressed tablets and their properties. Processes involved in the production of tablets; Tablets excipients; Defects in tablets; Evaluation of tablets; Physical standards including Disintegration and Dissolution. Tablet coating-Sugar coating; film coating, enteric coating and microencapsulation (Tablet coating may be dealt in an elementary manner).

15. Processing of Capsules—Hard and soft gelatin capsules; different sizes of capsules; filling of capsules; handling and storage of capsules. Special applications of capsules.

16. Study of immunological products like sera, vaccines, toxoids and their preparations.

Contents

1

Introduction to Different Dosage Forms

A drug may be defined as an agent, intended for use in the diagnosis, mitigation, treatment, cure or prevention of disease in man or in other animals. Drugs are rarely administered in their original pure state. They are administered in different dosage forms after converting them into a suitable formulation. Every dosage form is a combination of the drug and different kinds of non-drug components called "additives". The additives are used to give a particular shape to the formulation, to increase its stability and also to increase its palatability as well as to give more elegance to the preparation.

Importance of Dosage Forms

Transformation of drug into different dosage forms is done for the following reasons:

1. To provide a safe and convenient delivery of accurate dosage.
2. Many dosage forms can be easily identified from their distinct colour, shape or identifying markings.
3. To protect the drug substance from oxidation, hydrolysis, and reduction *e.g.* coated tablets and sealed ampoules.
4. To protect the drugs from the destructive effect of gastric juice (Hydrochloric acid) of the stomach after oral administration *e.g.* enteric coated tablets.
5. To conceal the bitter, salty or obnoxious taste or odour of a drug substance *e.g.* capsules, coated tablets and flavoured syrups etc.
6. To provide for the insertion of the drug into one of the body cavities *e.g.* rectal or vaginal suppositories.
7. To provide for the optimum drug action through inhalation therapy *e.g.* inhalation aerosols and inhalants.

DOSAGE FORMS

- SOLID DOSAGE FORMS
  - UNIT DOSAGE FORM
    - Tablets
    - Capsules
    - Powders
    - Pills
  - BULK
    - INTERNAL
      - FINE POWDERS
      - GRANULES & EFFERVESCENT GRANULES
    - EXTERNAL
      - Dusting powders
      - Insufflations
      - Dentifrices (Tooth powders)
      - Snuffs
- LIQUID DOSAGE FORMS
  - MONOPHASIC
    - EXTERNAL
      - Liniments
      - Lotions
      - Gargles
      - Throat paints
      - Mouth washes
      - Sprays
      - Eye lotions
      - Eye drops
      - Nasal drops
    - INTERNAL
      - Syrups
      - Eiixirs
      - Linctus
      - Drops
  - BIPHASIC
    - Emulsions
    - Suspensions
- SEMI-SOLID DOSAGE FORMS
  - EXTERNAL
    - Ointments
    - Creams
    - Pastes
    - Jellies
  - INTERNAL
    - Suppositories
    - Pessaries

8. To provide the maximum drug action from topical administration sites *e.g.* creams, ointments, ophthalmic preparations and E.N.T. (Ear, Nose and Throat) preparations.
9. To provide sustained released action through controlled released mechanism, *e.g.* sustained released tablets, capsules and suspensions.
10. To provide liquid dosage form of the drugs soluble in a suitable vehicle *e.g.* solutions.
11. To provide liquid preparation of the drugs which are insoluble or unstable in different vehicles *e.g.* suspensions.
12. To provide the drugs within body tissues *e.g.* injections.

▩ CLASSIFICATION OF DOSAGE FORMS ▩

Dosage forms may be classified on the basis of physical form of the final product which are as under:

1. Solid dosage form
2. Liquid dosage form
3. Semi-solid dosage form

▩ SOLID DOSAGE FORMS ▩

The solid dosage forms are available mostly in unit dosage forms (consisting of doses which are taken by numbers) such as tablets, capsules, pills, cachets or powders. When drugs are to be administered orally in dry state, tablets and capsules are the most convenient dosage form. They are effective and patients have no problem in their handling, identification and administration. Some solids are packed and supplied in bulk. The bulk forms meant for internal use are supplied either as granules or fine powder. The bulk powders meant for external use are dusting powders, insufflations, snuffs and tooth powders.

Powders are the solid dosage form of medicament, which are meant for internal or external use. They are available in crystalline or amorphous form. The powders are generally used in the following forms:

1. Bulk powder for internal use *e.g.* fine powders or granules
2. Bulk powder for external use *e.g.* snuffs, dusting powders tooth powders and insufflation.
3. Simple and compound powders for internal use.
4. Powders in the form of compressed tablets and tablet triturates.
5. Powders enclosed in cachets and capsules.

Dusting Powders

These are meant for external application to the skin and are generally applied in a very fine state of subdivision to avoid local irritation. Hence, dusting powders should be passed through a 80 sieve to enhance their effectiveness.

Dusting powders are of two types:

(*i*) Medical

(*ii*) Surgical

Medical dusting powders are used mainly for superficial skin conditions whereas surgical dusting powders are used in body cavities and also on major wounds as a result of burns and umbilical cords of infants. Surgical dusting powders must be sterilised before their use, whereas medical dusting powders must be free from dangerous pathogenic micro-organisms.

Dusting powders are generally prepared by mixing two or more ingredients one of which must be either starch, kaolin or talc as one of the ingredients of the formulation. Talc and kaolin are more commonly used because these are chemically inert. However, since such ingredients are readily contaminated with pathogenic bacteria, these must be sterilised dry heat method (160° for 2 hours) before their use..

The dusting powders are mainly used for their antiseptic, astringent, absorbent, antiperspirant and antipruritic action.

Insufflations

These are medicated dusting powders meant for introduction into the body cavities such as nose, throat, ears and vagina with the help of an apparatus known as "Insufflator". It sprays the powder into a stream of finely divided particles all over the site of application. The following difficulties are however generally faced while using the insufflators:

(*i*) It is difficult to obtain a measured quantity of the drug as a uniform dose.

(*ii*) It gets blocked when it is slightly wet or the powder used is wet.

Insufflations should be in finely divided powders so that a stream of fine particles of medicaments gets applied to the site of application. Nowadays the insufflations are available in the form of pressure aerosols. These are used for the administration of potent drugs. This method has the advantage of excellent control of dose through metered valves. Moreover, it also protects the product from external environment.

The insufflations are used to produce a local effect, as in the treatment of ear, nose and throat infection with antibiotics or to produce a systemic effect from a drug that is destroyed in the gut.

Snuffs

These are finely divided solid dosage forms of medicament which are inhaled into nostrils for its antiseptic, bronchiodilator and decongestion action.

Dentifrices (Tooth powders)

These are applied with the help of a tooth brush for cleaning the surface of the teeth. They contain a suitable detergent or soap, some abrasive substance and a suitable flavour. The abrasive agents such as calcium sulphate, magnesium carbonate, sodium carbonate and sodium chloride are used in fine powder. A strong abrasive substance should however not to be used as it may damage the tooth structure.

The commonly used formula of dentifrice is as follows.

DENTIFRICE (NF XI)

Hard soap, in fine powder	50 g
Precipitated calcium carbonate	935 g
Saccharin sodium	2 g
Peppermint oil	4 ml
Cinnamon oil	2 ml
Methyl salicylate	8 ml

Triturate the saccharin sodium, the oils and methyl salicylate with about one half of the precipitated calcium carbonate and mix the soap with the remaining portion of the precipitated calcium carbonate. Mix the two powders thoroughly and then pass it through a fine sieve.

Granules

The bitter, nauseous and unpleasant powders cannot be given in tablet form or in a capsule because a large number of them are required to be taken as a single dose. These powders are not given in liquid form because of stability problem. Such medicaments are given in the form of granules.

The solid medicaments are mixed with sweetening, flavouring and colouring agent. A suitable granulating agent is added to moisten the powder so as to form a coherent mass. The coherent mass is passed through sieve number 10 to make granules. Dry the granules in an hot air oven at a temperature no exceeding 60°C. The dry granules are passed through sieve number 20. The dry granules are supplied in single-dose sachets which are dissolved in water before taking.

Now-a-days, various antibiotics like erythromycin, ampicillin, phenoxymethyl penicillin etc., which are unstable in solution are prepared in the dry granular form in which drug is mixed with suspending, sweetening, flavouring, colouring and granulating agents. The granules are prepared and packed in a special type of bottles with a specific direction on its label for the patient to add specific amount of freshly boiled and cooled water to dissolve it or shake well to form a homogenous solution. The label should also state the time limit within which the reconstituted preparation should be consumed.

Effervescent Granules

The effervescent granules are the specially prepared solid dosage form of medicament, meant for internal use. They contain a medicament mixed with citric acid, tartaric acid and sodium bicarbonate. Sometimes saccharin or sucrose may be added as a sweetening agent. Before administration, the desired quantity is dissolved in water, the acid and bicarbonate react together producing effervescence. The carbonated water produced from the release of carbon dioxide serves to mask the bitter and saline taste of drugs. Moreover, carbon dioxide stimulates the flow of gastric juice and helps in the absorption of medicament.

Methods of preparation There are two methods of preparation of effervescent granules.

1. Heat method
2. Wet method

Heat method A large porcelain or stainless steel evaporating dish is placed over the boiling water bath. The dish must be sufficiently hot before transferring the powder into it, to ensure rapid liberation of the water of the crystallisation from the citric acid. If heating of the dish is delayed, the powder which is added to it, will heat up slowly and the liberated water of crystallisation will go on evaporating simultaneously. As a result, sufficient water will not be available to make a coherent mass.

The water needed for granulation is provided from two sources:

(*i*) From water of crystallisation of citric acid. The citric acid contains one molecule of water of crystallisation which is liberated during heating.

(*ii*) The water produced from the reactions of citric acid and tartaric acid with sodium bicarbonate.

$$\underset{\text{Sodium bicarbonate}}{3NaHCO_3} + \underset{\text{Citric acid}}{C_6H_8O_7.H_2O} \xrightarrow{\Delta} \underset{\text{Sodium citrate}}{C_6H_5Na_3O_7} + 3CO_2 + 3H_2O$$

$$\underset{}{2NaHCO_3} + \underset{\text{Tartaric acid}}{C_4H_6O_6} \xrightarrow{\Delta} \underset{\text{Sodium tartarate}}{C_4H_4Na_2O_6} + 2CO_2 + 2H_2O$$

Generally, heating stage takes 1 to 5 minutes. The damp mass is then passed through a sieve to prepare the granules of suitable size, dried in an oven at a temperature not exceeding 60°C and then packed in an air tight container.

Wet method In this method, the mixed ingredients are moistened with a non-aqueous liquid (*e.g.* Alcohol) to prepare a coherent mass which is then passed through a No. 8 sieve and dried in an oven at a temperature not exceeding 60°C. The dried granules are again passed through the sieve to break the lumps which may be formed during drying. The dried granules are packed in air tight containers.

Tablets

These are solid dosage forms of medicament or medicaments which are prepared by moulding or by compression. Certain excipients are also added to the medicaments in the formulation of tablets. The compressed tablets are prepared in bulk by the large-scale production methods. (Detail is given in the chapter, "Processing of Tablets")

Capsules

The capsules are solid unit dosage form in which one or more medicaments and inert substances are enclosed within a small shell, generally prepared from a suitable form of gelatin. Depending on their formulation, the gelatin capsule shell may be hard or soft. (Detail is given in the chapter, "Processing of Capsules")

Pills

Pills are small rounded solid dosage forms containing medicament and are intended to be administered orally. The medicaments are mixed with excipients to form a firm plastic mass. The mass is rolled to uniform pill pipe, which is cut into a number of pills. These are rounded to form pills of uniform size and shape. Pills are spherical in shape and are produced by rolling them under wooden pill rounder. The pills are sometimes coated with varnish, silver leaf, gold leaf to improve the finish, mask the unpleasant tastes and increase stability.

In olden days pills were preferred because of their spherical shape which can be easily swallowed. But now the pills are outdated preparations because of a number of disadvantages such as:

1. The disintegration time of pills is uncertain. The freshly prepared pills disintegrate readily as compared to the old dried pills.

The dried pills are less soluble and sometimes pass through G.I.T. without disintegration.

2. It is difficult to prepare pills of a uniform size.
3. It is not possible to prepare pills of a uniform weight.

■ LIQUID DOSAGE FORMS ■

Liquid stage forms are meant for internal, parenteral or external use. They are available in monophasic or biphasic forms.

MONOPHASIC LIQUID DOSAGE FORMS

Monophasic liquid dosage forms are represented by true or colloidal solution. The component of the solution which is present in a large quantity is known as "solvent", whereas the component present in a small quantity is termed as "solute". Water is mainly used as solvent for majority of monophasic liquid dosage forms. A solution is homogenous because the solute is in an ionic or molecular form of subdivision. In case of colloidal solutions, the solute are present as aggregates although they cannot be seen by the naked eye or under ordinary microscope. Monophasic liquid dosage forms are available as:

1. Liquids for internal use *e.g.* syrups, elixirs, linctus, drops and draughts.
2. Liquids for external use, which are of two types:
   (*a*) Liquids to be applied to the skin *e.g.* liniments and lotions etc.
   (*b*) Liquids meant for body cavities *e.g.* gargles, throat paints, mouth washes, eye drops, eye lotions, ear drops, nasal drops, sprays and inhalations.

Syrups ■

Simple syrup is a saturated solution of sucrose in purified water. The concentration of sugar is 66% *w/w*. The syrups are sweet viscous preparations. The syrups containing medicinal substances are called "Medicated syrups" and those containing aromatic or flavoured substances are known as "Flavoured syrups".

Syrups are very commonly used for the following reasons:

1. Syrups retards oxidation because it is partly hydrolysed into reducing sugars, such as, lavulose and dextrose.
2. It prevents decomposition of many vegetable substances. Syrups have high osmotic pressure which prevents growth of bacteria, fungi and moulds which are the chief causes of decomposition in solutions of vegetable matter.

3. They are palatable. Due to the sweetness of sugar it is a valuable vehicle for the administration of nauseous substances.

The syrups may be divided into two groups:—

(*a*) Syrups prepared by simple solution or admixture *e.g.* syrups, syrup ginger, syrup orange and syrup lemon.

SYRUP I.P.

Sucrose	667 g
Purified water, sufficient to produce	1000 g

Add sucrose to purified water and heat it to dissolve sucrose with occasional stirring. Cool it and add more of purified water to make the required weight.

GINGER SYRUP I.P.

Strong ginger tincture	50 ml
Syrup, sufficient to produce	1000 ml

Mix.

(*b*) Syrups made by a process of extraction *e.g.* Tolu syrup.

TOLU SYRUP I.P.

Tolu balsam	12.5 g
Sucrose	660.0 g
Purified water sufficient to produce	1000.0 g

Add boiling purified water to the Tolu balsam contained in a tared vessel. Cover the vessel lightly and boil the contents gently for half an hour, stirring frequently. Add purified water to adjust the specified weight. Cool, filter the solution and add sucrose. Heat on a water-bath to dissolve the sucrose. Finally add sufficient purified water to produce the required volume.

Syrups are now used for formulating antibiotics, antihistaminics, sedatives, antitussives, vitamins and bitter or saline drugs.

Elixirs

Elixirs are sweet aromatic preparations and are usually coloured. The main ingredients of elixirs are ethyl alcohol (4-40%), water, glycerin or propylene glycol, flavouring agent, syrup and some suitable preservative. The medicated elixirs usually contain some very potent drug, such as, antibiotics, antihistamines or sedatives. The flavouring elixirs are used as flavours and vehicles. The following are examples of commonly used elixirs:

PIPERAZINE CITRATE ELIXIR I.P.

Piperazine citrate	180 g
Chloroform spirit	5 ml
Glycerin	100 ml
Syrup	500 ml
Purified water, sufficient to produce	1000 ml

Dissolve the piperazine citrate in part of the purified water. Add the orange oil, glycerin, syrup, chloroform spirit and sufficient purified water to produce the required volume.

PHENOBARBITONE ELIXIR I.P.

Phenobarbitone	400 mg
Alcohol 90%	40 ml
Compound orange spirit	2.5 ml
Glycerol	40.0 ml
Amaranth solution	1.0 ml
Purified water, sufficient to produce	100 ml

Dissolve the phenobarbitone in alcohol 90%. Add the compound orange spirit before adding the glycerol and amaranth solution. Add sufficient quantity of water to make the required volume.

Linctuses

Linctuses are viscous liquid and oral preparations that are generally prescribed for the relief of cough. They contain medicaments which have demulcent, sedative or expectorant action. Linctuses should be taken in small doses, sipped and swallowed slowly without diluting it with water in order to have the maximum and prolonged effect of medicaments.

Simple syrup is generally used as a vehicle for most of the linctuses. Tolu syrup is preferred in certain cases because of its aromatic odour and flavour. Moreover, it is believed to have a mild expectorant action *e.g.*

CODEINE LINCTUS B.P.C.

Codeine phosphate	3 g
Lemon syrup	200 ml
Benzoic acid solution	20 ml
Chloroform spirit	20 ml
Water	20 ml
Compound tartrazine solution	10 ml
Syrup to make	1000 ml

Weigh codeine phosphate and dissolve it in water, heat gently, if required. Add benzoic acid solution, compound tartrazine solution and chloroform spirit. Add the lemon syrup and adjust the volume by adding more of syrup.

Drops

These are liquid preparations meant for oral administrations. The oil soluble vitamins, such as, vitamin A and D concentrates in fish-liver oil are presented as drops for administration. Since these preparations contain potent medicaments, the dose must be measured accurately. The following two methods are commonly used for this purpose:

(*a*) Use of a dropper which is accurately graduated in fractions of a millilitre.

(*b*) Use of a pre-calibrated dropper in which the number of drops equivalent to the prescribed dose of the particular preparation being administered is known.

The size of the drops from the medicine dropper depends on factors, such as, surface tension, viscosity, density and temperature of the liquid.

Liniments

Liniments are liquid and semi-liquid preparations meant for application to the skin. Liniments are usually applied to the skin with friction and rubbing of the skin. The liniments may be alcoholic or oily solutions or emulsion. Alcohol helps in the penetration of medicaments into the skin and also increases its counter-irritant or rubefacient action. Arachis oil is used in some liniments which spread more easily on the skin. Soap is also included as ingredients in some of the liniments which helps in easy application of liniment on the skin.

Generally, liniments contain medicaments possessing analgesic, rubefacient, soothing and counter-irritant or stimulating properties.

A liniment should not be applied to broken skin because it may cause excessive irritation.

The following are some of the liniments which are official in Pharmacopoeia of India.

CAMPHOR LINIMENT

Camphor	200 g
Arachis oil	800 g

Dissolve the camphor in the arachis oil in a closed vessel.

AMMONIATED CAMPHOR LINIMENT

Camphor	125 g
Eucalyptus oil	5 ml
Ammonia solution strong	250 ml
Alcohol (90%) sufficient to produce	1000 ml

Dissolve the camphor and eucalyptus oil in 600 ml of alcohol 90%. Add the ammonia solution strong gradually with frequent shaking into it. sufficient alcohol 90% to produce the required volume.

TURPENTINE LINIMENT

Soft soap	90 g
Camphor	50 g
Turpentine oil (freshly rectified)	650 ml
Purified water, sufficient to produce	1000 ml

Mix the soft soap with 100 ml of purified water. Prepare a solution of the camphor in the freshly rectified turpentine oil. Gradually add the camphor solution to the soap mixture with trituration till a thick creamy emulsion is formed. Add sufficient purified water to produce the required volume. Mix it thoroughly.

SOAP LINIMENT

Soft soap	80 g
Camphor	40 g
Lemon grass oil	15 ml
Purified water	170 ml
Alcohol (90 per cent), sufficient to produce	1000 ml

Dissolve the soft soap, camphor, and lemon grass oil in 600 ml of alcohol (90 per cent). Add the purified water and sufficient alcohol (90 per cent) to produce the required volume. Set aside for a week and filter.

Lotions

Lotions are liquid preparations meant for external application without friction. They are applied direct to the skin with the help of some absorbent material, such as, cotton wool or gauze soaked in it. Lotions may be used for local action as cooling, soothing or protective purposes. They are generally prescribed for antiseptic action. *e.g.* calamine lotion.

CALAMINE LOTION I.P.

Calamine	150 g
Zinc oxide	50 g
Bentonite	30 g
Sodium citrate	5 g
Liquefied phenol	5 ml
Glycerin	50 ml
Rose water, of commerce, sufficient to produce	1000 ml

Dissolve sodium citrate in about 700 ml of rose water. Triturate the calamine, zinc oxide and bentonite with a solution of the sodium citrate. Add the liquefied phenol and the glycerin. Add rose water in sufficient quantity to produce the required volume.

Alcohol is sometimes included in aqueous lotions for its cooling and soothing effect *e.g.* salicylic acid lotion. In salicylic acid and mercuric chloride lotion acetone is used as a vehicle. The preparation is used for scalp conditions.

SALICYLIC ACID LOTION B.P.

Salicylic acid	2.0 g
Castor oil	1.0 ml
Alcohol (90 per cent) to make	100 ml

Dissolve salicylic acid in 3/4th of alcohol 90%. Add castor oil. Add more of alcohol 90% to make final volume.

Gargles

Gargles are aqueous solutions used to prevent or treat throat infections. They are usually available in concentrated form with direction for dilution with warm water before use. They are brought into intimate contact with the mucous membrane of the throat and are allowed to remain in contact with it for a few seconds, before they are thrown out of the mouth . They are used to relieve soreness in mild throat infection. Phenol or thymol is generally present in small concentration for its antibacterial activity. Potassium chlorate is also included in gargles for its weak astringent effect to tone up a relaxed throat. It also stimulates secretion of saliva which relieves dryness *e.g.* phenol gargles, potassium chloride and phenol gargles.

POTASSIUM CHLORATE AND PHENOL GARGLES B.P.C.

Potassium chlorate	30.0 g
Patent blue V	0.009 g
Liquefied phenol	15.0 ml
Water sufficient to make	1000 ml

Dissolve the potassium chlorate in warm water. Cool and add liquefied phenol. Add the dye solution, filter and make up the volume.

Mouth Washes

These are aqueous solutions with a pleasant taste and odour used to make clean and deodorise the buccal cavity. Generally, they contain antibacterial agents, alcohol, glycerin, sweetening agents, flavouring agents and colouring agents.

SODIUM CHLORIDE MOUTH-WASH, COMPOUND B.P.C.

Sodium chloride	15 g
Sodium bicarbonate	10 g
Peppermint water to produce	1000 ml

ZINC SULPHATE AND ZINC CHLORIDE MOUTH-WASH B.P.C.

Zinc sulphate	20 g
Zinc chloride	10 g
Dilute hydrochloric acid	10 ml
Compound tartrazine solution	10 ml
Chloroform water to produce	1000 ml

Dissolve the zinc sulphate and zinc chloride in water. Add dilute hydrochloric acid to make a clear solution. Add compound tartrazine solution. Add chloroform water to make the required volume.

Throat Paints

Throat paints are viscous liquid preparations used for mouth and throat infections. Glycerin is commonly used as a base because, being viscous, it adheres to mucous membrane for a long period and it possesses a sweet taste.

IODINE PAINT COMPOUND (MANDL'S PAINT) B.P.C.

Potassium iodide	25.0 g
Iodine	12.5 g
Alcohol (90%)	40.0 ml
Water	25.0 ml
Peppermint oil	4.0 ml
Glycerin to produce	1000.0 ml

Dissolve the potassium iodide in water. Add the iodine and stir until completely dissolved. Dissolve peppermint oil in alcohol 90% in a small container and then transfer it into the iodine solution. Mix well. Add glycerin and mix thoroughly. Add more of glycerin to make the required volume. The preparation is to be stored in a cool place since iodine is volatile in nature.

Sprays

Sprays are preparations of drugs in media which may be aqueous, alcoholic or glycerin. They are applied to the mucous membrane of nose or throat with an atomiser. The throat-sprays must be sprayed from a special type of atomiser known as 'nebuliser', which removes large droplets by a baffling system. Only fine droplets are required so that they may reach the lungs.

ADRENALINE AND ATROPINE SPRAY COMPOUND B.P.C.

Adrenaline acid tartrate	8.0 g
Atropine methonitrate	1.0 g
Papaverine hydrochloride	8.0 g
Sodium metabisulphite	1.0 g

Chlorobutol	5.0 g
Propylene glycol	50.0 ml
Purified water, freshly boiled and cooled to make	1000 ml

Prepare freshly boiled and cooled purified water. Dissolve separatrely the adrenaline acid tartrate, atropine methonitrate and sodium metabisulphite in this water. Mix the three solutions. Dissolve the papaverine hydrochloride in the mixture. Prepare the solution of chlorobutol in propylene glycol and add the solution to the above mixture. Filter if necessary and adjust to volume through the filter.

Inhalations

These are liquid preparations containing volatile substances and are used to relieve congestion and inflammation of the respiratory tract. The inhalations containing the volatile substances which are volatile at room temperature may be placed on an absorbent pad or handkerchief to inhale therefrom. In other cases inhalations are added to hot, but not boiling water (about 65°C) and vapours are inhaled for about 10 minutes.

BENZOIN INHALATION B.P.C.

Benzoin crushed	100 g
Prepared storax	50 g
Alcohol (95 per cent) to produce	1000 ml

It is prepared by macerating the benzoin and the prepared storax with alcohol 95% for 24 hours. Filter and pass sufficient of the alcohol through the filter to produce the required volume.

MENTHOL AND EUCALYPTUS INHALATION B.P.C.

Light magnesium carbonate	70 g
Menthol	20 g
Eucalyptus oil	100 ml
Water to produce	1000 ml

Dissolve the menthol in eucalyptus oil and add light magnesium carbonate and sufficient water to produce the required volume.

Nasal Drops

These are solutions of drugs that are instilled into the nose with a dropper. These are usually aqueous and not oily drops, since the latter inhibit the movement of cilia in the nasal mucosa and if used for long periods, may reach the lungs and cause lipoid pneumonia.

Nasal drops should be isotonic having neutral pH and viscosity similar to nasal secretions by using methyl cellulose.

EPHEDRINE NASAL DROPS B.P.C.

Ephedrine hydrochloride	0.5 g
Chlorobutol	0.5 g
Sodium chloride	0.5 g
Water to produce	1000 ml

Dissolve the ephedrine hydrochloride, chlorobutol and sodium chloride in water. Cool, filter if necessary. Add more water on filter to make the required volume.

Eye Drops

These are sterile solutions or suspensions of drugs that are instilled (put in by drops) into the eye with a dropper. The eye drops are usually made in aqueous vehicle. It should be sterile, isotonic with lachrymal secretions, buffered and free from foreign particles to avoid irritation to the eye. A suitable preservative like phenyl mercuric nitrate (0.002%), benzalkonium chloride (0.01%) and chlorhexidine acetate (0.01%) may be used to prevent bacterial or fungal growth. Eye drops usually contain substances having antiseptic, anti-inflammatory, anaesthetic and miotic properties.

The eye drops are generally prepared by dissolving the medicament in the aqueous vehicle containing one of the prescribed antimicrobial substances and any other preservative specified in the individual monograph. The solution is clarified by filtration and transferred to the final containers, which are then closed to exclude micro-organisms. The sterilisation is done by autoclaving or by heating with bactericide at 98ºC to 100ºC for 30 minutes or by filtration through bacteria proof filter.

The eye drops should be packed in neutral glass containers or in a suitable plastic container. The glass droppers are made of neutral glass. The teats are made of rubber which are compatible with the antimicrobial substance to be used in the formulation.

The following precautions are required to be observed while using eye drops:

1. If the dropper is separate, always hold it with its tip down.
2. Never touch the dropper surface.
3. Never rinse the dropper.
4. Never use eye drops that have changed colour.
5. When the dropper is at the top of the bottle, avoid contaminating the cap when removed.
6. After instillation of drops, do not close eyes tightly or blink more often than usual as this may remove the medicine from the place where it is needed.

Eye Lotions

These are the aqueous solutions used for washing the eyes. The eye lotions are supplied in concentrated form and are required to be diluted with warm water immediately before use. Eye lotions should be isotonic and free from foreign particles to avoid irritation to the eye. They are required to be prepared afresh and should not be stored for more than two days as the lotion may get contaminated with micro-organisms. Two examples of eye lotion are given below:

SODIUM CHLORIDE EYE LOTION

Sodium chloride	9 g
Purified water to produce	1000 ml

SODIUM BICARBONATE EYE LOTION

Sodium bicarbonate	35 g
Purified water to produce	1000 ml

Ear Drops

These are solutions of drugs that are instilled into the ear with a dropper. These are generally used for cleaning the ear, softening the wax and for treating the mild infections. The solution is generally prepared in water, glycerin, propylene glycol or dilute alcohol. However, vehicles like glycerin and propylene glycol are preferred.

SODIUM BICARBONATE EAR-DROPS B.P.C.

Sodium bicarbonate	5 g
Glycerin	30 ml
Purified water to produce	100 ml

Dissolve sodium bicarbonate in water. Add the glycerin and sufficient of the water to produce the required volume, and mix. The ear-drops should have been prepared recently.

PHENOL EAR-DROPS B.P.C.

Phenol glycerin	40 ml
Glycerin to produce	100 ml

BIPHASIC LIQUID DOSAGE FORMS

The liquids which consist of two phases are known as biphasic liquids *e.g.* emulsions and suspensions. In general both the phases are liquid, while in suspensions the finely divided solids are dispersed in a liquid which acts as a continuous phase.

Emulsions

An emulsion is a biphasic liquid preparation containing two immiscible liquids, one of which is dispersed as minute globules into the other. The liquid which is converted into minute globule is called the 'dispersed phase' and the liquid in which the globules are dispersed is called the 'continuous phase'. Normally, two immiscible liquids cannot be dispersed for a long period. So, an emulsifying agent is added to the system. It forms a film around the globules in order to scatter them indefinitely in the continuous phase, so that a stable emulsion is formed.

The emulsions are of two types:

(*a*) *Oil in Water type (o/w) emulsion*, in which oil is in the dispersed phase whereas water is in the continuous phase. The *o/w* type emulsions are preferred for internal use. In these emulsions, gum acacia, tragacanth, methyl cellulose, saponins synthetic substances and soaps formed from monovalent bases like Na^+, K^+ and NH_4^+ are used as an emulsifying agent.

(*b*) *Water in Oil type (w/o) emulsion*, in which water is in the dispersed phase whereas oil is in continuous phase. The wool fat, resins, beeswax and soaps formed from divalent bases like Ca^{++}, Mg^{++} and Zn^{++} are used as an emulsifying agent. The *w/o* emulsions are mainly used externally as lotions or creams.

The following tests are done for distinguishing between *o/w* and *w/o* emulsions:

(*i*) *Dilution test*—The emulsion is diluted with water. In case the emulsion remains stable after its dilution, it is *o/w* emulsion. The *w/o* emulsion breaks on its dilution with water but remains stable when diluted with oil.

(*ii*) *Dye test*—The scarlet red dye is mixed with the emulsion. Place a drop of the emulsion on a microscope slide, cover it with a cover-slip, and examine it under a microscope. If the disperse globules appear red and the "ground" colourless, the emulsion is *o/w* type. The reverse condition occurs in *w/o* type emulsion *i.e.* the disperse globules appear colourless in the red "ground".

(*iii*) *Conductivity test*—Water is a good conductor of electricity, whereas oil is non-conductor of electricity. The conductivity test can be performed by dipping a pair of electrodes connected through a low voltage bulb in the emulsion. If the bulb glows on passing the electric current, the emulsion is *o/w* type, because water is in the continuous phase. In case the bulb does not glow, the emulsion is *w/o* type, because oil is in the continuous phase.

(iv) *Fluorescence test*—Certain fixed oils possess the physical property of fluorescing in the presence of ultraviolet radiation. On microscopic examination of emulsion under ultraviolet radiation, the whole field fluorescence indicates that oil is present in continuous phase (w/o type emulsion) and droplets fluorescence indicates that oil is present in disperse phase (o/w type emulsion)

The emulsions are of three types according to their use. These are:

(*a*) Emulsions for oral administration.
(*b*) Intravenous emulsions.
(*c*) Emulsions for external application.

Emulsions for oral administration These are generally *o/w* type emulsions, and are used for administration of medicinal oils. The emulsification helps to mask the disagreeable taste and the "oily" feel of the medicinal oil and thus increases its palatability *e.g.* liquid paraffin emulsion.

LIQUID PARAFFIN EMULSION I.P

Liquid paraffin	500.0 ml
Indian gum, in powder	125.0 g
Tragacanth, in powder	5.0 g
Sodium benzoate	5.0 g
Vanillin	0.5 g
Glycerin	125.0 ml
Chloroform	2.5 ml
Purified water sufficient to produce	1000 ml

Triturate the liquid paraffin and chloroform with the Indian gum, the tragacanth and the vanillin. Add in one quantity 250 ml of purified water and triturate until a creamy emulsion is formed. Add the glycerin and the sodium benzoate, dissolve in 50 ml of purified water. Add sufficient purified water to produce 1000 ml. Mix.

Intravenous emulsion The oil soluble sex hormones, vitamin A, D and K are administered as intravenous injections. The emulsified oils are also injected as diagnostic aids. These emulsions should have small globule size and must be sterile.

Emulsions for external use The emulsions for external application may be both *o/w* or *w/o* type but *o/w* type emulsion is preferred. When a drug is emulsified its rate of penetration through the skin may get reduced. It helps to prolong the action of a drug. Generally the emulsions for application to the skin are semi-solid at room temperature and are considered to be an excellent vehicle.

Suspensions

The suspensions are the biphasic liquid dosage form of medicament in which finely divided solid particles are dispersed in a liquid or semi-solid vehicle. The solid particles act as disperse phase whereas liquid vehicle acts as the continuous phase. Suspensions are generally taken orally or by parenteral route. They are also used for external applications.

These days many suspensions are supplied as dry powders which are converted into suspensions by adding the specified amount of a vehicle before use. This is done to ensure the stability of the suspension *e.g.*

Ampicillin for oral suspensions I.P.
Barium sulphate for suspensions I.P.
Insulin zinc suspension (amorphous)
Insulin zinc suspension (crystalline)

An ideal suspension must possess the following properties:

(1) It should settle slowly and should be readily re-dispersed on gentle shaking of the container.

(2) The particle size of the suspension remains fairly constant throughout its long period of undisturbed standing.

(3) The suspension should pour readily and evenly from its container.

(4) It should be free from large particles which spoil its appearance, give a gritty taste to oral preparations and also cause irritation to sensitive tissues when applied externally.

The suspensions are classified into four main classes according to its pharmaceutical use. These are:

(a) Oral suspensions
(b) Parenteral suspensions
(c) Ophthalmic suspensions
(d) Suspensions for external use

Oral suspensions These suspensions are to be consumed by the patient by oral route. Oral suspensions generally contain flavouring and sweetening agents to mask the bitter taste of the drug. They are also made palatable by using a suitable derivatives of drugs e.g., chloramphenicol palmitate suspension is prepared to mask the bitter taste of the chloramphenicol.

Parenteral suspensions The suspensions which are administered by parenteral route are called parenteral suspensions. The particle size of the drug of these suspensions should be such that it can be easily pass through the needle of the syringe. The viscosity of these suspensions should not interfere with its flow through the syringe needle. These suspensions should be sterilized.

Ophthalmic suspensions These are not commonly used as compared to eye-drops. These are prepared only in those cases, when the drug is insoluble in the desired solvent or unstable in liquid form. The particle size of the eye suspensions should be fine enough so that it should be non-irritant to the eye. These suspensions should be isotonic, having desired viscosity and sterilised.

Suspensions for external use These suspensions are meant for external use e.g., lotions, inhalations, ear drops etc. These suspensions contain very small particles to avoid grittiness.

The suspensions are also classified as flocculated and non-flocculated suspensions. The suspensions are said to be flocculated, when the individual particles are in contact with each other and form a network like structure. Whereas in case of non-flocculated suspensions, the individual particle exists as a separate entity.

All suspensions should be packed in containers having adequate airspace above the liquid to permit adequate shaking. The oral suspensions should be packed in wide mouth bottles to permit prompt removal of the suspension. The suspensions should be stored in tight containers, protected from freezing, excessive heat and light. The suspension should be shaken before its use to ensure a uniform distribution of solid in the vehicle, thereby giving a uniform and proper dosage.

SEMI-SOLID DOSAGE FORMS

Semi-solid dosage forms are mainly meant for external application *e.g.* ointments, creams, pastes, jellies etc. The suppositories are also included in this category although these are unit dosage forms.

Ointments

Ointments are semi-solid preparations meant for application to the skin or mucous membrane. They usually contain a medicament or medicaments dissolved, suspended or emulsified in the ointment base. They may contain a suitable antimicrobial preservative. The ointments are mainly used as protective or emollient for the skin. The medicated ointments are meant for action on epidermis or for action on deeper layers of cutaneous tissues or to penetrate deep and release medicaments to body fluids.

The ointments which are meant for application to the eye are called 'Ophthalmic Ointments'. These ointments are sterile and free from irritation. In the preparation of these ointments, the yellow soft paraffin is used instead of white soft paraffin; the reason for this being that white soft paraffin may contain small traces of the bleaching agent which are generally left over after bleaching the yellow soft paraffin. Hence, the white soft paraffin may cause irritation to the eye.

While selecting a suitable ointment base, the factors such as the action desired, nature of the medicament to be incorporated and the stability of an ointment are to be considered. An ideal ointment base should possess the following properties:

(1) It should be inert, odourless and smooth.

(2) It should be physically and chemically stable.

(3) It should be compatible with the skin and with the incorporated medicaments.

(4) It should be of such a consistency that it spreads and softens when applied to the skin with stress.

(5) It should not retard healing of the wound.

(6) It should not produce irritation or sensitisation of the skin.

There is no single ointment base which possesses all the qualities of an ideal ointment base. So it becomes necessary to use more than one ointment base in the preparation of ointments. The ointment bases are classified into:

1. Oleaginous bases
2. Absorption bases
3. Emulsion bases
4. Water soluble bases.

Oleaginous Bases

These bases consist of water soluble hydrocarbons, vegetable oils, animal fats and waxes. The constituents of hydrocarbon bases are soft paraffin, hard paraffin and liquid paraffin. The animal fat includes lard. The vegetable oils are used chiefly in ointments to lower the melting point or to soften bases of higher consistency.

These bases serve to keep the medicaments in prolonged contact with the skin and also act as occlusive dressings. They have a low capacity to absorb water and are used chiefly for their emollient effects.

These bases are losing their importance now a days for the following reasons:

1. They are greasy.
2. They are sticky and are difficult to remove both from skin and clothing.

3. They retain body heat which may produce an uncomfortable feeling of warmth.
4. They do not help in the absorption of medicaments.

Absorption Bases

These bases are generally anhydrous substances which have the property of absorbing (emulsifying) considerable quantities of water but still retaining their ointment-like consistency. The absorption bases are of two types:

(*i*) Non-emulsified bases
(*ii*) Water in oil emulsions

The non-emulsified bases absorb water and aqueous solutions producing *w/o* emulsions *e.g.* wool fat (*anhydrous lanolin*), wool alcohol, bees wax and cholesterol. The water in oil emulsions are capable of absorbing more water and have the properties of non-emulsified bases *e.g.* hydrous wool fat (*lanolin*).

These bases are used as vehicles for aqueous liquids or as solutions of medicaments.

Emulsion Bases

These bases are semisolid or have a cream-like consistency. Both *o/w* and *w/o* emulsions are used as ointment base. The oil in water type of emulsion bases are more popular because these can be easily removed from the skin or clothes by washing with water. The *w/o* type of bases are greasy and sticky *e.g.* compound benzoic acid ointment (*Whitfield's ointment*) and zinc undecenoate ointment are prepared by using the emulsifying ointment. The emulsifying ointment is prepared from emulsifying wax, white soft paraffin and liquid paraffin.

Water-Soluble Bases

These are commonly known as "greaseless ointment bases". The water-soluble bases consist of water soluble ingredients, such as, polyethylene glycol polymers which are popularly known as carbowaxes. The carbowaxes are water soluble, non-volatile and inert substances. These are available in varying consistencies depending upon their molecular weights. The poly-ethylene glycols 400, 1500, 4000 and 6000 are most commonly used in pharmacy. By mixing different carbowaxes, ointments of varying consistencies can be obtained.

The following are examples of some of the important and commonly used ointments which are official:

EMULSIFYING OINTMENT I.P.

Emulsifying wax	300 g
White soft paraffin	500 g
Liquid paraffin	200 g

Melt the emulsifying wax and white soft paraffin. Add the liquid paraffin. Stir until it attains room temperature.

COMPOUND BENZOIC ACID OINTMENT B.P.C.
(WHITFIELD'S OINTMENT)

Benzoic acid, in fine powder	60 g
Salicylic acid, in fine powder	30 g
Emulsifying ointment	910 g

Triturate the benzoic acid and the salicylic acid with a portion of the emulsifying ointment until smooth ointment is made. Gradually incorporate the remainder of the ointment.

SIMPLE OINTMENT I.P.

Wool fat	50 g
Hard paraffin	50 g
Cetostearyl alcohol	50 g
White/Yellow soft paraffin	850 g

Melt together. Stir until cold.

AMMONIATED MERCURY OINTMENT I.P.

Ammoniated mercury, finely powdered	25 g
Simple ointment	975 g

Triturate the ammoniated mercury with a portion of the simple ointment until smooth ointment is prepared. Add the remaining simple ointment and mix thoroughly.

SULPHUR OINTMENT I.P.

Sublimed sulphur, finely sifted	100 g
Simple ointment	900 g

WOOL ALCOHOLS OINTMENT I.P.

Wool Alcohols	60 g
Hard paraffin	240 g
White soft paraffin *or* Yellow soft paraffin	100 g
Liquid paraffin	600 g

Melt all the ingredients. Stir until cold.

SALICYCLIC ACID OINTMENT I.P.

Salicylic acid, finely sifted	20 g
Wool alcohols ointment	980 g

Melt the wool alcohol ointment. Add the salicylic acid and stir until cold.

IODINE OINTMENT, NON STAINING

Iodine	50 g
Arachis oil	150 ml
Yellow soft paraffin	a sufficient quantity

Shake the iodine with the arachis oil at room temperature until dissolved, and maintain the solution at 50ºC, with occasional stirring, until the brown colour disappears. Determine the concentration of iodine present by doing the assay. Add sufficient of the yellow soft paraffin, previously heated to 40ºC to produce ointment having iodine content between 4.75 to 5.25 per cent. Pour the mixed mass into a warm container and allow to cool without stirring to prevent air being entrapped in the ointment.

Creams

These are viscous semi-solid emulsions which are meant for external use. The creams are of two types, aqueous and oily creams. In case of aqueous creams, the emulsions are oil-in-water type and in case of oily creams, emulsions are water in oil type. The oil-in-water type cream is relatively non-greasy. In aqueous creams, the emulsifying anionic, cationic and non-ionic waxes, polysorbates and triethanolamine soaps are used as emulsifying agents. The oily creams are generally prepared with emulsifying agents, such as, wool fat, wool alcohols, beeswax and calcium soaps. A suitable preservative is generally added in aqueous creams which have the tendency to bacterial and fungal growth.

Creams should be stored and supplied in well-closed containers which prevent evaporation and contamination. Collapsible tubes of metal or suitable plastic should be used for storage of creams.

The following are some of the formulae of creams.

HYDROCORTISONE CREAM B.P.C.

Hydrocortisone, in ultra-fine powder	10 g
Cetomacrogol emulsifying ointment	300 g
Chlorocresol	1 g
Purified water, freshly boiled and cooled	689 g

Dissolve the chlorocresol in water with the aid of gentle heat. Melt the cetomacrogol emulsifying ointment on a water bath. Add the chlorocresol solution at the same temperature, stir until cold. Mix hydrocortisone with it.

NEOMYCIN CREAM B.P.C.

Neomycin sulphate	5.0 g
Cetomacrogol emulsifying ointment	300.0 g
Chlorocresol	1.0 g
Disodium edetate	0.1 g
Purified water, freshly boiled and cooled	693.9 g

Dissolve the chlorocresol and the disodium edetate in about 650 ml of water with the aid of gentle heat. Melt the cetomacrogol emulsifying ointment on a water-bath. Add the aqueous solution at the same temperature and stir until cold. Incorporate the neomycin sulphate dissolved in the remaining part of the water.

Pastes

Pastes are semi-solid preparations intended for external application to the skin. They differ from ointment as they contain a high proportion of finely powdered medicaments, such as zinc oxide, calcium carbonate, starch *etc*. These substances make the paste very thick and stiff. Moreover pastes are less greasy than ointments. The stiffness property of paste makes them useful as protective coatings. They are used mainly as antiseptic, protective or soothing dressings which are often spread on lint before being applied.

Pastes should be stored and supplied in containers made of materials which do not allow absorption or diffusion of the contents.

Jellies

Jellies are transparent or translucent, non-greasy, semi-solid preparations mainly used for external application to the skin. These are also used for lubricating catheters, surgical gloves and rectal thermometers. The substances like gelatin, starch, tragacanth, sodium alginate and cellulose derivative are used in the preparation of jellies. These are now becoming popular for contraceptive purposes and contain surfactants to enhance the supermicidal properties of the jelly.

Suppositories

Suppositories are semisolid dosage form of medicament for insertion into body cavities other than mouth. They may be inserted into rectum, vagina or nasal cavity. The medicament is incorporated into the suppository base and product is formulated in such a way that they will either melt or dissolve in the body cavity fluid to release the medicament. Suppositories are available in different shapes, sizes and weights. Suppositories are used to produce local, systemic and mechanical action.

The various types of suppository bases are used to prepare suppositories, so that they can retain its shape and firmness during storage and administration. They should melt or dissolve in body cavity fluids, when inserted into the body cavity. Now-a-days suppositories are prepared by cold compression method.

The suppositories are required to be stored in a cool place so that they can retain their shape at the room temperature.

Pessaries

They are meant for introduction into the vagina. They are larger than rectal suppositories and vary in weight from 4 to 8 gramme or more. The pessaries may be conical, wedge shaped or rod shaped. Now-a-days special shaped suppositories are manufactured and are supplied with applicators to facilitate insertion into the vagina.

The pessaries are also available as tablets and capsules and are known as vaginal tablets and capsules respectively.

Pessaries should be stored in a cool place.

NEW DRUG DELIVERY SYSTEM

Drugs are administered with the main aim of curing a patient of his or her disease. Drugs are never administered in their pure form but are converted into a suitable formulation so that its onset and intensity of action as well as total duration of action can be checked according to the need. With the advancement of pharmaceutical sciences, new concepts have evolved various modern dosage forms and methods of their administration. Some of the modern dosage forms are:

1. Implants
2. Films and strips
3. Liposome drug carriers
4. Controlled drug delivery modules
5. Erythrocytes
6. Nanoparticles
7. Prodrugs.

IMPLANTS

The hypodermic tablets are placed under the skin by a minor surgery in order to release drugs over prolonged periods of time. Now the magnetically controlled implants have been developed which can be opened or closed at will in order to release or stop the drug. The implants which are in capsule form, consist of a body and a cap. It can be opened by placing a magnet on the skin and moving it in the desired direction. These implants are placed in the upper thigh at a depth of 5 mm. These implants are useful in hormone therapy. When AlNicor rod magnet is taped over the skin immediately above the capsule, it will remain open and release the medicament but the capsule gets closed as soon as the magnet is removed.

FILMS AND STRIPS

These are meant for topical application for slow release of drug over predetermined period of time. The films and strips which are becoming popular these days are:

1. Zero order release films
2. Buccal strips
3. Spray bandages

Zero Order Release Films

These films are called "laminates", and are meant for topical applications. Nitroglycerin laminates are prepared by mixing propylene glycol with about 1% carbopol resin. The mixture is neutralised with sodium hydroxide solution and then 0.1% of nitroglycerin is added. It is then placed between polythene sheets 5 × 5 cm and its edges are sealed by heat. It is then placed on a pressure sensitive adhesive sheet of 5.5 × 5.5 cm so that it can be properly adhesive to the skin. Such laminates release the drug (*nitroglycerin*) slowly into circulation for about 12 hours. Similarly pilocarpine films are prepared from acrylates and methacrylates.

Buccal Strips

The buccal and sublingual tablets are now replaced with buccal strips. These strips consist of a thin absorbent base of fabrics, filter paper and cotton *etc*. The buccal strips are prepared by immersing a long piece of fabric made from polyamide fibres into a molten mixture of carbowaxes and dissolved or dispersed drug (around 20%). The fabric is then cooled and cut into small pieces (ideal dimension is 2 × 1 cm). The buccal strip is made in contact with buccal mucosa for about 15 minutes and then it is removed and discarded.

Spray Bandages

These bandages are prepared by spraying the solution of drug in polylactide (polymer of lactic acid anhydride). A 2% solution of purified lactide polymer is made in chloroform and the drug in the concentration of 0.01% to 90% is dissolved or dispersed in it. Such solution is then packed in an aerosol container having a suitable propellant, such as, CF_2Cl_2 (Dichloro-difluro methane). When this solution is sprayed, it will be a comfortable bandage which can be simply washed off with warm water.

LIPOSOME DRUG CARRIERS

There are several carriers in our body which transport bio-chemicals from one part of the body to an other *e.g.* proteins, enzymes etc. Liposomes are phospholipids which can transport both hydrophilic and hydrophobic drugs. Large multilamellar vesicles (LMV), small unilamellar vesicles (SUV) and large unilamellar vesicles (LUV) are some of the liposomes which are known today. By modifying the method of preparation, it is possible to prepare different liposomes. The small drug molecules get trapped in liposomes, whereas large drug molecules can also make hydrophobic or electrostatic bonding with it. Liposomes are sometimes mixed with cholesterol or ergosterol to change the permeability of liposomes to solute molecules.

Applications Liposomal drugs have wide therapeutic applications, some of which are as follows:

1. Used in diseases caused by intracellular parasites *e.g.* malaria, tuberculosis and amœbiasis.
2. Liposome entrapped insulin is active orally and can be replaced by intramuscular administration of insulin.
3. Liposomes can be used to transport functional DNA/RNA molecules into cells.
4. Liposomes can be used to transport radio-pharmaceuticals and immunological products.
5. Liposomal daunomycin has longer duration of action than free daunomycin which is used in the treatment of neoplasia.
6. Liposome entrapped actinomycin-D and nitrogen mustard are more effective than the parent drug.

CONTROLLED DRUG DELIVERY MODULES (CDDM)

Controlled drug delivery modules are devices which are formed by embedding the drug within a polymeric matrix so that it gets released slowly to the body over a very long period of time. The polymeric matrices used to hold the drug reversibly are polyethylenes, silicone elastomers and cellulose esters. The drug-polymer complex may be formulated into tablet, capsule or any other suitable formulation. These controlled drug delivery modules are punctured before administration with laser beam to make a small orifice of a few microns in diameter for the release of the drug. The drug is released from these modules by diffusion, osmosis or chemical reaction.

Controlled drug delivery modules can be applied to the skin, implanted subcutaneously or inserted into various body cavities. The CDDM has an advantage because there is an unattended drug delivery without any patient intervention.

ERYTHROCYTES

Erythrocytes have also been tried in order to achieve controlled release of drugs. The life span of an erythrocyte is about 120 days. Erythrocytes can allow a drug to circulate in the body for a long time which helps in the slow release of drug in serum. When the drug is encapsulated in eryhthrocytes, the drug gets leaked out of its cell over to prolonged period of time. Moreover, it can be sent to the specified sites.

Resealed erythrocytes are prepared by putting them into a hypotonic medium, so that they can be swollen. The aqueous solution of the drug is added to the medium so that the drug gets into erythrocytes through the open pores. When the isotonicity is adjusted the erythrocytes shrink, thus encapsulating the drug within them. These erythrocytes may be suspended in normal saline solution for preparing injections.

Resealed erythrocytes technique as drug carrier is very promising but it is difficult to arrange a large quantity of these erythrocytes. The techniques can be used on commercial scale only if erythrocytes are made available in test tubes.

Applications

1. Resealed erythrocytes of urease have been used in kidney failure to degrade serum urea.
2. Resealed erythrocytes of asparaginase have shown good results in asparaginase dependent leukaemia.
3. Resealed erythrocytes of methotrexate and adrianycin have been tried in cancer therapy. It has shown good results.
4. Resealed erythrocytes of prednisolone have shown good results to prolong the antiinflammatory action.

NANOPARTICLES

It is based on colloidal drug delivery system. The particle size of this system is in nanometer range *i.e.* 200-500 mm. That is why they are called nanoparticles. The system consists of a drug and a carrier to deposit the drug at the target site. The carriers used are naturally occurring macromolecules like human serum albumin, bovine serum albumin and other substances like gelatin, casein and ethylcellulose.

The method of preparation of nanoparticles is similar to coacervation phase separation used in microencapsulation except that it is in quite controlled manner. An aqueous solution of natural macromolecules is prepared and drug is mixed in it. In case the drug is hydrophobic, it is dissolved in a small quantity of organic solvents and mixed with the carrier, taking precautions that the drug may not be precipitated. The system is then desolvated in controlled manner by adding a solvent competing solute like sodium sulphate or alcohol. This results in the formation of colloidal particles in nanometer range. These nanoparticles may be hardened, isolated and dried for storage. Nanoparticles can be dispersed in aqueous system.

Applications

1. Flourescein isothiocyanate (FITC) nanoparticles have been used to incorporate cytotoxic agents into tumour cells in cancer chemotherapy.
2. Nanoparticles along with biological maker like immunoglobulins can be used to target the drugs to very specific sites.
3. In nuclear medicine 99 m Technitium nanoparticles are used to study the morphology, blood flow and functions of various organs of the body.

PRODRUGS

The compounds which undergo biotransformation before showing desired pharmacological activity are called prodrugs or proagents. Prodrugs are generally the esters or amides of parent drugs. The prodrugs are useful in improving the solubility, stability, bioavailability of drugs, masking the unpleasant taste and odour of the parent drug and reducing the drug toxicity.

Applications

1. Chloramphenicol palmitate, the prodrug of chloramphenicol is used in the preparation of paediatric suspension because it has no bitter taste.
2. Procaine-penicillin G and Benzathine-penicillin G are prodrugs of penicillin G which shows resistance to hydrolysis as compared to the parent drug.

3. Testosterone cypionate the prodrug of testosterone is long-acting in comparison to the parent drugs when injected in an oil base.
4. Clindamycin 2-palmitate the prodrug of clindamycin has no bitter taste of the parent drug.
5. Clindamycin 2-phosphate the prodrug of clindamycin cause little pain and irritation at the site of injection when given by I/m route as compared to its parent drug.

REVISION QUESTIONS

I. Very short answer type questions

1. Define the term 'Unit dosage form'.
2. Why drugs are not given in their original pure state?
3. Give a few examples of preparations covered under the solid dosage form.
4. What do you know about "Dusting Powders"?
5. What are the main ingredients of dentifrices?
6. Why pills are outdated preparations?
7. Why is it necessary to use sterilised talc and kaolin in preparing dusting powders?
8. Give three examples of monophasic liquid dosage form meant for internal use.
9. Give five examples of monophasic liquid dosage form meant for body cavities.
10. Why is glycerine used as a base in throat paints?
11. Give a list of preparation covered under biphasic liquid dosage forms.
12. Name the emulsifying agents used in the preparations of w/o and o/w emulsions.
13. Why are additives needed in preparing different dosage form?
14. Why is emulsifying agent required in preparing an emulsion?
15. Name some of the modern dosage forms.

II. Short answer type questions

16. Write the importance of dosage forms.
17. Name the preparations which are covered under bulk powders meant for external use. Write in brief about dusting powders.

18. Describe briefly the solid dosage forms
19. How are effervescent granules prepared?
20. Define 'Syrup'. Why syrup is preferred?
21. How will you distinguish w/o and o/w emulsions?
22. What precautions should be taken while using eye drops?
23. What are the qualities of an ideal suspension?
24. Write the advantages and disadvantages of pills.
25. Mention the qualities of an ideal ointment base.
26. What are precautions to be taken while using eye drops?
27. Give the importance of erythrocytes in new drug delivery system.
28. Write the applications of liposomal drugs.
29. Define "Prodrugs". What are its applications?
30. Why is white soft paraffin not used in ophthalmic ointments?

III. Long answer type questions

31. How will you classify different dosage forms? Write the importance of dosage form.
32. Define 'Solid Dosage Forms'. How will you classify solid dosage forms? Write in brief about dentifrices and effervescent granules.
33. What are 'Monophasic liquid dosage form? Write in detail about syrups and elixirs.
34. What are 'emulsions'? State the different types of emulsions and also how will you distinguish them?
35. What are "ointments'? Classify different ointment bases used in the preparation of ointments. Describe briefly each base.
36. What are the preparations covered under biphasic liquid dosage forms? How will you differentiate between emulsion and suspension?
37. Define "creams". How it differs from ointments? Write in brief about creams.
38. Give a brief account of liposome drug carriers. Write its applications.
39. How erythrocytes help in controlled release of drugs? Write its applications.
40. Give the method of preparation of any two of the following:
    (*a*) Tolu syrup (*b*) Terpin hydrate elixir
    (*c*) Codeine linctus (*d*) Turpentine liniment

(*e*) Calamine lotion (*f*) Iodine paint compound
(*g*) Ephedrine nasal drops (*h*) Sodium bicarbonate ear drops

41. Define the following terms.
   (*a*) Elixirs (*b*) Gargles
   (*c*) Emulsions (*d*) Syrups
   (*e*) Eye drops (*f*) Linctuses
   (*g*) Nasal drops (*h*) Insufflations
   (*i*) Mouthwashes (*j*) Suspension
42. Explain briefly:
   (*a*) Nanoparticles (*b*) Erythrocytes
   (*c*) Prodrugs (*d*) Films and strips
   (*e*) Liposomes drugs carriers
43. Differentiate between the following:
   (*a*) Dusting powder and insufflations
   (*b*) Syrups and Elixirs
   (*c*) Gargles and Mouthwashes
   (*d*) Eye drops and Eye lotions
   (*e*) Ointment and Cream
   (*f*) Paste and Jellies
44. Write short notes on:
   (*a*) Emulsions (*b*) Insufflations
   (*c*) Effervescent granules (*d*) Ointments
   (*e*) Creams (*f*) Dusting powders
   (*g*) Dentifrices (*h*) Inhalations

IV. Objective type questions

A. Completion type questions.

Fill in the blanks with suitable word/words.

45. Simple syrups is ________ solution of ________ in water having sucrose concentration ________ .
46. Soap is included in liniments because it helps in ________ of the liniment on skin.
47. ________ is used to introduce the medicated dusting powder into the body cavities.
48. Dusting powder should be passed through a ________ sieve to enhance its ________ .
49. In olden days pills were preferred because of their ________ shape so that they could be easily ________ .
50. The emulsions meant for external use should be ________ type.

51. The implants are useful in ________ therapy.
52. The throat sprays are sprayed from a special type of ________ known as ________ .
53. In case of aqueous creams, the emulsions used are of ________ type and in oily creams these are of ________ type.

B. Matching type questions

54. Match the items of *Column I* with appropriate items in *Column II*.

Column I		*Column II*
A. Linctuses	(*i*)	are sweet aromatic preparations.
B. Liniments	(*ii*)	are liquid preparation meant for external application without friction.
C. Elixirs	(*iii*)	are viscous liquid preparation meant for the relief of cough.
D. Inhalations	(*iv*)	are inhaled into nostrils for their bronchio-dilator and decongestion action.
E. Lotions	(*v*)	are liquid and semi-liquid preparations meant for application to skin with friction.
F. Snuffs	(*vi*)	are liquid preparations containing volatile substances used to relieve congestion of respiratory tract.

KEY

45. saturated, sucrose, 66.7% *w/w*
46. easy application
47. Insufflator
48. 85, effectiveness
49. spherical, swallowed
50. *o/w*
51. Hormone
52. Atomiser, Nebuliser
53. *o/w*, *w/o*
54. A(*iii*), B(*v*), C(*i*), D(*vi*), E(*ii*), F(*iv*)

2

Introduction to Pharmacopœias

The term Pharmacopœia comes from the Greek word 'Pharmakon' meaning 'drug' and 'Poiein' meaning 'make', and the combination means any recipe or formula or other standard required to make or prepare a drug.

The term 'Pharmacopœia' was first used in 1580 in a book on drug standards printed in Bergamo, Italy. After that a number of national pharmacopœias were published by various European Pharmacopœias—the London, the Edinburgh and the Dublin pharmacopœia were official throughout the kingdom. Each pharmacopœia described different strength and method of preparation for the same preparation. Hence there was a lot of confusion. To overcome this difficulty, the first British Pharmacopœia came into existence in 1864.

In the United States, the first pharmacopœia was published in December 1820 both in English and in Latin. Later on a National Formulary was also published in addition to U.S.P. (United States Pharmacopœia). The object of the first U.S.P. was to select from substances the ones which possess medicinal power, converted them into preparations of suitable composition in order to enhance their power to the maximum advantage.

The first International Pharmacopœia was published by the World Health Organisation in 1951 (Volume I) and in 1955 (Volume II). The object of this was to provide a uniform list which would avoid the confusion caused by different national standards, strengths and names especially for the use of travellers who might need to use the same prescription in different countries.

HISTORY OF THE PHARMACOPŒIA OF INDIA

The Government of India through its letter No. 2338 H(C)/43 dated 26 January, 1944, directed the Drugs Technical Advisory Board to list the drugs in use in India, which are not mentioned in British Pharmacopœia and also recommend the standards to be prescribed to maintain uniformity and the chemical tests to be used to establish identity and purity. The

Government of India published the Indian Pharmacopœial List in 1946, as a supplement to the British Pharmacopœia. The term "List" in the title was "misleading" in that, the book not only contained a list of drugs which were of substantial medicinal value but also laid down standards.

The Indian Pharmacopœial List contained about 180 monographs and a number of appendices prepared on the lines of the British Pharmacopœia.

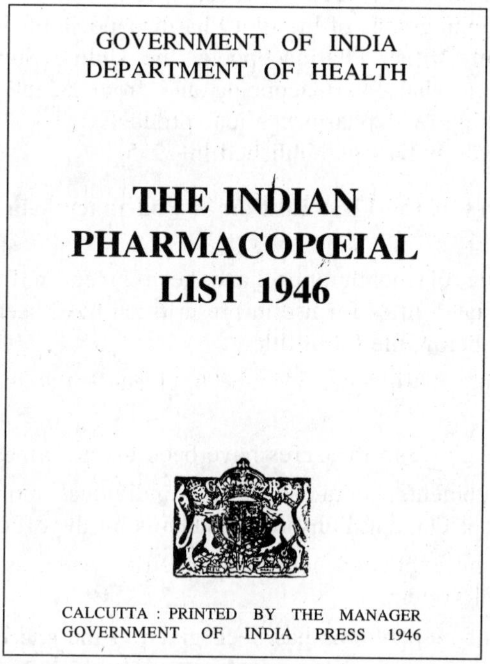

GOVERNMENT OF INDIA
DEPARTMENT OF HEALTH

THE INDIAN PHARMACOPŒIAL LIST 1946

CALCUTTA : PRINTED BY THE MANAGER
GOVERNMENT OF INDIA PRESS 1946

Title page of the Indian Pharmacopœial List 1946

Approximately 100 monographs were on vegetable drugs growing in India and on their galenicals. The drugs of plant origin such as artemesia, bael, berberis, cannabis, ispaghula, kaladana, kurchi, myrobalan, picrorhiza, punarnava, rauwalfia, vasaka etc. were included in it. Similarly several oils such as ajowan, cassia, chaulmoogra, neem and pudina were included in it. The appendices gave detail for a number of determinations referred to in the monograph.

The Pharmaceuticals and Drug Research Committee of the Council of Scientific and Industrial Research decided in February 1947 to compile a "Brochure" to highlight the information and clinical uses of the important indigenous drugs of India. Later on it was decided to prepare a "Codex" instead of Brochure on the lines of the British Pharmaceutical

Codex. The first Indian Pharmaceutical Codex was published in 1953. The Codex consisted of two parts. The first part carried about 190 general monographs on natural products and drugs of vegetable and animal origin, and a few chemicals. The second part consisted of formulary of galenicals and other preparations.

After the publication of the Indian Pharmacopoeial List, the Government of India constituted Indian Pharmacopoeial Committee in 1948, in compiling the monographs of the first Pharmacopoeia of India. The help was taken from British Pharmacopoeia, the United States Pharmacopoeia, the Interntional Pharmacopoeia and from scientific institutions interested in drugs and pharmaceutical products. The first edition of Pharmacopoeia of India was published in 1955.

Salient Features of the First Edition of Pharmacopœia of India (1955)

1. The title of monographs have been given in Latin language. Abbreviated titles for use in prescription have been given immediately below the Latin title.
2. The English title has also been given below the abbreviation title.
3. The weights and measures have been given in metric system.
4. All statements contained in the individual monographs have been considered as constitute standards for the official substances.
5. Doses are expressed both in the metric system as well as in the imperial system.
6. A list of preparations has been given at the end of some of the monographs.
7. The temperature has been expressed in Celsius thermometric scale.
8. The descriptive terms (very soluble, freely soluble, sparingly soluble, slightly soluble, very slightly soluble, practically insoluble) have been used where the exact solubility of a pharmacopœial substance is not known.

After the publication of first edition of Pharmacopoeia of India, Indian Pharmacopoeial Committee was reconstituted. The Committee compiled a supplement to the first edition of the Indian Pharmacopoeia which was published in 1960. The Indian Pharmacopoeial committee appointed the sub-committes and working groups to facilitate the compilation work of second edition of the Pharmacopoeia of India. The second edition of the Pharmacopoeia of India was published in 1966 and later on its supplement was published in 1975.

Salient Features of the Second Edition of Pharmacopœia of India

1. The titles of monographs have been changed from Latin to English.
2. The words of the title have been transposed to give the name of the drug first *e.g.* Injection of Aminophylline has been changed to Aminophylline Injection.
3. Doses are expressed in the metric system only.
4. Solubility is expressed in parts of solvent per unit part of solute.
5. The preparations of a drug have been given immediately after the monograph on the parent drug.
6. The test for sterility has been modified to provide for detection of fungi in addition to aerobic and anaerobic bacteria.
7. New analytical techniques such as non-aqueous titrimetry, column chromatography have been included.
8. In the monographs of "Tablets" and "Injections", a new sub-heading "Usual Strength" has been given to represent the strength of the tablet or injection in which it should be generally marketed.

The Government of India, Ministry of Health and Family Welfare, reconstituted the Indian Pharmacopoeial Committee in 1979, for the preparation of the third edition of Pharmacopoeia of India. To facilitate the compilation work of third edition of Pharmacopoeia of India, sub-committees and working groups were constituted by the Indian Pharmacopoeial Committee. The third edition of Pharmacopoeia of India was published in 1985 by the Government of India.

Salient Features of the Third Edition of Pharmacopœia of India (1985)

1. The new analytical techniques such as Flame Photometry, Flurometry, Electrophoresis and Photometric Haemoglobinometry have been introduced as official method for certain chemical analysis.
2. Dissolution Test has been introduced in the case of certain tablets.
3. Disintegration Test has been amended by modifying the design of the apparatus and method of testing.
4. A microbial limit test has been prescribed for certain pharmaceutical aids and oral liquid preparations.
5. The Pyrogen Test has been revised to make the test less time-consuming than the previous method.

6. Gas Liquid Chromatography has been recognised as an alternative method for the determination of alcohol concentration in various preparations.
7. The test for determination of viscosity has been modified by the introduction of other methods involving the use of Ostwald Viscometer.
8. The new appendix on "Water for Pharmaceutical Use" has been introduced to clearly indicate the different official standard in respect of purified water, water for injection and sterile water for injection.
9. Some of the drugs have been renamed in this edition *e.g.* 'Acetylsalicylic Acid' has been changed to 'Aspirin'.
10. Many drugs have been omitted from the third edition and many new drugs have been included in the third edition.

The Government of India, Ministry of Health and Family Welfare reconstituted the Indian Pharmacopoeial Committee for a period of five years in 1991, for the preparation of the fourth edition of Pharmacopoeia of India.

The Committee appointed the subcommittees and working groups in order to expedite the preparation of the new edition of the Indian Pharmacopœia.

The Monographs, Appendices and General Notes as prepared by the "Working Group" and finalised by the Committee were then published in the form of fourth edition of the Pharmacopœia of India in 1996 by the Government of India.

Salient Features of the Fourth Edition of Pharmacopœia of India (1996) ▩

1. It contains 1149 monographs and 123 appendices and available in two volumes.
2. The computer-generated structural formulae have been introduced.
3. Some titles have been changed to include the more commonly accepted names in India. *e.g.* Hyoscine Hydrobromide for Scopolamine Hydrobromide
4. Infra-red and ultra-red absorption spectrophotometric tests for identification of drug substance have been introduced as alternative tests to the classical chemical tests. The infra-red reference spectra of a number of drug substances has been included in an appendix.

5. The high performance liquid chromatography (HPLC) has been widely used as a method to analyse many formulations which can otherwise be analysed only by more difficult and less accurate method *e.g.* biological assay of Insulin has been replaced by HPLC.
6. The test for bacterial endotoxins as a more suitable substitute for the test for pyrogens has been introduced for some articles.
7. A number of general monographs *e.g.* eye drops, eye ointments, nasal preparations, oral liquids, pessaries, suppositories etc. have been included.
8. A quantitative method for determining particulate matter in injectable preparations has been replaced by the qualitative test of the previous edition. The test is applicable to injectable solutions that are supplied in containers with 100 ml or more.
9. The specific biological assays and tests provided for vaccines; hormones, blood products and enzymes have been transferred from an appendix to the individual monographs.
10. In the monographs for Oral Rehydration Salts (ORS), ORS-Bicarbonate formula has been dropped due to its stability problem, whereas ORS-Citrate formula recommended by WHO is retained.

After the publication of fourth edition of the Indian Pharmacopoeia in 1996, an addendum was published in 2000. In view of rapid developments in the field of pharmaceutical sciences and technology it becomes necessary to update the official compendium frequently. Addendum 2002 was published to incorporate the latest developments made in pharmaceutical sciences. The numbering of pages in this Addendum is continuous with that of Volume I and II of Indian Pharmacopoeia 1996 and Addendum 2000. The following changes are made:—

1. A number of tests and standards in monographs have been amended and replaced with old monographs.
2. The test on bacterial endotoxins replaces the pyrogen test.
3. A new appendix on 'residual solvent' has been incorporated to monitor the content of organic volatile impurities that are used or produced in the manufacture of an active pharmaceutical substance, excipient or medicinal product.
4. An appendix on HPLC has been replaced by a revised version covering ion chromatography.
5. Monographs of a number of anti-retroviral activities and their formulations have been introduced in this Addendum.

6. Monographs on vaccines for Hepatitis B and that for Rabies have been revised.

Government of India, Ministry of Health and Family Welfare, constituted the Indian Pharmacopoeia Commission (IPC) on 22nd March 2005. The commission had its headquarters in the Central Indian Pharmacopoeia Laboratory (CIPL), Sector-23, Raj Nagar,Ghaziabad, U.P. The Indian Pharmacopoeia Commission had the following three tier structure:—

General Body	19 members
Governing Body	8-10 members
Scientific Body	15-23 members

Along with this various expert committees were also made to prepare various monographs. The fifth edition of Pharmacopoeia of India was published in 2007.

Salient Features of the Fifth Edition of the Indian Pharmacopoeia (2007)

1. The Indian Pharmacopoeia 2007 is presented in three volumes. Volume I contains the general notes, preface, the structure of the IPC, Introduction and general chapters. Volume II deals with the general monographs on drug substances, dosage forms and pharmaceutical aids. Volume III contains monographs on drug substances, dosage forms, pharmaceutical aids, vaccines and immunosera for human use, herbs and herbal products, blood and blood related products, biotechnology products and veterinary products.
2. General chemical tests for identification have been almost eliminated and more specific infra-red and ultra-violet spectrophotometric tests have been given.
3. The test for pyrogens involving the use of animals has been virtually eliminated. The test for bacterial endotoxins has been introduced.
4. The test for abnormal toxicity is now confined to certain vaccines.
5. The use of chromatographic methods has been extended in assays to large number of pharmaceutical products.
6. Labelling and storage are featured at the end of a monograph.
7. The general monographs for dosage forms of active pharmaceutical ingredients are grouped together at the beginning of Volume II followed by the monographs for active pharmaceutical ingredients, pharmaceutical aids and individual dosage forms, all in alphabetical order.

8. Monographs for other articles of a special nature such as vaccines and immunosera for human use, herbs and herbal products, blood and blood related products, biotechnology products and veterinary products are given in separate section in Volume III.
9. Limit of bacterial contamination has been introduced for controlling the microbial quality of all medicinal products.
10. Analytical methods are in general in harmony with those adopted internationally for monitoring the quality of drugs.

The 6th edition of Indian Pharmacopoeia was published in 2010 by Indian Pharmacopoeia Commission.

Salient Features of the Sixth Edition of Pharmacopoeia of India (2010) ▩

1. The Pharmacopoeia is presented in three volumes:—
   (*i*) Volume I contains notices, structure of IPC, acknowledgement, introduction and general chapters.
   (*ii*) Volume II contains general notice, general monograph on dosage forms, monograph on drug substances, dosages forms and pharmaceutical aids (A to M)
   (*iii*) Volume III contains monographs on dosage forms (N to Z) followed by monographs on vaccines, and immunosera for human use, herbs and herbal products, blood and blood related products, biotechnology products and veterinary products.
2. The Pharmacopoeia has 2000 monographs, 287 new monographs and more than 600 monographs has been updated.
3. A new chapter of liposomal products is introduced and monograph of Liposomal Amphotericin B Injection is included in it.
4. A chapter on microbial contamination is also updated to a great extent to harmonise with prevailing international requirements.
5. The scope of the Pharmacopoeia has been extended to include products of biotechnology, indigenous herbs and herbal products, veterinary vaccines and anti-retroviral drugs and formulations.
6. A chapter on NMR is in Appendices
7. The standards for new drugs and drugs used under National Health Programmes are added in this edition.
8. General chemical tests for identification for an article have been almost eliminated and more specific infra-red and ultra-violet spectrophotometric tests have been given emphasis.

9. Most of the existing assays and related substances tests are upgraded by liquid chromatographic methods in view to harmonise with other International Pharmacopoeia.
10. The test for pyrogens involving the use of animals have been virtually eliminated.
11. The test for abnormal toxicity is now confined to certain vaccines.
12. The tests for bacterial endotoxins introduced in the previous editions is now applicable to more items.
13. The number of monographs of excipients, anti-cancer drugs, herbal products and anti-retroviral drugs have been increased in this edition.
14. The drugs as well as their formulations not in use are omitted from this edition.

The 7th edition of the Indian Pharmacopoeia has been published by the Indian Pharmacopoeia commission in 2014 on behalf of the Government of India, Ministry of Health and Family Welfare.

Salient Features of the Seventh Edition of Indian Pharmacopoeia (2014)

1. The Indian Pharmacopoeia 2014 is presented in four volumes.
2. I.P. 2014 incorporates 2548 monographs of drugs out of which 577 are new monographs consisting of APLS, excipients, dosage forms and herbal products etc.
3. Many chapters have been revised in Appendices.
4. The monograph on water for injection in bulk and purified water are also upgraded to harmonise with prevailing international requirements.
5. General chemical tests for identification of an article have almost eliminated and more specific infra-red and ultra-violet spectrophotometric and HPLC tests have been given emphasis.
6. The test for pyrogens involving the use of animals has been replaced with Bacterial Endotoxin test.
7. More essential oils monographs, crude herbal drugs and their extracts have been incorporated.
8. 19 monographs on radio-pharmaceutical preparations along with chapter on radio-pharmaceuticals have been added in volume-III of this edition.

9. A separate volume for veterinary monographs as volume IV of this edition of Indian Pharmacopoeia has been designed to those concerned with the quality control of veterinary medicines.
10. A general chapter on cell cultures for the production of veterinary vaccines.
11. Standards for new drugs and drugs used under National Health Programmes are added and the drugs as well as their formulations not in use now-a-days are omitted from this edition.

List of Pharmacopœias and Some of the Standard Reference Books of Common Use in India

1. Indian Pharmacopœia (I.P.)
2. British Pharmacopœia (B.P.)
3. United States Pharmacopœia (U.S.P.)
4. European Pharmacopœia
5. International Pharmacopœia
6. Japanese Pharmacopœia
7. Martindale Extra Pharmacopœia
8. British Pharmaceutical Codex (B.P.C.)
9. Pharmaceutical Codex
10. Merck Index
11. British National Formulary
12. United States National Formulary
13. National Formulary (N.F.)
14. United States Dispensatory
15. Indian Pharmaceutical Codex (I.P.C.)
16. National Formulary of India (N.F.I.) 1960, 1966, 1979, 2011

REVISION QUESTIONS

I. Very short answer type questions

Answer the following questions in brief.

1. In which year was the first British Pharmacopœia published?
2. Give the year of publication of the first U.S.P.
3. In which year did the first Pharmacopœia of India come out?
4. How many monographs are there in the Indian Pharmacopœial List?
5. When was the first International Pharmacopœial List published?
6. Who were the publishers of the International Pharmacopœia?
7. When was the Indian Pharmacopœial List published?
8. In which years the various editions of the Pharmacopœia of India come out?

9. When was the first Indian Pharmaceutical Codex published?
10. When was the term "Pharmacopœia" used for the first time?

II. Short answer type questions ■

11. Define the term "Pharmacopœia".
12. Name the various pharmacopœias commonly used in India.
13. Name the various standard reference books on pharmacy in common used in our country.
14. Give the reasons for the publication of International Pharmacopœia by W.H.O.
15. Why did publication of Indian Pharmacopœial List in 1946 become necessary?

III. Long answer type questions ■

16. Describe in detail the various stages which ultimately led to the development of first Pharmacopœia of India.
17. Give the salient features of the second edition of Pharmacopœia of India.
18. What are the salient features of the third edition of Pharmacopœia of India?
19. Write the salient features of fifth edition of Indian Pharmacopoeia 2007.
20. Give, in brief, the history of the Pharmacopœia of India.
21. Write the salient features of sixth edition of Indian Pharmacopoeia 2010
22. Give the main features of seventh edition of Indian Pharmacopoeia 2014
23. What are the features of Indian Pharmacopoeia 2014 which helps to harmonise with prevailing international requirements?

IV. Objective type questions ■

A. Completion type questions (Fill in the blanks with suitable word/words)

24. The term Pharmacopœia was first used in______ in a book on _______ printed in _________.
25. The first U.S.P. was published in ________ both in _______ and______ languages.
26. The Indian Pharmacopœial List was published in ___________as a supplement to ____________.

27. The first International Pharmacopœia was published by__________ in____________ (Volume I) and in ______________ (Volume II).

28. The dissolution test has been introduced in ________ edition of Pharmacopœia of India.

B. Matching type questions

29. Match the items of *Column I* with the appropriate items of *Column II*.

Column I	*Column II*
A. Pharmacopœia	(*i*) modified in 3rd edition of I.P.
B. British Pharmacopœia	(*ii*) in two volumes in 1950, and in 1955.
C. Disintegration Test	(*iii*) term has been derived from Greek word.
D. Pyrogen Test	(*iv*) 1960
E. The supplement to first edition of I.P. was published	(*v*) is published after every five years.
F. International Pharmacopœia was published	(*vi*) is less time consuming in 3rd edition of I.P.

C. Multiple type questions (*Choose the correct answer*)

30. The new edition of British Pharmacopœia is published after every:
    (1) 4 years (2) 5 years
    (3) 6 years (4) Alternate year

31. The first edition of the Pharmacopœia of India was published in:
    (1) 1947 (2) 1955
    (3) 1966 (4) 1946

32. The supplement to second edition of the Pharmacopœia of India was published in:
    (1) 1981 (2) 1975
    (3) 1985 (4) 1966

33. The first U.S.P. was published in:
    (1) English (2) Latin
    (3) French (4) English and Latin

34. The Indian Pharmacopœial List was published as a supplement to:
    (1) British Pharmacopœia (2) U.S.P.
    (3) Pharmacopœia of India (4) I.P.C.

KEY

1. 1864
2. 1820
3. 1955
4. 180
5. 1950 Vol I, 1955 Vol II
6. W.H.O.
7. 1946
8. 1955, 1966, 1985, 1996, 2007, 2010, 2014
9. 1953
10. 1580
24. 1580, drug standards, Italy
25. December 1820, English and Latin
26. 1946, The British Pharmacopoeia
27. WHO, 1950, 1955
28. Third
29. A(iii), B(v), C(i), D(vi), E(iv), F(ii)
30. (2)
31. (2)
32. (2)
33. (4)
34. (1)

3

Metrology

There are two systems of weights and measures:

1. Imperial System
2. Metric System

IMPERIAL SYSTEM

It is an old system but still a large number of old physicians write the prescription in accordance with this system. So the pharmacist should be familiar with this system.

Measurement of Weight in Imperial System

The Imperial system is divided into two parts for the purpose of measurement of weight. These are:

(*a*) Avoirdupois system
(*b*) Apothecaries system

Avoirdupois System In this system the "pound" is the standard unit for weighing and all measures of mass are derived from the Imperial Standard Pound (Lb), thus:

TABLE 3.1

1 Lb	= 16 oz (avoir)
1 Lb	= 7000 grains
1 oz (avoir)	= 7000/16
	= 437.5 grains

Apothecaries System This system is also known as the Troy system. The grain is the standard weight in this system and all other weights are derived from it.

TABLE 3.2

20 grains (gr)	= 1 scruple (→)
60 grains	= 1 drachm (ʒ)
480 grains	= 1 ounce (℥) (apothe)

8 drachms	=	1 ounce (apothe)
12 ounces	=	1 pound (Lb) (apothe)
5760 grains	=	1 pound (apothe)

Measurement of Capacity in Imperial System ■

The standard units for capacity is the same in both the avoirdupois and the apothecaries systems. The 'gallon' is the standard unit and all other measures of capacity are derived from it.

TABLE 3.3

1 gallon (c)	=	160 fluid ounces
1/4th of a gallon	=	1 quart
1/8th of a gallon	=	1 pint (o)
1/160th of a gallon	=	1 fl ounce (℥)
1/8th of a fl ounce	=	1 fl drachm (ʒ)
1/60th of a fl drachm	=	1 minim (m)
1 quart	=	40 fl ounces
1 pint	=	20 fl ounces
1 fl ounce	=	480 minims
1 fl drachm	=	60 minims

■ METRIC SYSTEM ■

The metric system is used in the Indian pharmacopœia for the measurement of weight and capacity.

Measurement of Weight in Metric System ■

A 'kilogram' is the standard unit for measurement of weight and all other measures are derived from it.

TABLE 3.4

1 Kilogram (Kg)	=	1000 grams (g)
1 Hectogram (hg)	=	100 grams
1 Decagram (dag)	=	10 grams
1 Decigram (dg)	=	0.1 gram
1 Centigram (cg)	=	0.01 gram
1 Milligram (mg)	=	0.001 gram
1 Microgram (μg or mcg)	=	0.000,001 gram
1 Gram (g)	=	1000 mg

Measurement of Capacity

A 'litre' is the standard unit for measurement of capacity and all measures of capacity are derived from it.

1 Litre (lt) = 1000 millilitre (ml)

CONVERSION TABLES

The Pharmacopœia of India uses only the Metric system in formulae, but the prescriptions are still written in the Imperial system by many an old time physicians. So a conversion tables (given below) is used by the pharmacists.

TABLE 3.5

(*i*) **Weight Measures**

1 Kilogram (Kg) = 2.2 Lb (pound)
30 g = 1 ounce (℥)
450 g = 1 pound (avoir)
1 g = 15 grains
60 mg = 1 grain

(*ii*) **Capacity Measures**

1000 ml = 1 quart
500 ml = 1 pint
30 ml = 1 fluid ounce
4 ml = 1 fluid drachm
1 ml = 15 minims
0.06 ml = 1 minim

TABLE 3.6
Conversion Table for Domestic Measures

Domestic measure	*Metric system*	*Imperial system*
1 drop	0.06 ml	1 minim
1 teaspoonful	4.00 ml	1 fluid drachm
1 desert spoonful	8.00 ml	2 fluid drachm
1 tablespoonful	15.00 ml	4 fluid drachm
2 tablespoonful	30.00 ml	1 fluid ounce
1 wine glassful	60.00 ml	2 fluid ounce
1 teacupful	120.00 ml	4 fluid ounce
1 tumblerful	240.00 ml	8 fluid ounce

PERCENTAGE CALCULATIONS

The pharmacopœia has expressed "per cent" in defining standards according to circumstances, with any one of the four different meanings. These are:

1. Per cent *w/w* (Percentage Weight in Weight), expresses the number of grammes of the active substance in 100 grammes of product.
2. Per cent *w/v* (Percentage Weight in Volume), expresses the number of grammes of the active substance in 100 millilitres of product.
3. Per cent *v/v* (Percentage Volume in Volume), expresses the number of millilitres of the active substance in 100 millilitres of product.
4. Per cent *v/w* (Percentage Volume in Weight), expresses the number of millilitres of the active substance in 100 grammes of product.

The strength of solution of solids in liquids is expressed as percentage weight in volume, of liquid in liquid as percentage volume in volume and of gases in liquids as percentage weight in weight.

COMMON FORMULAE USED IN PERCENTAGE CALCULATIONS

1. Preparation of 1% *w/v* solution in the imperial system

(*a*) Solid – 1 gr
Solvent, to produce 110 m

(*b*) Solid – 4.375 gr
Solvent, to produce 1 fluid ounce

(*c*) Solid – 35 gr
Solvent to produce 8 fluid ounce

The formula (*a*) above should be used when the volume of the solution required is small and the strength of the solution required is weak. The formulae (*b*) and (*c*) should be used in other cases.

2. Preparation of 1% *w/v* solution in metric system

Solid – 1 g
Solvent, to produce 100 ml

3. Preparation of percentage solution by diluting the concentrated solution

$$\text{Strength of dilute solution} = \frac{\text{Strength of concentrate}}{\text{Degree of dilution}}$$

$$\text{Volume of stronger alcohol to be used} = \frac{\text{Volume required} \times \text{Percentage required}}{\text{Percentage used}}$$

$$\text{Weight of stronger acid to be used} = \frac{\text{Weight required} \times \text{Percentage required}}{\text{Percentage used}}$$

Wherever possible the metric system should be used even if a quantity is demanded in the imperial system. The calculations are made using convenient metric quantities. In case it is necessary to transpose a formula from the metric to the imperial system, the following relationship may be applied.

Solid	1 g	1 oz (avoir)	4.375 gr	1 gr
Solvent to produce	100 ml	100 fl oz	1 fl oz	100 m

There are two rules which may be applied:

Rule 1— g may be read as oz avoir
ml may be read as fl oz

Rule 2— g may be read as grain.
ml may be read as minim after adding 10 per cent to the figure.

Rule (1) is applied for large batches and Rule (2) is applied for small batches.

Weight in Volume (*w/v*) Solutions

The following are some of the examples which show the calculations meant for making *w/v* solution:

Example 1 Calculate the quantity of dextrose required to prepare 1 fl oz of a 10% solution.

Calculation This is a solution of solid in a liquid, hence it is a *w/v* solution. The volume of the solution prepared is small.

By applying the formula:

4.375 gr, in 1 fl oz, are required to make a 1% *w/v* solution

4.375 × 10 gr, in 1 fl oz, are required to make a 10% *w/v* solution
= 43.75 gr
≅ 44 gr (because it is difficult to weigh fraction of a grain)

So, 44 gr of dextrose when dissolved in water to make 1 fl oz, produces 1% *w/v* solution.

Example 2 Calculate the quantity of dextrose required to prepare 8 fl oz of a 5 per cent solution.

Calculation In this case, the volume of the solution prepared being large, the following formula is applicable for calculating the amount of dextrose required to prepare 5% of 8 fl oz solution.

35 gr, in 8 fl oz are required to make a 1% solution

35 × 5 gr (= 175 gr), in 8 fl oz, are required to make a 5% solution

Therefore, 175 gr of dextrose is dissolved in water and diluted to 8 fl oz will produce a 5% *w/v* solution.

Example 3 Calculate the quantity of potassium permanganate required to prepare 1 pint of 1 in 400 solution.

Calculation In this case, the volume of the solution prepared being large, the following formula is applicable:

35 gr, in 8 fl oz, are required to make 1% (1 : 100) solution

$\frac{35 \times 100}{400}$ gr in 8 fl oz, are required to make 1 : 400 solution

$\frac{35 \times 100 \times 20}{400 \times 8}$ gr in 20 fl oz, are required to make 1 : 400 solution

$= 22.8$ gr

So 23.0 gr of potassium permanganate is dissolved in water to produce 20 fl oz to make 1 : 400 solution.

Example 4 Calculate the quantity of sodium chloride required to prepare 600 ml of a 0.9% solution.

Calculation

1 g, with solvent to produce 100 ml makes 1% *w/v* solution

1 × 0.9 g, with solvent to produce 100 ml makes 0.9% *w/v* solution

$\frac{0.9 \times 600}{100}$ g, with solvent to produce 600 ml makes 0.9% *w/v* solution

$= 5.4$ g

Hence 5.4 g of sodium chloride is dissolved in water to produce 600 ml makes 0.9% *w/v* solution

Sometimes the solutions are supplied in a concentrated form with directions for making an appropriate dilution. In such cases, the strengths are generally stated as parts of the dissolved substance in parts of solution *e.g.* 1 : 400, 1 : 2500 and 3 : 1000 etc.

Mistakes are often made in converting strengths expressed in this form to percentages. The following table, however, helps in avoiding any mistake.

TABLE 3.7

1 in 100	=	100/100 per cent	=	1%
1 in 400	=	100/400 per cent	=	0.25%
1 in 600	=	100/600 per cent	=	0.166%
1 in 1,000	=	100/1,000 per cent	=	0.1%
1 in 2,000	=	100/2,000 per cent	=	0.05%
1 in 2,500	=	100/2,500 per cent	=	0.04%
3 in 1,000	=	3 × 100/1,000 per cent	=	0.3%
4 in 5,000	=	4 × 100/5,000 per cent	=	0.08%
2 in 10,000	=	2 × 100/10,000 per cent	=	0.02%

Example 5 How many tablets, each containing 8.75 gr of mercuric chloride will be required to make one quart of a 0.05 per cent solution?

Calculation 35 gr, in 8 fl oz, are required to make 1% *w/v* solution

35 × 0.05 gr in 8 fl oz, are required to make 0.05% *w/v* solution

$$\frac{35 \times 0.05 \times 40}{8} \text{ gr in 40 fl oz, are required to make 0.05\% } w/v \text{ solution}$$

$$= 8.75 \text{ gr}$$

8.75 gr of mercuric chloride is present in one tablet. So, 0.05 per cent solution of mercuric chloride is prepared if one tablet is dissolved in water to produce one quart.

Example 6 Prepare 8 oz of a solution so that two teaspoonful diluted to a quart, will make 1 in 2,500 solution.

Calculation

$$1 \text{ in } 2{,}500 \text{ solution} = \frac{1 \times 100}{2{,}500} \text{ per cent} = 0.04 \text{ per cent}$$

In such cases, the calculation involves two steps:

Step 1—To find out how many grains will be required to make a quart of 0.04 per cent solution.

Step 2—Every two teaspoonful of the 8 oz of a strong solution must contain the required number of grains calculated in step 1. So, it must be multiplied by the number of two teaspoonful present in 8 fl oz.

35 gr, in 8 fl oz will make a 1% *w/v* solution

35 × 0.04 gr in 8 fl oz, will make a 0.04% *w/v* solution

$\frac{35 \times 0.04 \times 40}{8}$ gr in 40 fl oz, will make a 0.04% *w/v* solution

= 7.0 gr

Therefore, 7.0 gr must be present in every 2 teaspoonfuls of the solution.

1 oz = 8 teaspoonful

8 oz = 64 teaspoonful

2 teaspoonful contains = 7.0 gr

64 teaspoonful contains = $\frac{7.0 \times 64}{2}$ = 224.0 gr

So 224.0 gr is dissolved in water to produce 8 oz.

Example 7 Calculate the number of grains required to make 12 oz, so that 1 tablespoonful diluted to half a pint will make 0.04 per cent solution.

Calculation (½ pint = 10 fl oz) The calculation involves two steps:

Step 1 — To find out how many grains will be required to make half a pint of 0.04 per cent solution

Step 2 — Every 1 tablespoonful of 12 oz of a strong solution must conain the required number of grains calculated in step 1. So, it must be multiplied by the number of 1 tablespoonful present in 12 ft oz.

35 gr, in 8 fl oz will make 1% w/v solution

$\frac{35 \times 0.04 \times 10}{8}$ gr, in 10 fl oz, will make 0.04% w/v solution

= 1.75 gr

Therefore 1.75 gr must be present in every 1 tablespoonful of the solution

1oz = 2 tablespoonful

12 oz = 24 tablespoonful

1 tablespoonful contains 1.75 gr

24 tablespoonful contains 1.75 × 24 = 42 gr

So, 42 gr is dissolved in water to produce 12 oz

Example 8 Prepare 5 oz of a solution so that 1 tablespoonful to 1 quart makes 1 in 500 solution.

Calculation (1 quart = 40 fl oz)

1 in 500 = 100/500 = 0.2%

1 quart = 40 fl oz

35 gr, in 8 fl oz, will make a 1% *w/v* solution
35 × 0.2 gr, in 8 fl oz, will make a 0.2% *w/v* solution

$$\frac{35 \times 0.2 \times 40}{8} \text{ gr, in 40 fl oz, will make a 0.2\% } w/v \text{ solution}$$

$$= 35 \text{ gr}$$

So, 35 gr must be contained in every tablespoonful.

1 oz = 2 tablespoonfuls
5 oz = 10 tablespoonfuls

Therefore, 35 × 10 gr = 350 gr must be contained in 5 oz (10 table spoonful)

Sometimes concentrated percentage solutions are supplied and labelled with directions for preparing weaker percentage solutions.

Example 9 Calculate the number of grains required to make 8 oz of a 4 per cent solution and label with directions for preparing a quart of a 1 in 2,000 solution.

Calculation

Ist Step—Calculation for preparing 8 oz of a 4 per cent solution

35 gr, in 8 fl oz, will make a 1 per cent solution.

35 × 4 gr, in 8 fl oz will make a 4 per cent solution = 140 g

140 gr is dissolved in water and diluted to 8 oz.

IInd Step—The volume of the prepared solution required to make a quart of a 1 in 2,000 solution

Strength of concentrated solution = 4%
Strength of dilute solution 1 in 2,000 = 100/2000 = 1/20 = 0.05%

$$\text{Degree of dilution} = \frac{\text{Strength of concentrate}}{\text{Strength of dilute solution}} = \frac{4}{0.05} = 80 \text{ times}$$

Quantity of concentrated solution required = 40/80 = 1/2 oz
1/2 oz = 1 tablespoonful

1 tablespoonful to be diluted to a quart to make 1 in 2000 solution.

Alternative method:
Strength of dilute solution = 0.05%
Strength of concentrate solution = 4%
Volume of dilute solution to be prepared = 1 quart = 40 oz
Volume of strong solution required = ?

By applying the following formula:

$$\text{Volume of stronger solution required} = \frac{\text{Volume of dilute solution} \times \text{Percentage of dilute solution}}{\text{Percentage used}}$$

$$= \frac{40 \times 0.05}{4}$$

$= 0.5$ oz

$= ½$ oz $= 1$ tablespoonful

So, 1 tablespoonful of 4% solution is diluted to a quart make 1: 2000 solution

Example 10 How much of a 5 per cent will be required to prepare 600 ml of a 1 in a 800 solution?

Calculation Strength of concentrated solution = 5%

Strength of dilute solution = 1:800 = 100/800 = 1/8 = 0.125%

$$\text{Degree of dilution} = \frac{\text{Strength of concentrate}}{\text{Strength of dilute solution}} = \frac{5}{0.125} = 40 \text{ times}$$

Quantity of concentrated solution required = 600/40 = 15 ml

15 ml = 1 tablespoonful

So 1 tablespoonful of 5% solution to be diluted to 600 ml to produce 1 : 800 solution.

Alternative method:

Strength of dilute solution = 0.125%

Strength of concentrate solution = 5%

Volume of dilute solution to be prepared = 600 ml

Volume of concentrate solution required = ?

By applying the following formula:

$$\text{Volume of stronger solution required} = \frac{\text{Volume of dilute solution} \times \text{Percentage of dilute solution}}{\text{Percentage used}}$$

$$= \frac{600 \times 0.125}{5}$$

$= 15$ ml

15 ml = 1 tablspoonful

Therefore, 1 tablespoonful of 5% solution is diluted to 600 ml to prepare 1:800 solutions

Example 11 Prepare 100 ml of a solution of mercuric chloride of which one part diluted with three parts of water makes a 1 in 4,000 solution.

Calculation Strength of concentrated solution = ?

Strength of dilute solution = 1 in 4,000

1 in 4,000 = 100/4,000 = 0.025%

Degree of dilution = 1 + 3 = 4 times

$$\text{Strength of dilute solution} = \frac{\text{Strength of concentrate}}{\text{Degree of dilution}}$$

$$0.025 = \frac{\text{Strength of concentrate}}{4}$$

$$0.025 \times 4 = \text{Strength of concentrate}$$
$$= 0.1\%\ w/v$$

1 g, in 100 ml, will make a 1% *w*/*v* solution.
0.1 g, in 100 ml, will make a 0.1% *w*/*v* solution.

So, 100 mg is dissolved in water to produce 100 ml solution.

Example 12 Prepare 100 ml of a solution of potassium permanganate of which one part diluted with four parts of water makes 1 in 2500 solution.

Calculation Strength of concentrated solution = ?
Strength of dilute solution = 1 in 2,500
1 in 2,500 = 100/2,500 = 0.04%
Degree of dilution = 1 + 4 = 5 times

By applying the formula:

$$\text{Strength of dilute solution} = \frac{\text{Strength of concentrate}}{\text{Degree of dilution}}$$

$$0.04 = \frac{\text{Strength of concentrate}}{5}$$

$$0.04 \times 5 = \text{strength of concentrate}$$
$$= 0.2\%\ \text{w/v}$$

1 g in 100 ml, will make a 1% w/v solution
0.2 g in 100 ml, will make a 0.2% w/v solution

So, 200 mg of potassium permanganate is dissolved in water to produce 100 ml of solution

Example 13 Prepare 400 ml of a 5 percent solution and label with a direction for preparing 2 litre quantities of a 1 in 2,000 solution.

Calculation

Strength of concentrate = 5 per cent

Strength of dilute solution = 1 in 2,000

= 100/2,000

= 0.05%

Degree of dilution = ?

By applying the formula:

$$\frac{\text{Strength of concentrate}}{\text{Degree of dilution}} = \text{Strength of dilute solution}$$

$$\frac{5}{\text{Degree of dilution}} = 0.05$$

∴ Degree of dilution = 5/0.05 = 100 times

Volume of the solution to be prepared = 2 litre

= 2,000 ml

Therefore, dilute solution is obtained by diluting

2,000/100 = 20 ml of concentrated solution to 2 litre.

Alternative method:

Strength of dilute solution = 0.05%

Strength of concentrate solution = 5%

Volume of dilute solution to be prepared = 2 litre

Value of concentrate solution required = ?

By applying the following formula

$$\text{Volume of stronger solution required} = \frac{\text{Volume of dilute solution} \times \text{Percentage of dilute solution}}{\text{Percentage used}}$$

$$= \frac{2000 \times 0.05}{5}$$

$$= 20 \text{ ml}$$

Therefore dilute solution is prepared by diluting 20 ml of concentrate solute to 2 litre.

Example 14 Prepare 500 ml of a 1 in 4000 solution from the 1 in 800 solution.

Calculation

Strength of concentrate 1 in 800 = 100/800 = 0.125%

Strength of dilute solution 1 in 4000 = 100/4000 = 0.025%

By applying the formula:

$$\frac{\text{Strength of concentrate}}{\text{Degree of dilution}} = \text{Strength of dilute solution}$$

$$\frac{0.125}{\text{Degree of dilution}} = 0.025$$

$\therefore$ Degree of dilution = 0.125/0.025

= 5 times

Volume of solution to be prepared = 500 ml

Therefore, dilute solution is obtained by diluting 500/5 = 100 ml of 1 in 800 solution to 500 ml.

Alternate method:

Strength of dilute solution = 0.025%

Strength of concentrate solution = 0.125%

Volume of dilute solution to be prepared = 500 ml

Volume of concentrate solution required = ?

$$\text{Volume of stronger solution required} = \frac{\text{Volume of dilute solution} \times \text{Percentage of dilute solution}}{\text{Percentage used}}$$

$$= \frac{500 \times 0.025}{0.125}$$

$$= 100 \text{ ml}$$

Therefore, 500 ml of 1:4000 solutions is prepared by diluting 100 ml of 1:800 solution to 500 ml

Weight in Weight (*w/w*) Solutions

Normally percentage solutions of solids in liquids are not made *w/w* unless it is specially required for the reason that:

1. Solutions are generally administered by volume, hence it is convenient to prepare solution by volume.
2. Equal volumes of all *w/v* solution of the same strength contain the same amount of solute.

3. Equal volumes of *w/w* solutions of the same strength do not contain the same quantity of solute, because of the difference in the specific gravities of the liquids acting as the solvent. Example 13, illustrate this type of difficulty.

Example 15 Prepare 100 ml of phenol glycerin I.P.

Calculation I.P. 66 formula is:

Phenol = 160 g
Glycerin = 840 g

Phenol glycerin contains phenol ≅ 16.0 per cent *w/w* of glycerin.

Weight per ml of glycerin = 1.252 to 1.257
= 1.26

So for preparing 100 ml of phenol glycerin
the quantity of glycerin required = 100 × 1.26 = 126 g

$$\text{Quantity of phenol required} = \frac{160 \times 126}{840} = 24 \text{ g}$$

For preparing 100 ml of phenol glycerin I.P., the formula becomes:

	I.P. Formula	*Quantity required for 100 ml*
Phenol	160 g	24 g
Glycerin	840 g	126 g

Volume in Volume (*v/v*) Solutions

The percentage solution of liquids in liquids is made volume in volume. The general formula in the metric system is:

Liquid solute	1 ml	} for 1% *v/v* solution
Solvent to produce	100 ml	

Alcohol Dilution

The dilute alcohols are made from 95% alcohol which contain 95 parts by volume of ethyl alcohol and 5 parts by volume of water. Hence it is a volume in volume (*v/v*) percentage solution.

When alcohol gets mixed with water the following changes take place:

1. There is contraction of volume.
2. There is rise in temperature.
3. There is turbid appearance in the solution, because solubility of air is more in alcohol than in water. When alcohol is diluted with water, minute bubbles of air get evolved from the alcohol and make the turbid appearance.

When alcohol is diluted with water it is necessary to cool the mixture to about 20°C and then final volume is made up.

The following examples illustrate the method of calculating alcohol dilutions.

Example 16 Prepare 400 ml of 45 per cent alcohol from 95 per cent alcohol.

Calculation

Volume required = 400 ml
Percentage of alcohol required = 45
Percentage of alcohol used = 95

By applying the formula:

$$\text{Volume of stronger alcohol to be used} = \frac{\text{Volume required} \times \text{Percentage required}}{\text{Percentage used}}$$

$$= \frac{400 \times 45}{95} = \frac{3600}{19}$$

$$= 189.47 \text{ ml}$$

$$\cong 190 \text{ ml}$$

190 ml of 95% alcohol is diluted with water to produce 400 ml. The strength of dilute alcohol will be 45%.

Example 17 Prepare 8 oz of 60% alcohol from 95 per cent alcohol.

Calculation

Volume required = 8 oz
Percentage of alcohol required = 60
Percentage of alcohol used = 95

By applying the formula:

$$\text{Volume of stronger alcohol to be used} = \frac{\text{Volume required} \times \text{Percentage required}}{\text{Percentage used}}$$

$$= \frac{8 \times 60}{95} = \frac{96}{19}$$

$$= 5.05$$

$$\cong 5 \text{ oz}$$

5 oz of 95% alcohol is diluted with water to make 8 oz of 60% alcohol.

Example 18 Prepare 600 ml of 60% alcohol from 95 percent alcohol.

Calculation Volume required = 600 ml
Percentage of alcohol required = 60
Percentage of alcohol used = 95

By applying the formula:

$$\text{Volume of stronger alcohol to be used} = \frac{\text{Volume required} \times \text{Percentage required}}{\text{Percentage used}}$$

$$= \frac{600 \times 60}{95} = \frac{36000}{95} \text{ ml}$$

$$= 379 \text{ ml}$$

Therefore 379 ml of alcohol 95% is diluted with water to produce 600 ml. The strength of dilute solution will be 60%.

MISCELLANEOUS PERCENTAGE SOLUTIONS

Sometimes a request for dilution of acids (acetic acid) and other compounds (ammonia and formaldehyde) is made. As some of the percentage dilutions may be of two types, so great care must be taken to find out which type of dilution is required. The following are few examples to illustrate it.

Example 19 Prepare and submit 250 ml of an 8.25 per cent solution of acetic acid

Calculation The solution can be prepared in two ways:

Method 1—Considering acetic acid is the official name of an acid of defined strength, the request may be taken as to prepare a solution containing 8.25 per cent of the official acid. Acetic acid is a liquid so the solution must be supplied in *v/v*.

8.25 ml of acetic acid diluted to 100 ml = 8.25% *v/v* of acetic acid

$\frac{8.25 \times 250}{100}$ ml of acetic acid diluted to 250 ml = 8.25% *v/v* of acetic acid = 20.6 ml

So, 20.6 ml of acetic acid is diluted to 250 ml with water to produce 8.25 per cent *v/v* acetic acid.

Method 2—Considering acetic acid I.P. contains 33 percent *w/w* of real acid, the solution is required to prepare in *w/w* and not in *v/v*.

Weight per ml of acetic acid is 1.04.

So weight of 250 ml of acetic acid will be = 250 × 1.04 = 260 g

The calculation in this case is same as that used for alcohol dilution *i.e.*,

$$\text{Weight for stronger acid required} = \frac{\text{Weight required} \times \text{Percentage required}}{\text{Percentage used}}$$

$$= \frac{260 \times 8.25}{33} = 65 \text{ g}$$

Thus the formula becomes:

Acetic acid I.P.	65 g
Water	195 g
	260 g

So, 65.0 g of Acetic acid I.P. is diluted with 195.0 g of water to produce 8.25% *w/w* acetic acid.

Example 20 Prepare and submit 200 ml of a solution containing 4 per cent of formaldehyde.

Calculation The solution can be prepared in two methods.

Method 1—4% of formaldehyde means a solution containing 4% *v/v* of the official solution. The calculation can be made as:

4.0 ml of official formaldehyde solution diluted to 100 ml = 4% *v/v* of formaldehyde

$\frac{4 \times 200}{100}$ ml of official formaldehyde solution diluted to 200 ml = 4% *v/v* of formaldehyde

(= 8 ml)

So 8.0 ml of formaldehyde is diluted to 200 ml with water to produce 4% *v/v* of formaldehyde solution.

Method 2—Formaldehyde solution I.P. contains 34 to 38 g of formaldehyde in 100 g *i.e. w/w* solution. This means the 4% solution is required to prepare in *w/w* and not in *v/v*.

Wt. per ml of formaldehyde solution I.P. is about 1.08 g

Therefore, weight of 200 ml of formaldehyde solution will be

$$= 200 \times 1.08 \text{ g}$$
$$= 216 \text{ g}$$

The calculation can be made as:

$$\text{Weight of stronger formaldehyde solution to be used} = \frac{\text{Weight required} \times \text{Percentage required}}{\text{Percentage used}}$$

$$= \frac{216 \times 4}{36} = 24.0 \text{ g}$$

Thus the formula becomes:

Formaldehyde solution I.P. = 24.0 g

Purified water sufficient to produce 216.0 g. It will produce 4% *w/w* of formaldehyde solution.

Example 21 Prepare and submit 400 ml of cetrimide solution B.P. from strong cetrimide solution B.P.

Strong cetrimide solution B.P. contains 40% w/v cetrimide. Cetrimide solution B.P. is a 1% w/v solution.

Calculation Strength of concentrated solution = 40% w/v
Strength of dilute solution = 1 % w/v

Volume of the cetrime solution to be prepared = 400 ml

By applying the following formula:

$$\text{Volume of stronger solution required} = \frac{\text{Volume of dilute solution} \times \text{Percentage of dilute solution}}{\text{Percentage used}}$$

$$= \frac{400 \times 1}{40}$$

$$= 10 \text{ ml}$$

Therefore 10 ml of strong cetrimide solution is required to be diluted to 400 ml with water to make cetrimide solution.

ALLIGATION METHOD IN CALCULATIONS

When the calculation involves mixing of two similar preparations of different strengths, to produce a preparation of intermediate strength, the alligation method may be used. The method is recommended for the purpose of checking the calculations.

For calculation purpose, the figures are written as given below:

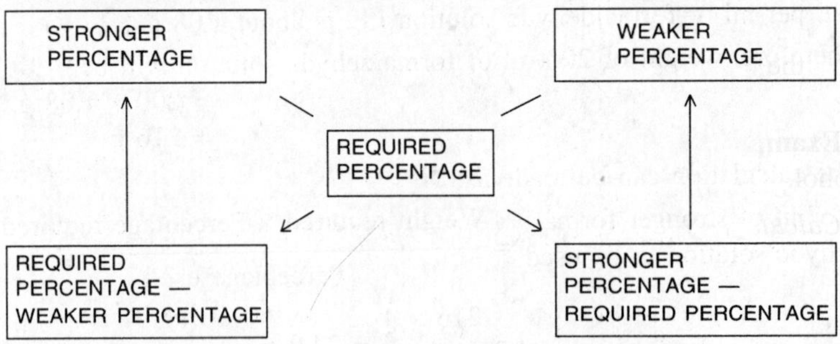

The following example illustrates the use of this method:

Example 22 Prepare 500 g of dilute acetic acid from acetic acid I.P.

Calculation Acetic acid I.P. = 33% *w/w* of Acetic acid

Dilute acetic acid = 6% *w/w* of Acetic acid

Let x be the number of grams of 33% acetic acid required, then as per question:

$$\frac{33}{100} \times x + \frac{0}{100}(500 - x) = \frac{6}{100} \times 500$$

$$33x + 0\,(500 - x) = 3000$$

$$33x + 0 = 3000$$

$$33x = 3000$$

$$x = 91 \text{ g}$$

Number of grams of 33% acetic acid required = 91 g

Number of grams of water required = 500 – 91 = 409 g

Therefore, 91.0 g of 33% acetic acid is required to be mixed with 409 g of water to produce 500 g of 6% dilute acetic acid.

The above calculation can be checked by alligation method.

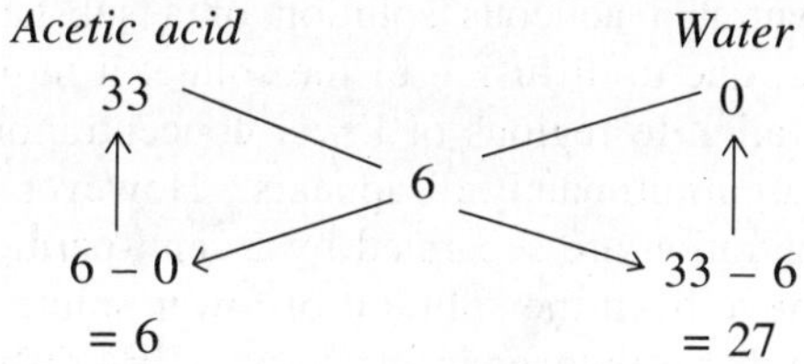

This means that 6 parts by weight of acetic acid 33% *w/w* when mixed with 27 parts by weight of water it will produce 33 parts by weight of dilute acetic acid 6%. Therefore, for preparing 500 g of dilute acetic acid,

the quantity of 33% acid required = $\frac{500 \times 6}{33}$ = 91 g

the quantity of water required = $\frac{500 \times 27}{33}$ = 409 g

Example 23 Prepare 600 ml of 70 per cent alcohol from 95% alcohol.

Calculation Percentage of alcohol required = 70

Percentage of alcohol used = 95

By using allegation method:

Alcohol		*Water*
95		0
	70	
70 – 0		95 – 70
= 70		= 25

70 parts of 95% alcohol and 25 parts of water will produce the required percentage alcohol

$$\text{Quantity of 95\% alcohol required} = \frac{600 \times 70}{95}$$

$$= 442.10 \text{ ml}$$

$$\text{Quantity of water required} = \frac{600 \times 25}{95}$$

$$= 157.90 \text{ ml}$$

ISOTONIC SOLUTIONS

When a concentrated aqueous solution of a substance is placed in contact with water, due to diffusion of the solute, it moves from regions of higher concentration to regions of lower concentration, so that differences in concentration ultimately disappears. However, if two solutions of different concentration are separated by a semi-permeable membrane, the solvent will move from the solution of lower solute concentration to the solution of higher solute concentration. This diffusion of solvent through a membrane is called "Osmosis". The excess of solvent molecules passing in one direction creates a pressure called 'Osmotic pressure'. Osmotic pressure is directly proportional to the number of solute units. It is also proportional to the gram molecular concentration.

The membranes which allow solvent molecules to pass through but resist the passage of dissolved substances, are called 'Semi-permeable membranes'. The blood cells are enclosed in a semi-permeable membrane and they strictly follow the principle of osmosis.

Solutions having the same osmotic pressure are called 'Iso-osmotic'. It is not necessary that solutions which are iso-osmotic will also be isotonic. If a red blood cell is in contact with a solution that has the same osmotic pressure as that of blood plasma, the cell wall will neither swell nor shrink *i.e.*, it will retain its tone and therefore the solution is said to be 'Isotonic'.

To determine whether or not a solution is isotonic with erythrocytes, it is necessary to determine the concentration of the solute at which the cells retain their normal size and shape. The parenteral solutions and ophthalmic solutions need adjustment to iso-osmoticity and iso-tonicity.

The solutions which are not having the same osmotic pressure are called 'Paratonic'. While comparing a solution with the one of known osmotic pressure, those which exert a greater pressure are called 'Hypertonic' and those with a lower pressure are called 'Hypotonic'. Blood plasma contains 0.88% of inorganic salts, mainly sodium chloride, which make the main contribution to osmotic pressure.

A solution containing 0.9% of sodium chloride is, therefore, practically isotonic with blood plasma and is regarded as standard. A solution containing more than 0.9% sodium chloride is called 'hypertonic' and one containing less than that is called 'hypotonic'.

General Principles for Adjustment to Isotonicity

(1) *Solutions for i/v injection* : Approximate isotonicity is always desirable.

(2) *Solutions for s/c injection* : Isotonicity is needed but it is not essential, since they are injected into fatty tissues and not in blood stream.

(3) *Solutions for i/m injection* : The aqueous solutions should be slightly hypertonic to promote rapid absorption.

(4) *Solutions for intra-cutaneous injection* : The parenteral preparations which are meant for diagnostic purpose should be isotonic in order to avoid the false reaction.

(5) *Solutions for intra-thecal injection* : These must be isotonic, because the volume of C.S.F. (cerebro spinal fluid) is only 60 to 80 ml. Hence, a small volume of a paratonic solution will disturb the osmotic pressure and may cause vomiting and other side-effects.

(6) *Solutions used for nasal drops* : Isotonicity is needed, since paratonic solution may cause irritation.

(7) *Solutions used as eye drops and eye lotion* : Eye lotion should be isotonic with lachrymal secretion, since a large volume is brought in contact with the eye. Eye drops may not be isotonic, because only a small volume is used which quickly get diluted by the lachrymal secretion.

CALCULATIONS FOR SOLUTIONS ISO-OSMOTIC/ ISOTONIC WITH BLOOD AND TEARS

The following are some of the methods by which the calculations are made for solutions meant for iso-osmotic with blood and tears:

1. Method based on freezing point data.
2. Method based on molecular concentration.
3. Graphic method based on vapour pressure and freezing-point depression.
4. Method based on sodium chloride equivalent.

1. Method based on Freezing-Point Data

There are certain physical properties of solutions known as 'colligative properties' which are independent of the nature of the dissolved substances. These colligative properties are:

1. Osmotic pressure
2. Depression of freezing-point

Determination of the depression of freezing point is simpler and more accurate than direct measurement of osmotic pressure. So, this property of the solution is used to compare osmotic pressures.

The temperature at which blood plasma and tears freeze is –0.52°C. This means that the dissolved substances contained in them depress the freezing point 0.52°C below that of pure water. So, any other solution which freezes at –0.52°C will have the same osmotic pressure as blood plasma and tears.

The hypotonic solutions have a freezing-point higher than that of blood plasma and tears. For example, a 1% *w/v* solution of boric acid freezes at –0.288°C as given in Table 3.8.

TABLE 3.8

Freezing-Point of a 1 per cent *w/v* Solution of Substances Commonly Used in Injections and Ophthalmic Solutions

S. No.	*Name of the substance*	*Freezing point*
1.	Adrenaline acid tartrate	– 0.098 °C
2.	Amethocaine hydrochloride	– 0.109 °C
3.	Apomorphine hydrochloride	– 0.080 °C
4.	Atropine methonitrate	– 0.100 °C
5.	Atropine sulphate	– 0.074 °C
6.	Benzalkonium chloride solution B.P.C.	– 0.046 °C
7.	Boric acid	– 0.288 °C

S. No.	Name of the substance	Freezing point
8.	Calcium chloride, $2H_2O$	– 0.298 °C
9.	Calcium gluconate	– 0.091 °C
10.	Carbachol	– 0.205 °C
11.	Chlorbutol	– 0.138 °C
12.	Cocaine hydrochloride	– 0.090 °C
13.	Dextrose, anhydrous	– 0.101 °C
14.	Dextrose (Monohydrate)	– 0.91 °C
15.	Emetine hydrochloride	– 0.058 °C
16.	Ephedrine hydrochloride	– 0.165 °C
17.	Ethanolamine	– 0.306 °C
18.	Flourescein sodium	– 0.181 °C
19.	Homatropine hydrobromide	– 0.097 °C
20.	Hyoscine hydrobromide	– 0.068 °C
21.	Lignocaine hydrochloride	– 0.130 °C
22.	Magnesium sulphate	– 0.094 °C
23.	Morphine hydrochloride	– 0.086 °C
24.	Morphine sulphate	– 0.079 °C
25.	Neostigmine bromide	– 0.127 °C
26.	Neostigmine methylsulphate	– 0.115 °C
27.	Papaverine hydrochloride	– 0.061 °C
28.	Pethidine hydrochloride	– 0.125 °C
29.	Phenobarbitone sodium	– 0.135 °C
30.	Physostigmine salicylate	– 0.090 °C
31.	Pilocarpine nitrate	– 0.132 °C
32.	Potassium chloride	– 0.439 °C
33.	Procaine hydrochloride	– 0.122 °C
34.	Quinine hydrochloride	– 0.077 °C
35.	Silver nitrate	– 0.190 °C
36.	Sodium biocarbonate	– 0.38 °C
37.	Sodium chloride	– 0.576 °C
38.	Sodium citrate	– 0.178 °C
39.	Sodium metabisulphite	– 0.386 °C
40.	Sodium nitrite	– 0.48 °C
41.	Sulphacetamide sodium	– 0.132 °C
42.	Urea	– 0.341 °C
43.	Zinc sulphate	– 0.086 °C

In order to make this solution isotonic, an adjusting substance must be added to produce the freezing point to –0.52°C. The general formula for calculation for solutions to be made iso-osmotic with blood serum is as follows:

$$\text{Percentage } w/v \text{ of adjusting substance needed} = \frac{0.52 - a}{b}$$

where a = Freezing-point of the un-adjusted solution
b = Freezing-point of a 1% *w/v* solution of the adjusting substance.

(*Note*—Each solute exerts its effect on the freezing-point independently of the other solute present in the solution. Hence, if a solution contains more than one solute, then the value of "*a*" will be the sum of their depressions.)

Example 24 Find out the proportion of procaine hydrochloride which will yield a solution iso-osmotic with blood plasma.

(*Given* : The freezing-point of a 1% *w/v* solution of procaine hydrochloride is –0.122°C)

Calculation By applying the formula:

$$\text{Percentage } w/v \text{ of procaine hydrochloride required} = \frac{0.52 - 0.00}{0.122}$$

$$= 4.26\% \ w/v$$

Example 25 Find the concentration of sodium chloride required to make a 1 per cent solution of boric acid, iso-osmotic with blood plasma.

(*Given* : The freezing-point of 1% *w/v* solution of boric acid is –0.288°C. The freezing-point of 1% *w/v* solution of sodium chloride is –0.576°C)

Calculation By applying the formula:

$$\text{Percentage } w/v \text{ of sodium chloride required} = \frac{0.52 - 0.288}{0.576}$$

$$= 0.402\% \ w/v$$

Example 26 Find the concentration of sodium chloride required to make a 1.5 per cent solution of cocaine hydrochloride iso-osmotic with blood plasma.

(*Given* : The freezing point of 1% *w/v* solution of cocaine hydrochloride is –0.09°C. The freezing-point of 1% *w/v* solution of sodium chloride is –0.576°C)

Calculation By applying the formula:

$$\text{Percentage } w/v \text{ of sodium chloride required} = \frac{0.52 - (0.09 \times 1.5)}{0.576}$$

$$= 0.668\% \ w/v$$

Sometimes a solution has to be prepared of such a strength that, on dilution with a specified volume of water, it will be iso-osmotic with tissue fluids.

Example 27 Find the amount of sodium chloride to be included in 100 ml of 0.5 per cent solution of zinc sulphate so that, on dilution with an equal quantity of water, it will be iso-osmotic with tissue fluids.

(*Given* : The freezing-point of 1% *w/v* solution of zinc sulphate is –0.086°C. The freezing-point of 1% *w/v* solution of sodium chloride is – 0.576°C)

Calculation It can be done in three different ways.

Method (1)—Calculation based on twice the freezing-point for lachrymal secretion.

Therefore, the general formula becomes:

$$\text{Percentage of adjusting substance} = \frac{(2 \times 0.52) - a}{b}$$

By applying the above formula:

$$\text{Percentage of sodium chloride required} = \frac{(2 \times 0.52) - (0.5 \times 0.086)}{0.576}$$

$$= \frac{1.04 - 0.043}{0.576} = \frac{0.997}{0.576}$$

$$= 1.73\ \%w/v$$

Therefore, the quantity of sodium chloride in 100 ml of zinc sulphate required will be 1.73 g.

Method (2)—Calculation based on the diluted solution *i.e.* calculate the amount of sodium chloride required for 200 ml of a 0.25 per cent solution instead of 100 ml of 0.5 per cent solution.

$$\text{Percentage of sodium chloride required} = \frac{0.52 - (0.25 \times 0.086)}{0.576}$$

$$= \frac{0.52 - 0.0215}{0.576} = \frac{0.4985}{0.576}$$

$$= 0.865 \text{ per cent}$$

The quantity of sodium chloride required for 200 ml solution

$$= 2 \times 0.865 = 1.73 \text{ g}$$

Method (3)—Calculate in the normal way ignoring the dilution and add to the result 0.9 g of sodium chloride *i.e* 0.9% of 100 ml

$$\text{Percentage of sodium chloride required} = \frac{0.52 - (0.5 \times 0.086)}{0.576}$$

$$= \frac{0.52 - 0.043}{0.576} = 0.83\%$$

In 0.83% of 100 ml solution the quantity of sodium chloride = 0.83 g

Therefore, total quantity of sodium chloride required = 0.83 + 0.9
= 1.73 g

Example 28 Find the concentration of sodium chloride required to make 50 ml of isotonic solution containing 0.5% ephedrine hydrochloride and 0.5% chlorobutol.

(*Given* : Freezing point of 1% *w/v* solution of ephedrine hydrochloride is –0.165°C. Freezing point of 1% *w/v* solution of chlorobutol is –0.138°C)

Calculation As the concentration of ephedrine hydrochloride in the preparation is 0.5% *w/v*, the depression in freezing-point of ephedrine hydrochloride = 0.165 × 0.5 = 0.0825°C.

As the concentration of chlorobutol in the preparation is 0.5% *w/v*, the depression in freezing-point of chlorobutol = 0.138 × 0.5 = 0.069°C

Therefore, total depression in freezing-point of both the substances will be = 0.0825 + 0.069 = 0.1515

$$\text{Percentage } w/v \text{ of sodium chloride required} = \frac{0.52 - 0.1515}{0.576}$$

$$= 0.644\%$$

Weight of sodium chloride required to make 100 ml of solution = 0.644 g

Weight of sodium chloride required to make 50 ml of solution = 0.322 g

2. Method Based on Molecular Concentration

Molecular concentration means the number of units *i.e.* molecules or ions or both present in a solution. A solution containing one gram molecule of a non-ionising solute in 22.4 litres at normal temperature and pressure (NTP) has an osmotic pressure of one atmosphere. So, a solution containing one gram molecule in 1 litre (a mole solution) will have an osmotic pressure of 22.4 atmosphere.

The osmotic pressure of blood plasma and lachrymal secretion is approximately 6.7 atmosphere.

$$\text{Hence molarity of these fluids} = \frac{6.7}{22.4} = 0.3 \text{ M (approx.)}$$

Therefore, a 0.3 M solution of any non-ionising solution will be iso-osmotic with blood plasma and tears. This knowledge may be used to calculate the concentrations of un-ionised medicaments needed to produce iso-osmotic solutions by using the following formula:

$$W = 0.3 \text{ M}$$

where W = Concentration required in g per litre
M = Molecular weight of the solute

If the solute ionises in solution, the following formula is used:

$$W = \frac{0.3 \text{ M}}{N}$$

where N = Number of ions produced from each molecule of the solution assuming that dissociation is complete

Example 29 Find the proportion of dextrose needed to form a solution iso-osmotic with blood plasma.

Calculation Molecular weight of dextrose = 180

Dextrose is non-ionising substance

Hence the formula used is : W = 0.3 M

$$W = 0.3 \times 180$$
$$= 54.0 \text{ g/litre}$$
$$\textit{Or } W = 5.4 \text{ g/100 ml}$$

Example 30 Find the concentration of sodium chloride required to produce a solution iso-osmotic with blood plasma.

Calculation Molecular weight of sodium chloride = 58.5

Sodium chloride is ionising substance and it gets dissociates into 2 ions.

Hence, the following formula is used.

$$W = \frac{0.3 \text{ M}}{N}$$

$$= \frac{0.3 \times 58.5}{2} = 8.8 \text{ g per litre}$$

$$\textit{Or } W = 0.88 \text{ g per 100 ml}$$

Those solutions which are not iso-osmotic, can be made so by adding a suitable adjusting substance, such as, sodium chloride or dextrose in order to produce a total concentration of solutes equivalent to a. 0.3 M concentration of a non-ionising solute. In such cases, the calculation is done in three steps:

1. To find out Effective Molar Concentration (EMC).
2. Subtract it from 0.3 to obtain the effective molar concentration of the adjusting substance.
3. The value is converted to g per litre.

Example 31 Find the proportion of sodium chloride required to make a 1% solution of a cocaine hydrochloride iso-osmotic with blood plasma.

Calculation

Step 1 : Molecular weight of cocaine hydrochloride = 339.5

Cocaine hydrochloride is ionising substance and it gets dissociated into 2 ions.

By applying the formula:

$$W = \frac{0.3\ M}{N}$$

Let C is the effective molar concentration (EMC).

Substituting C for 0.3 in the formula

$$W = \frac{C \times M}{N}$$

where W is the concentration required in g/litre = 10 g/litre

$$10 = \frac{C \times 339.5}{2}$$

$$C = 20/339.5 = 0.059 \text{ g/litre.}$$

Step 2 : Effective molar concentration of adjusting substance *i.e.* sodium chloride = 0.3 – 0.059

= 0.241 g/litre

Step 3 : Required concentration of sodium chloride is

$$W = \frac{0.241 \times M}{N}$$

Molecular weight of sodium chloride = 58.5

Sodium chloride is dissociated into 2 ions

$$W = \frac{0.241 \times 58.5}{2} = 7.01 \text{ g/litre}$$

Or W = 0.7 g/100 ml *i.e.* 0.7% *w/v*

Generally, an error occurs in both the methods of calculation, particularly, when ionising substances are used. Moreover, in more concentrated solutions osmotic pressure and freezing-point depression are not strictly proportional to the concentration. So, the error increases with the concentration. To get accurate result, the graphic method based on vapour pressure and freezing-point depression or method based on sodium chloride equivalents is used.

3. Graphic Method based on Vapour Pressure and Freezing-Point Depression ▪

In this method the solutions of various concentrations of sodium chloride are prepared and their freezing-points are determined with accuracy. A graph is prepared from this data by taking percentage concentration against freezing points. Such graphs are prepared for each medicament. From these graphs the percentage of adjusting substances required to make any percentage of medicament isotonic with blood plasma or body fluids can be determined.

4. Method based on Sodium Chloride Equivalents ▪

It is based on a factor called the 'sodium chloride equivalents' which can be used to convert a specified concentration of medicament to the concentrate of sodium chloride which will produce the same osmotic effect. Sodium chloride equivalent can be calculated from the following formula.

$$\text{Sodium chloride equivalent of a medicament} = \frac{\text{Freezing-point depression produced by a solution of a medicament}}{\text{Freezing-point depression produced by a sodium chloride solution of the same strength}}$$

These days, a table is also available in which information on over 250 medicaments is given with regard to their sodium chloride equivalents at various concentrations (0.5, 1, 2, 3, 4, 5 per cent *w/v*). Table 3.9 also includes the freezing-point depressions of some of the solutions at various concentrations, which are given in bracket.

The percentage of sodium chloride required for adjustment to isotonicity can be calculated using the following formula:

$$\text{Percentage of sodium chloride for adjustment to isotonicity} = 0.9 - \left[\text{Percentage strength of medicament solution} \times \text{sodium chloride equivalent of medicament}\right]$$

TABLE 3-9

Sodium Chloride Equivalents and Freezing Point Depression

(The Freezing Point Depressions are given in brackets)

S. No.	*Medicament*	*Strength of solution (% w/v)*					*Per cent w/v iso-osmotic with body fluids*
		0.5	*1*	*2*	*3*	*5*	
1.	Ammonium chloride	1.16 (0.331°)					0.8
2.	Boric acid	0.52 (0.146°)	0.50 (0.283°)				1.9
3.	Dextrose anhydrous	0.18 (0.050°)	0.18 (0.100°)	0.18 (0.205°)	0.18 (0.310°)	0.18 (0.516°)	5.05
4.	Ephedrine hydrochloride	0.32 (0.087°)	0.30 (0.169°)	0.29 (0.331°)	0.28 (0.489°)		3.2
5.	Glycerin	0.36 (0.104°)	0.35 (0.202°)	0.35 (0.403°)			2.6
6.	Hyoscine hydrobromide	0.12 (0.234°)	0.12 (0.068°)	0.12 (0.135°)	0.12 (0.201°)	0.12 (0.333°)	7.85
7.	Methoxamine hydrochloride	0.28 (0.078°)	0.26 (0.148°)	0.25 (0.281°)	0.24 (0.416°)		3.82
8.	Morphine sulphate	0.16 (0.046°)	0.14 (0.078°)	0.12 (0.131°)	0.11 (0.178°)	0.09 (0.258°)	
9.	Potassium chloride	0.76 (0.219°)	0.76 (0.439°)				1.19
10.	Potassium nitrate	0.58 (0.163°)	0.56 (0.323°)				1.62
11.	Procaine hydrochloride	0.24 (0.065°)	0.21 (0.122°)	0.20 (0.227°)	0.19 (0.327°)	0.18 (0.515°)	5.05
12.	Silver nitrate	0.33 (0.095°)	0.33 (0.190°)	0.33 (0.380°)			2.74
13.	Sodium chloride	1.00 (0.289°)	1.00 (0.576°)				0.9
14.	Sodium metabisulphite	0.7 (0.206°)	0.67 (0.389°)				1.38

Example 32 Calculate the percentage of sodium chloride required to make 1% *w/v* solution of procaine hydrochloride iso-osmotic with blood plasma.

Calculation

Sodium chloride equivalent of 1% procaine hydrochloride = 0.21

Strength of procaine hydrochloride = 1% *w/v*

∴ Percentage of sodium chloride for adjustment to isotonicity

$$= 0.9 - (1 \times 0.21)$$
$$= 0.9 - 0.21 = 0.69$$

Example 33 Calculate the percentage of anhydrous dextrose required to make a 1% solution of ephedrine hydrochloride iso-osmotic with body fluids.

Calculation

Sodium chloride equivalent of 1% ephedrine hydrochloride = 0.30
Strength of ephedrine hydrochloride = 1% *w/v*

∴ Percentage of sodium chloride for adjustment to isotonicity

$$= 0.9 - (1 \times 0.3)$$
$$= 0.9 - 0.3$$
$$= 0.6$$

When solution is made iso-osmotic with body fluids by adding an adjusting substance other than sodium chloride, the above value is divided by the sodium chloride equivalent of the adjusting substance.

Equivalent percentage of anhydrous dextrose = 0.6/0.18 = 3.3

Example 34 Calculate the percentage of sodium chloride necessary to make an injection containing 2% procaine hydrochloride iso-osmotic with blood plasma.

Calculation

Sodium chloride equivalent of 2 per cent
Procaine hydrochloride = 0.20
Strength of procaine hydrochloride = 2% *w/v*

∴ Percentage of sodium chloride for adjustment $= 0.9 - (2 \times 0.20)$

$$= 0.9 - 0.40$$
$$= 0.50$$

REVISION QUESTIONS

1. Calculate the following: [*Hint* : See examples 1 to 5]
   (*a*) 4 oz of a 1 in 2000 solution [0.875 gr in 4 fl oz]
   (*b*) 6 oz of a 1 in 40 solution [65.62 gr in 6 fl oz]
   (*c*) 8 oz of a 1 in 800 solution [4.3575 gr in 8 fl oz]
   (*d*) 1 pint of a 0.9% sodium chloride solution [78.75 gr in 20 fl oz]
   (*e*) 1 pint of a 1 in 80 solution of mercuric chloride [109.375 gr in 20 fl oz]

(*f*) How many tablets, each containing 8.75 gr of mercuric chloride, will be required to make half a gallon of a 1 in 500 solution? [8 tablets]

(*g*) How many tablets, each containing 8.75 gr of Mercuric chloride, will be required to make one pint of a 0.2 per cent solution. [2 tablets]

2. Calculate the number of grains required to make:

[*Hint* : See examples 6 & 7]

(*a*) 4 oz, so that 2 teaspoonful diluted to a pint will make 1 in 1000 solution [140 gr]

(*b*) 12 oz, so that 3 teaspoonful diluted to a quart will make 1/8 per cent solution [700 gr]

(*c*) 8 oz, so that 1 tablespoonful to half a gallon makes 1 in 500 solution [1120 gr]

(*d*) 8 oz, so that 3 teaspoonful diluted to a pint will make 0.0625 per cent solution [116.66 gr]

(*e*) 12 oz, so that 1 tablespoonful diluted to half a pint will make 0.04 per cent solution [42 gr]

3. Calculate the number of grains required to make:

[*Hint*: See examples 7 to 14]

(*a*) 8 oz, of a 10% solution and label with a direction for preparing a pint of 1 : 400 solution

[350 gr, 1 tablespoonful to be diluted to a pint]

(*b*) 16 oz, of a 20% solution and label with direction for preparing 2 gallon of 1 in 1600 solution

[1400 gr, 2 tablespoonful to be diluted to 2 gallon]

(*c*) 12 oz, of a 20% solution and label with direction for preparing half a gallon of 1 in 400 solution

[1050 gr, 2 tablespoonful to be diluted to half a gallon]

(*d*) How much of 8 per cent solution of mercuric chloride will be required to prepare 1 pint of 1 in 1000 solution? [4200 minims]

(*e*) Prepare 100 ml of a solution of potassium permanganate of which one part diluted with four parts of water makes 1 in 2500 solution [0.2% *w/v*]

(*f*) Prepare 200 ml of a solution of zinc sulphate of which one part diluted with four parts of water makes 1 in 5000 solution

[0.1% *w/v*]

4. Calculate the quantity of 95% alcohol required to make:

[*Hint* : See examples 16 to 18]

(*a*) 1 pint of 40% alcohol [8 oz]

(*b*) 1 quart of 45% alcohol [19 oz]

(*c*) 6 oz of 75% alcohol [5 oz]

(*d*) 500 ml of 20% alcohol [105 ml]

5. Calculate the quantity of 60% alcohol required to make:

[*Hint* : See examples 16 to 18]

(*a*) 500 ml of 20% alcohol [166.66 ml]

(*b*) 1 litre of 45% alcohol [750.0 ml]

(*c*) 500 ml of 30% alcohol [250.0 ml]

(*d*) 400 ml of 40% alcohol [266.66 ml]

6. How much 90 per cent alcohol will be required to make:

[*Hint* : See examples 16 to 18]

(*a*) 700 ml of 20% alcohol [155.5 ml]

(*b*) 600 ml of 60% alcohol [400 ml]

(*c*) 1 litre of 40% alcohol [444.44 ml]

(*d*) 250 ml of 70% alcohol [194.44 ml]

7. What concentration of cocaine hydrochloride will yield a solution iso-osmotic with blood plasma? (Given the freezing point of 1% *w/v* solution of cocaine hydrochloride is –0.090°C). [*Hint* : See example 24; 5.77% *w/v*]

8. What concentration of lignocaine hydrochloride will yield a solution iso-osmotic with blood plasma? The freezing-point of a 1% *w/v* solution of lignocaine hydrochloride is –0.091°C. [*Hint* : See example 24; 5.71% *w/v*]

9. Find the concentration of sodium chloride required to make a 1 per cent solution of cocaine hydrochloride iso-osmotic with blood plasma. The freezing-point of a 1% *w/v* solution of cocaine hydrochloride is –0.090°C. [*Hint* : See example 25, 0.746% *w/v*]

10. Find the concentration of sodium chloride required to make a 1 per cent solution of adrenaline acid tartrate iso-osmotic with blood plasma. The freezing-point of a 1% *w/v* solution of adrenaline acid tartrate is –0.098°C. [*Hint* : See the example 25; 0.732% *w/v*]

11. Find the concentration of boric acid required to produce a solution of iso-osmotic with lachrymal secretion. Molecular wt of boric acid is 62 and it is non-ionising. [*Hint* : See example 29; 1.86% *w/v*]

12. Find the concentration of dextrose required to produce a 1% solution of cocaine hydrochloride iso-osmotic with blood plasma. Molecular weight of dextrose is 180 and it is not ionising solute.

[*Hint* : See example 31; 4.3% *w/v*]

13. Find the concentration of sodium chloride required to make a 1.5 per cent solution of procaine hydrochloride iso-osmotic with blood plasma. The freezing point of 1% *w/v* solution of procaine hydrochloride is –0.122°C and that of sodium chloride is –0.576°C. [*Hint* : see example 27; 0.585% *w/v*]

14. Find the amount of sodium chloride to be included in 100 ml of a 0.3 per cent solution of zinc sulphate so that on dilution with an equal quantity of water it will be iso-osmotic with tissue fluids. The freezing-point of a 1% *w/v* solution of zinc sulphate is –0.086°C. [*Hint* : See ex. 27; 1.76 g]

15. Calculate the percentage of sodium chloride required to make a 1% solution of hyoscine hydrobromide iso-osmotic with body fluids. The sodium chloride equivalent of 1% hyoscine hydrobromide 0.12.

[*Hint* : See example 32, 0.78]

4

Packaging of Pharmaceuticals

After the manufacturing of drugs, it is essential that these should be stored properly. The stability of drug during its storage depends on so many factors and proper packaging is one of them. The pharmaceutical products are in direct contact with the containers and closures. So improper packing and poor quality of containers may lead to deterioration of the products.

Pharmaceutical container has been defined as a device that holds the drug and it may or may not be in direct contact with the pharmaceutical preparations. Closures are the devices by means of which containers can be opened and closed.

Qualities of a Good Container

1. It should be made of materials which can withstand wear and tear during normal handling.
2. The container must have a pharmaceutically-elegant appearance.
3. It should be so designed that a dose can be drawn from it conveniently.
4. The container must be neutral towards the material which is stored in it.
5. It should help in maintaining the stability of product against the environmental factors which cause its deterioration.
6. The material used for making of the container must be non-toxic.
7. It should be able to withstand changes in pressure and temperature. This is required in case of sterilisation of parenteral products along with its container and closure.
8. The container must not interact physically or chemically with the substance which it holds, so as to change the strength, quality or purity of the substance.
9. The container must be such that it can be labelled easily.

10. The closure of the container must be easily removable and replaceable.

▪ TYPES OF CONTAINERS ▪

Containers are divided into following types on the basis of their utility:

1. **Single dose containers** : These containers are used to supply only one dose of medicament and hold generally parenteral products *e.g.* ampoules and vials.

2. **Multi dose containers :** These containers allow the withdrawal of dose at various intervals without changing the strength, quality or purity of remaining portion. These containers hold more than one dose and are used for injectables *e.g.* vials.

3. **Light-resistant containers :** These containers protect the medicament from harmful effects of light. These containers are used to store those medicaments which are photo-sensitive.

4. **Well-closed containers :** A well-closed container protects the contents from loss during transportation, handling, storage or sale *etc.*

5. **Air-tight containers :** These are also called hermetic containers. These containers have air-tight sealing or closing. These containers protect the products from dust, moisture and air. Whereas air-tight sealed containers are used for injectables, air-tight closed containers are meant for the storage of other products.

6 **Tightly-closed containers :** These containers protect the contents from contamination by liquids, solids or vapours, from loss or deterioration of the material from effervescence, deliquescence or evaporation under normal condition of handling, storage and distribution. A tightly closed container must be capable of being tightly re-closed after use e.g. gas cylinder is a metallic tightly closed container designed to hold gas under pressure.

7. **Temper-evident containers :** These containers are fitted with a device or mechanism that reveals irreversibly whether the container has been opened.

8. **Aerosol containers :** These containers are used to hold aerosol products. These containers have adequate mechanical strength in order to bear the pressure of aerosol packing.

▪ MATERIALS USED FOR MAKING OF CONTAINERS ▪

The containers used for pharmaceutical products are usually made from the following basic materials:

1. Glass
2. Plastic
3. Metal
4. Paper and board

Glass

Glass containers are very commonly used in pharmaceutical packaging because of the following **advantages**:

1. They are transparent.
2. They are available in various shapes and sizes.
3. They can withstand the variation in temperature and pressure during sterilisation.
4. They are economical and readily available.
5. They can protect the photosensitive medicaments from light during their storage.
6. They are neutral after proper treatment.
7. They are impermeable to moisture and atmospheric gases.
8. They have good protection power.
9. They do not deteriorate with age.
10. They can be easily labelled.
11. They can be sealed hermetically or by removable closures

Disadvantages

1. Glass is fragile, so its containers are easily broken when dropped or knocked.
2. Glass containers are heavy, which increases the cost of its transportation from one place to another.
3. Glass containers may release alkali to aqueous preparations.

Composition of glass Glass is composed of sand, soda ash, lime stone and cullet. Cullet is broken glass that is mixed with the batch and acts as a fusion agent for the entire mixture. The composition of glass varies and it depends on the specific purpose for which it is used. Silicon, aluminium, boron, sodium, potassium, calcium, magnesium, zinc and barium are generally used in the preparation of glass.

Types of glass Glass of the following types are available commercially for making containers.

1. Lime-soda glass : It is composed of SiO_2 (75%), Na_2O (15%), CaO (10%) alongwith traces of K_2O, MgO and Al_2O_3. Lime-soda glass can be manufactured easily. Further, it is not so expensive. It is used for preparing containers which are meant for storage of solid medicaments. It is however not suitable as a container material for storage of parenteral products because:

(*i*) It liberates alkali in aqueous preparations.

(*ii*) On repeated use its surface loses some of its brilliance.

(*iii*) It is not resistant to sudden changes in temperature.

(*iv*) Flakes separate more easily as compared to other types of glass.

2. Borosilicate glass : It is composed of SiO_2 (80%), B_2O_3 (12%), Al_2O_3 (6%) and mixture of Na_2O, CaO and other oxides (2%). It is chemically more inert than lime-soda glass. It is a highly resistant glass.

3. Silicone-treated glass : Glass is treated with silicone so that it can be used for preparing containers to store alkali sensitive products.

4. Sulphured glass : It is a cheaper variety of glass used for construction of containers for parenteral products. The soda-lime glass is exposed to moist SO_2 at about 500°C to get sulphured glass. It does not liberate alkali.

5. Neutral glass : It is composed of SiO_2 (72-75%), B_2O_3 (7-10%), Al_2O_3 (4-6%), Na_2O (6-8%), BaO (2-4%) and K_2O (0.5-2%). It is resistant to alkalis, weather and can also withstand autoclaving. It is used for the preparation of multidose vials, transfusion bottles and ampoules.

6. Amber colour glass : Amber colour glass container is used for storage of photosensitive pharmaceutical products because it has the capacity to filter out U.V. radiations. It is obtained by adding C, S or Fe and MgO_2.

Some preparations are very sensitive to lead or arsenic. For such preparations only containers made from glass free from lead or arsenic should be used.

Containers for injectable preparations must be made from uncoloured glass. However, for substances which are highly sensitive to light coloured glass may be used but it should be transparent to permit visual inspection of its contents. The following types of glass are used for the preparation of containers meant for storage of parenteral preparations.

Type I glass : It is also called borosilicate glass or neutral glass. It offers a high hydrolytic resistance due to its chemical composition.

Type II glass : It is a soda-lime-silicate glass with high hydrolytic resistance as a result of an appropriate surface treatment with ammonium sulphate or sulphur dioxide. The containers made from this glass are suitable for most acidic and neutral aqueous preparations.

Type III glass : It is a soda-lime-silicate glass with only moderate hydrolytic resistance. The containers made from this glass are generally suitable for non-aqueous preparations for parenteral use, for powders for parenteral use (except for freeze-dried preparations) not for parenteral use.

Containers of Type II and Type III glass should be used once only. Containers for human blood and blood components must not be re-used.

Hydrolytic Resistance Glass

Glass containers should comply with the test for hydrolytic resistance as given in I.P. The test is carried on the unused containers. The number of containers to be examined and the volume of test solution to be used are given in the following Table 4-1.

TABLE 4-1

S. No.	*Normal capacity of container*	*Number of containers to be used*	*Volume of test solution to be used for titration*
1.	5 ml or less	at least 10	50.0 ml
2.	More than 5 ml, upto 30 ml	at least 5	50.0 ml
3.	More than 30 ml	at least 3	100.0 ml

Rinse each container at least twice with water at room temperature. Just before the test, rinse each container again with freshly distilled water. Fill the containers to the brim with freshly distilled water. Empty them and calculate the average overflow volume. In case of ampoules, fill them with freshly distilled water to its maximum volume. Fill bottles up to 90 per cent of their calculated overflow volume and cover them with borosilicate glass dishes which are previously rinsed with water. Place the containers in an autoclave and heat at temperature from 100°C to 121°C for twenty minutes and maintain the temperature of 121°C for sixty minutes. Cool the container and within one hour of removing from the autoclave carry out the titration by taking the specified quantity of test solution (as given in Table 4.2) into a conical flask. Add the required quantity of methyl red solution, titrate with 0.01 N hydrochloric acid. Repeat the titration using the same volume of freshly distilled water. The difference between the titration represents the volume of 0.01 N hydrochloric acid required by the test solution. Calculate the volume of 0.01 N hydrochloric acid required for each 100 ml of test solution.

The sample passes the test if the result is not greater than the volum given in Table 4-2.

TABLE 4-2

S. No.	*Capacity of container (corresponding to 90% average overflow volume)*	*Volume of 0.01 N HCl per 100 ml of test solution (ml)*	
		Type I or II glass	*Type III glass*
1.	Not more than 1 ml	2.00	20.00
2.	More than 1 ml but not more than 2 ml	1.80	17.60
3.	More than 2 ml but not more than 5 ml	1.30	13.20
4.	More than 5 ml but not more than 10 ml	1.00	10.20
5.	More than 10 ml but not more than 20 ml	0.80	08.10
6.	More than 20 ml but not more than 50 ml	0.60	06.10
7.	More than 50 ml but not more than 100 ml	0.50	04.80
8.	More than 100 ml but not more than 200 ml	0.40	03.80
9.	More than 200 ml but not more than 500 ml	0.30	02.90
10.	More than 500 ml	0.20	02.20

Plastic

Plastic containers are very commonly used in pharmaceutical packaging because of the following advantages:

1. They are light in weight and can be handled easily.
2. They are poor conductor of heat.
3. They have sufficient mechanical strength.
4. They can be transported easily.
5. They are unbreakable.
6. They are available in various shapes and sizes.
7. They are resistant to inorganic chemicals.
8. They have good protection power.
9. There are no changes of formation of flakes as it comes in glass containers.

However, plastic containers have certain **disadvantages** such as:

1. They are permeable to water vapour and atmospheric gases.
2. They cannot withstand heat without softening or distorting.
3. They may interact with certain chemical to cause softening or distortion.

4. They may absorb chemical substances, such as preservatives for solution.
5. They are relatively expensive.
6. Special type of gum or adhesive required for labelling

Composition of plastic Plastics are synthetic polymers of high molecular weight. Plastic is made from one or more polymers together with certain additives. The polymers commonly used are polyethylene polypropylene, polyvinyl chloride, polystyrene, polymethyl methoacrylate, polyethylene terephthalate and polytrifluroethylene. The additives included in plastic formulation are antioxidants, antistatic agents, colours, lubricants, plasticizers and stabilizers. The individual polymer has its own merits and demerits. Some of the polymers are described below:

1. Polyethylene (Polythene) : It is flexible, very light but tough plastic. It is impermeable to water vapour and does not deteriorate with age unless it is exposed to sunlight for a long period. It has high permeability to gases such as oxygen which can lead to deterioration of material stored in it. It has permeability to certain oils and preservatives. Its melting point being in the range of 110°C to 115°C, containers made from it can not be sterilised by heat. It is used for preparing bottles, tubings and heat sealable packaging films. High density polythene is a rigid plastic which has high resistance to oils. It has higher melting point and can be sterilised by autoclaving. It is used for preparing disposable syringes and containers for packaging of a number of pharmaceutical preparations.

2. Polyvinyl chloride (PVC) : It is less flexible, heavier and more permeable to water vapour as compared with normal polythene. It has high clarity and is not effected by sunlight. It is used for preparing eye-ointment tubes.

3. Polymethyl methoacrylate (PMMA) : It is a hard, strong but light, transparent plastic. It softens at about 100°C. It is used for preparing bottles and tubes.

4. Polystyrene : It is a hard, rigid, light material. It can be easily moulded into any shape. So it is used for preparing bottles, tubes, jars, boxes and syringes.

5. Polytetra fluoroethylene (PTFE) : It is translucent, opaque and possesses high resistance to solvents and chemicals. It is unchanged even at a temperature of 250°C.

6. Polypropylene : It is very much similar to high density polythene. It is very light and heat resistant. Its melting point is 170°C. It can be autoclaved repeatedly. It is used for preparing disposable syringes, tubings, squeeze bottles and packaging films.

7. Polyamides (Nylon) : It is very tough plastic having great amount of flexibility and heat resistance. Its melting point is about 200°C. It can be autoclaved repeatedly. Nylon has electro-negative polar centres and tends to attract several common preservatives such as phenol, parahydroxybenzoic acid and its esters. Nylon is used for the preparation of syringes, tubings and packaging films for surgical dressings and instruments.

8. Polycarbonate : It is transparent, has high impact strength and very good heat resistance. It is used in the preparation of surgical equipment.

Classification of plastics Plastics are classified into two groups according to their behaviour when heated:

(*i*) *Thermoplastic type* : This type of plastic gets softened to a viscous fluid on heating and hardens again on cooling. The hardness after cooling is influenced by the degree of cross linkage or inter-molecular attraction between the long chain molecules *e.g.* nylon, polystyrene and polymethyl methacrylate.

(*ii*) *Thermosetting type* : This type of plastic may become flexible but does not become fluid on heating. They are generally hard and brittle at room temperature because of a high degree of cross linking. They retain their shape even upto the temperature of decomposition *e.g.* phenol formaldehyde resins and urea formaldehyde resin.

The plastic used for packaging of pharmaceutical products should be tested for any extract coming out after treating it with acids, alkalies, water and organic solvents which are included in the formulation.

Metals

Metals are used for the construction of containers. The metals commonly used for this purpose are aluminium, tin plated steel, stainless steel, tin and lead.

The metal containers have the following **advantages**:

(1) They are sturdy.
(2) They are impermeable to light, moisture and gases.
(3) They can be made into rigid unbreakable containers by impact extrusion.
(4) They are light in weight as compared to glass containers.
(5) Labels can be printed directly on to their surface.

The metal containers have the following **disadvantages**:

(1) They are expensive.

(2) They may shed metal particles into the pharmaceutical product.

(3) They are not generally used for extemporaneous dispensing.

(4) They react with certain chemicals or drugs.

Aluminium, tin and lead are used for the construction of collapsible tubes. The collapsible tubes are available in different sizes. In pharmaceutical industry the collapsible tubes made from tin are preferred because they are compatible with a wide range of products. However, they are quite costly. The collapsible tubes made from aluminium are light in weight and are mostly used for tooth pastes and creams. These are less costly than collapsible tubes made from tin. Lead tubes are the cheapest among all metal collapsible tubes but are not used for pharmaceutical packing due to the risk of lead poisoning. If the product is not compatible with bare metal, the interior of the collapsible tube can be coated with wax-type formulation or with resin solutions. Wax linings are mostly used with water base products in tin tubes. The epoxides and vinyls are used as lining material for aluminium tubes which gives better protection to the product filled in it.

The metal containers are also used for bulk packaging of tablets, capsules, powders and food materials etc.

Metal foil may be used for wrapping individual suppositories or pessaries. However, it is mainly used in strip packaging or blister packaging.

Paper and Board ▒

Paper and board are used in various forms for packaging of pharmaceutical products. They are used for preparing outer containers, such as, cartons, boxes, envelopes and drums, to provide additional mechanical protection to other containers e.g. strip and blister packs of tablets, capsules, suppositories and pessaries may be packed in an outer paper board carton. Collapsible tubes of ointments, creams and gels as well as liquid medicines in sizes 500 ml and below, may be packed in an other paper board carton. Slide paper board boxes suitably lined may be used for extemporaneous dispensed suppositories, pessaries and powders.

▒ CLOSURES ▒

Closures are the devices by means of which containers can be opened and closed. Proper closing of the container is necessary because:

1. It prevents loss of material by spilling or volatilisation.
2. It avoids contamination of the product from dirt, microorganisms or insects.
3. It prevents deterioration of the product from the effect of the environment such as moisture, oxygen or carbon dioxide.

Types of closures : Closures are of the following types.

1. Plug type
2. Crown cap
3. Push-fit cap
4. Screw closures

1. Plug type : The closure of this type is a push-fit into the neck of the container *e.g.* cork or glass stopper. Nowadays the plastic stoppers are used instead of cork or glass stopper. Plastic stopper being unbreakable and flexible, is used to ensure a good fit into the container.

2. Crown cap : The cap is commonly used as crimped closure for beverage bottles.

3. Push-fit cap : These are simple slide fit over the neck of the container. These are made of plastic and are shaped in such a way that these must be stretched over the neck to fit on the container.

4. Screw closures : These are very commonly used. It consists of three components

(*i*) Cap
(*ii*) Wad
(*iii*) Liner

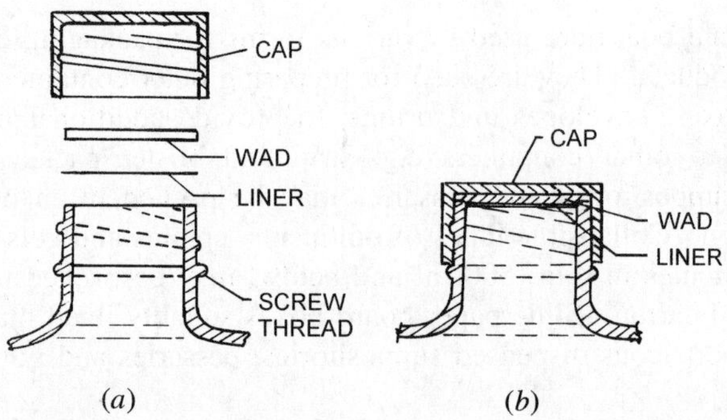

Fig 4-1 Components of the screw closure (*a*) separate (*b*) in position

Cap : It may be made of tin-plate or aluminium metal. Sometimes these caps are pre-formed and the container is closed simply by screwing the cap on the neck. Alternatively, a blank cap is dropped over the neck of the container and threads are formed in it with the help of a machine. Caps are also made of plastic material. Plastic caps are better than metal caps because they are capable of resisting corrosion and also do not contaminate the product.

Wad : It is a seal which prevents the contamination of the product. Wad should be inert and is made of such a material which does not absorb the product. Wads are made of rubber or silicone rubber. However, cork or cardboard wads are also commonly used.

Liner : It is made of metal foils, rubber, plastic films and paper impregnated with a suitable resin, wax or plastic.

MATERIALS USED FOR MAKING OF CLOSURES

The closures for containers meant for storage of pharmaceutical products are generally made from the following basic materials:

1. Cork
2. Glass
3. Plastic
4. Metal
5. Rubber

Cork Cork is obtained from the bark of oak tree. Cork is chemically inert and it does not impart any odour or flavour to the product. However, cork closures cannot be used for many liquid preparations because of danger of mould growth. Cork closures are rarely used nowadays. These have now been replaced by plastic or rubber closures.

Glass Glass closures are ideal but they mostly slip during transportation and handling. As such, these closures are mainly used for reagent bottles in laboratories.

Plastic Plastic closures are nowadays commonly used and they have mostly replaced old type of closures. They are available in various shapes and sizes. They are light in weight and are unbreakable. Plastic closures must be tested for any extractable matter contained in them and for their incompatibility with contents of the container. Plastic containers cannot however be made pilfer-proof unless a metal seal is employed.

Metal Metal closures are in common use these days. These closures are made from tin plate and aluminium. However, aluminium closures are preferred because of their ductability and also ease of conversion into desired shape. Tear-off closures can be easily made and have been satisfactory. Metal closures can be made pilfer-proof by using a liner.

Rubber Rubber is used mainly for the construction of closure meant for vials, transfusion fluid bottles, dropping bottles and as washers in many other types of products. In the natural rubber which is the latex of *Heavea braziliensis* the following additives are added to change its physical and chemical properties:

1. *Activators* such as zinc oxide, stearic acid and zinc stearate.
2. *Filters* such as asbestos, carbon black and calcium carbonate.
3. *Vulcanising agents* such as sulphur.
4. *Accelerators* such as thiazoles.
5. *Lubricants* such a talc and zinc stearate.
6. *Pigments* such as oxides and sulphides of antimony, cadmium and iron.
7. *Softeners* such as mineral oils and pine oil.

Rubber, whether natural or synthetic, must possess the following properties, in order to be used in pharmaceutical industry:

1. It should be soft.
2. It should be quite elastic.
3. It should not absorb medicament.
4. It should withstand the temperature and pressure of an autoclave.
5. It should be compatible with the ingredients of pharmaceutical formulation.
6. It should fulfil all the standards which are laid down by the pharmacopœia.
7. It should be impermeable to moisture and air.
8. It should release only negligible amount of undesirable substances.

Before using the rubber closures the tests such as extractive test, permeability test, compatibility test, fragmentation test and test for penetrability force must be performed.

AEROSOL PACKAGING

Aerosols may be defined as disperse phase system, in which very fine solid particles or liquid droplets get dispersed in the gas which acts as continuous phase. These are also called pressurised dosage form.

Advantages of Aerosols

1. The medicament can be delivered directly to the affected area such as burnt skin and wound. So it minimises the discomfort caused by mechanical or manual application.

2. Absence of air prevents oxidation of the product.
3. The hydrolysis of medicaments can be prevented.
4. Drugs can be given by oral inhalation.
5. The sterility of the products can be maintained.
6. The application of medicament is easier.
7. A fine mist is easily formed for inhalation purpose.
8. Manual contact with medicaments can be avoided.
9. Drugs given by oral inhalation do not pass through G.I.T. Hence its chances of decomposition are less.

Disadvantages of Aerosols

1. Aerosols are costly preparations.
2. Some of the propellants are very toxic.
3. The cooling effect of highly volatile propellants may cause discomfort on injured skin.
4. Lot of difficulties are faced in aerosol formulation when the drug is not soluble in propellant.

Classification of Aerosols

Aerosols may be classified as:

1. *Space sprays* : These are finely divided sprays having particle size upto 50 μ *e.g.* insecticides, disinfectants and room deodorizers.

2. *Surface coats* : These are also sprays but disperse particles are coarse with sizes upto 200 μ. They produce a wet coat when sprayed on a surface *e.g.* hair sprays, personal deodorant, powder sprays and topical medicament sprays.

3. *Foam* : These are produced by rapid expansion of propellants through an emulsion. Hence, the product comes out in the form of a foam or froth *e.g.* shaving cream and vaginal product.

Formulation of Pharmaceutical Aerosols

An aerosol formulation basically consists of a propellant and the medicaments to be propelled.

Propellant It develops a pressure in the container. Compressed gases such as carbon dioxide or nitrogen and liquified gases like methane or ethane can be used as propellants. Compressed gases are not commonly used. These days propellants like trichloro-fluoro-methane, dichloro-difluoro-methane, dichloro-tetrafluoro-ethane and difluoro-ethane are used in pharmaceutical aerosols.

The medicaments to be propelled may be solid or liquid. It may be soluble in the propellent or insoluble in it.

The various additives such as solvents, antioxidants, surface active agents and flavouring agents are also included in the formulation.

The propellants, medicaments and additives are filled into an aerosol container.

Aerosol system may be of two types:

1. Two phase system : Two phase system is employed in cases where the product is a solid insoluble in the propellant or it is solid or liquid which dissolve in it. In the first case solid is suspended in the propellant, so that aerosol system will have one liquid phase and gaseous phase is above it.

2. Three phase system : Three phase system is employed in cases where the product is immiscible with the propellant. The medicaments are dissolved in a liquid which does not mix with the liquefied propellant.

Containers used for Aerosols

Aerosol container can be divided into four parts:

1. Container : In pharmaceutical aerosol packaging, the containers are made from metal (such as tin plated steel, aluminium and stainless steel) glass and plastic. These containers can withstand high pressure.

2. Valves : The valves used should be such that it can be easily opened and closed. It should also deliver the content in the desired form. So three types of valves are used nowadays:

(*i*) Continuous spray valve
(*ii*) Metering valve
(*iii*) Foam valve

By using continuous spray valve, the medicament is expelled continuously as long as pressure is applied on the actuator. But by using metering valve, only a

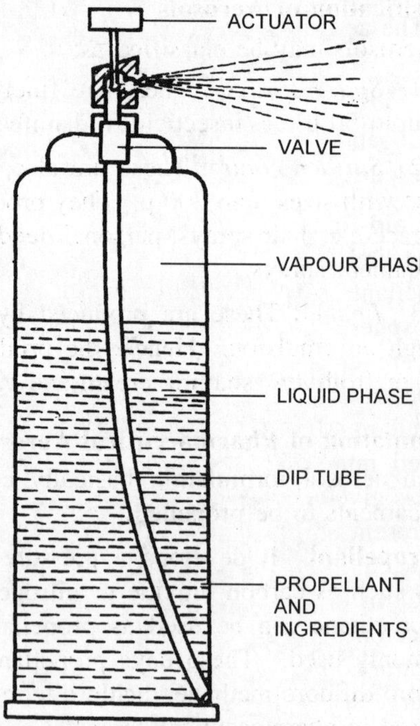

Fig.4-2 Aerosol container

definite quantity of medicament is expelled when actuator is pressed. If the contents of aerosol are required to come out in the form of a ball of foam, a foam valve is used in that case.

3. Actuator : Actuator is fitted on the valve stem. It helps in the easy opening and closing of the valve, whenever it is required. There are various types of actuators which can produce spray, fine mist or foam.

4. Dip tubes : The dip tubes are made from polyethylene or polypropylene. Dip tube is used for the following purposes:

(*i*) It conveys the liquid from the bottom of the container to the valve at the top.

(*ii*) It prevents the propellant to come out without dispensing the contents of the package.

The dip tube should be extended almost to the bottom of the container. In case the length of the dip tube is short, the contents of the aerosol container will not come out of it. However, if the dip tube is touching the bottom of the container, it will block the passage of liquid.

Packaging of Aerosols

The aerosol products can be filled in two ways:

(*i*) Cold-fill process

(*ii*) Pressure-fill process

Depending on the nature of the product concentrate, the aerosol can be filled by a cold filling or a pressure filling process.

Cold-fill process This process is used to fill metered aerosol products using a flurocarbon propellant. By lowering the temperature of a propellant below its boiling point, the propellant becomes liquid at atmospheric pressure. The active ingredients or concentrate and propellant are cooled to a low temperature of about –30° to –40°F. The concentrate is generally cooled to below 0° in order to reduce loss of propellant during the filling operation. The chilled concentrate is poured into the chilled container and propellant is added. Sufficient time is given for the propellant to partially vaporise, in order to expel the air present in the container. The valve is fitted on to the container which is placed into a water bath so that the contents are heated to 130°F (54°C) in order to check any leakage and strength of container. A dry ice-acetone bath is used to obtain the desired low temperature for laboratory scale preparation whereas refrigeration equipment is used for the large scale production of aerosols.

Pressure-fill process This process is used for filling aerosols containing hydrocarbon propellant. The product concentrate is placed into the container and the valve is sealed. The propellant is forced through the valve under pressure. After this the container is immersed in a water bath at 130°F (or 54°C) in order to check any leakage and strength of the container. It is essential that the air present in the container must be expelled before filling the contents into the aerosol container.

Applications of Aerosol Packaging

1. They are used for spray bandages and for application of drugs meant for topical use.
2. They are used for spray administration of drugs into various body cavities.
3. They are used for administration of drugs such as local anaesthetics, local antiseptic, local analgesics and anti-inflammatory drugs.
4. They are used to spray cosmetic preparations such as perfumes.
5. They are used to spray disinfectants, deodorizers and air sanitizers.

MODERN UNIT DOSE PACKAGING

Unit dose packaging of tablets and capsules has become very popular these days. The advantages of modern unit dose packaging are as under:

1. These are light weight.
2. These are temper resistant
3. The wastage is reduced.
4. These protect the solid dosage form from external environments.
5. These are hygienic.
6. These are child resistant.

However, modern unit dose packaging has certain disadvantages which are as under:

1. These are expensive.
2. Elderly patients may experience difficulty in use.
3. These packaging are not meant for dispensing purpose but mainly suitable for industry and hospital since lot of machinery is involved.

The following types of packaging are very common:

1. Blister package
2. Strip package
3. Bubble package
4. Sachet package
5. Oral liquid dispensers.

Blister package These consist of a lid and a blister (usually transparent). The blister package is formed by heat-softening of a sheet of thermoplastic resin and vacuum drawing the softened sheet of plastic into a contoured mould. After cooling, the sheet is released from the mould. The semi-rigid blister formed is filled with product (tablet or capsule) and lidded with a heat sealable backing material as shown in Fig. 4-3.

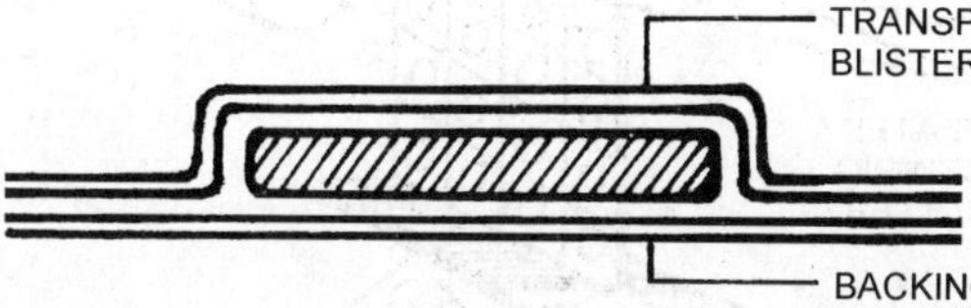

Fig. 4-3 Blister package

The lid material commonly used are aluminium foil and metallised polyester. The lid material has to satisfy certain criteria:

1. It should protect the pack material.
2. It acts as a barrier to moisture and atmospheric gases.
3. It must seal to the blister material and retain the medicament within the blister.
4. It should tear easily when blister content is pushed through it.
5. It should accept printing to label and identify the product.

The materials used for thermoformable blisters are polyvinyl chloride (PVC), polystyrene, polypropylene and combination of PVC and polyethylene. The blister material should have the following qualities:

1. It should act as barrier to moisture and atmospheric gases.
2. It should provide adequate protection to the medicament from abrasion.
3. It must soften without shrinking but stay soft without melting.
4. It should be flexible enough to allow removal of the contents.

Strip package It is commonly used for the packaging of tablets and capsules. A strip package is formed by feeding two webs of a heat-sealable flexible film through a heated crimping roller. As shown in Fig. 4-4 the product is dropped into the pocket formed before forming the final set of seals. A continuous strip of packets is formed which is cut to the desired number of packets in length. These are then packed into a folding carton. The product sealed between the two sheets of film usually has a seal around each tablet. The seal can be in a simple rectangular form or can be made to the shape of the product.

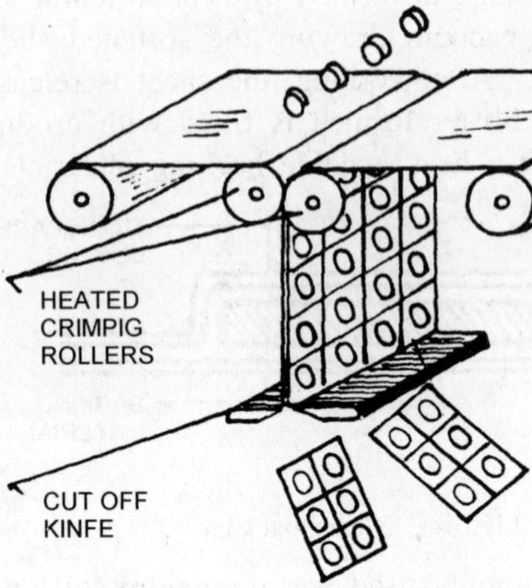

Fig. 4-4 Strip packaging system

The materials used for strip package are cellophane, polyester, polyethylene, polypropylene, polyvinyl chloride and saran.

Bubble package The bubble pack is usually formed by sandwiching the product between a thermoformable, heat-shrinkable plastic film and a rigid backing material. This is done by heat softening of the plastic film and withdrawal of vacuum from a packet into the film in a similar manner as it is done in blister package. The product is dropped into the pocket which is then sealed with a rigid material such as heat-seal-coated paper board.

Sachet package The sachet packs are invariably a laminated with aluminium foil serving as the centre core, besides a heat sealable plastic material as the product contact substance. Sachet are usually made in following three steps:—

1. Formation of the carrying pouch
2. Dosing with requisite product
3. Hermatically sealing process

Sachet packs are used for filling granules, creams, pastes, powders, liquids and even suppositories.

Oral liquid dispensers Nowadays oral liquids can be unit packaged in following ways:

1. A plastic pot sealed with a laminate, the laminate is torn off before use.

2. In a plastic syringe-type dispenser, the syringe is available in a number of sizes. The tip of the syringe is sealed by a small plastic ring.

Suppositories and enemas in plastic packs with rectal nozzles are now freely available in the market. Similarly unit packed eye ointments and drops are available for hospital use. Topical products packed in small sachets and tubes are also available these days. Effervescent granules and cough syrup are also available in sachets having one dose for the convenience of patients

■ REVISION QUESTIONS ■

I. Very short answer type questions ■

Answer the following questions briefly.

1. Write the basic qualities of neutral glass.
2. Why glass containers are not preferred these days?
3. Name the various containers which are prepared from glass.
4. Name different types of materials used for making of containers.
5. What are the different containers made from plastic?
6. Define the term "Cullet".
7. Name the different types of metals used in the construction of collapsible tubes.
8. What are the common polymers used in making plastic containers?
9. What do you know about "Unit dose packaging"?
10. What are different types of aerosols available in the market?

II. Short answer type questions ■

11. What are the different type of containers used in pharmaceutical industry?
12. Define "Containers". What are the basic materials used in making of containers?
13. What are the qualities of a good container?
14. Why hydrolytic resistant test is performed in glass containers?
15. Write the various types of aerosols which are commonly used.
16. Write the applications of aerosol packaging.
17. Why lime-soda glass is not used for storage of parenteral products?

18. Write the advantages and disadvantages of plastic containers.
19. How the aerosol products are filled into aerosol containers?
20. Define "moderate unit dose packaging". Write different types of such packaging which are commonly used.

III. Long answer type questions

21. Define "Pharmaceutical Containers". What are qualities of an ideal containers?
22. What are different types of containers commonly used in pharmacy? Write in brief about glass containers.
23. Write in brief about hydrolytic resistance test. Why it is necessary to perform this test on glass container meant for parenteral products?
24. What is the composition of glass? Describe in detail the different types of glass used for making of containers.
25. What is the composition of plastic? How will you classify plastic? Explain different types of plastic used for making containers.
26. Define "aerosols". How will you classify aerosols? Explain with the help of a diagram the various parts of aerosol packaging.
27. Explain the different methods of packing of aerosols. Write the advantages and disadvantages of aerosols.
28. Explain in detail the modern unit dose packaging.
29. Define the term "Closures". Write in detail about different types of closures commonly used in pharmaceutical industry.
30. Why plastic containers are more commonly used now-a-days? Write its demerits.

IV. Objective type questions

A. *Completion type questions (Fill in the blank with suitable word/words)*

31. __________ are used for storage of photosensitive pharmaceutical products.
32. Aerosol containers have good __________ in order to bear _______ of aerosol packing.
33. Air-tight containers are also called ________ containers.
34. The ________ and ________ are used as lining materials for collapsible tubes made from aluminium.
35. The cellophane sheets are used for__________ packaging of_________ and capsules.

36. Cork is obtained from the bark of_________ tree.

B. Matching type questions

37. Match the items of *Column I* with the appropriate items in *Column II*.

Column I	*Column II*
A. Containers	(*i*) highly resistant glass
B. Borosilicate glass	(*ii*) filter out U.V. radiation
C. Actuator	(*iii*) does not produce flakes
D. Plastic containers	(*iv*) helps in the easy opening and closing the valve.
E. Light resistant glass	(*v*) is a device that holds the drug

C. Multiple choice questions (Choose the correct answer)

38. Containers meant for storage of injectables are made of
    (1) Lime-soda glass (3) Type II glass
    (2) Neutral glass (4) Type I & II glass

39. Hydrolytic resistance test is performed on glass in order to find out
    (1) Mechanical strength (3) Alkali liberated by it
    (2) Quality (4) Limit of alkalinity liberated by it

40. Collapsible tubes made from lead is not used for pharmaceutical packing due to
    (1) Inferior metal (3) Soft in nature
    (2) Risk of lead poisoning (4) Not good in appearance

41. Air-tight sealed containers are used for
    (1) Tablets (3) Injectables
    (2) Capsules (4) Liquid preparations

KEY

31. Light resistant container/Amber colour glass container
32. Mechanical strength, pressure.
33. Hermetic
34. epoxides, vinyls
35. Strip, tablets
36. Oak
37. A(v), B(i), C(iv), D(iii), E(ii)
38. (4)
39. (4)
40. (2)
41. (3)

5

Size Reduction

Size reduction or comminution is the process of reducing drugs (vegetable and chemical substances) into smaller pieces, coarse particles or fine powder.

Importance of Particle Size Reduction

The process of size reduction is commonly employed in pharmaceutical industries due to the following reasons:

1. To increase the rate of solution in case of chemical substances, because reduction of the particle size increases the surface area for the action of solvent.
2. To allow the rapid penetration of the solvent (menstruum), in case of crude drugs for the extraction of active constituents from vegetable and animal drugs.
3. To get a uniform powder because particle size reduction helps in uniform mixing of drugs, required for preparing different formulations for administration.
4. To increase the rate of absorption of a drug. The smaller the particle size, the greater is the rate of absorption.
5. To improve the stability of certain pharmaceutical dosage form, such as suspensions. The rate of sedimentation decreases to a large extent by reducing the particle size of the drug.
6. To help in the process of separation of solids from liquids by filtration or by sedimentation. The rate of filtration or sedimentation depends upon the particle size.

Factors Affecting Size Reduction

The following factors affect the process of size reduction:

1. Hardness : The hardness of the material affects the process of size reduction. It is easier to break soft material to a small size than hard material.

2. Toughness : The crude drugs of fibrous nature or those having higher moisture content, are generally tough in nature. A soft but tough material may present more problem in size reduction, than a hard but brittle substance.

3. Stickiness : Stickiness causes a lot of difficulty in size reduction. This is due to the fact that material adheres to the grinding surfaces or sieve surface of the mill. It is difficult to powder a drugs of having gummy or resinous nature, if the method used for size reduction generates heat. Complete dryness of material may help to overcome this difficulty.

4. Material structure : Materials which show some special structure may cause problem during size reduction *e.g.* vegetable drugs which have cellular structure, generally produce long fibrous particles on its size reduction. Similarly a mineral substance having lines of weakness, produces flake like particles on its size reduction.

5. Moisture content : The presence of moisture in the material influences a number of its properties such as hardness, toughness or stickiness which in its turn affects the particle size reduction. The material should be either dry or wet. It should not be damp. The material having 5% moisture in case of dry grinding and 50% moisture in wet grinding does not create any problem.

6. Softening temperature : Waxy substances such as stearic acid or drugs containing oils or fats, become softened during the size reduction processes, if heat is generated. This can be avoided by cooling the mill.

7. Purity required : Various mills used for size reduction often cause the grinding surfaces to wear off and thus impurities come in the powder. If a high degree of purity is required, such mills must be avoided. Moreover, the mills should be thoroughly cleansed between batches of different materials in order to maintain purity.

8. Physiological effect : Some drugs are very potent. During their particle size reduction in a mill, dust is produced which may have an effect on the operator. In such cases, the enclosed mills may be used to avoid dust.

9. Ratio of feed size to product size : To get a fine powder in a mill, it is required that a fairly small feed size should be used. Hence it is necessary to carry out the size reduction process in several stages, using different equipment *e.g.* preliminary crushing followed by coarse powder and then fine grinding.

10. Bulk density : The output of the size reduction of material in a machine, depends upon the bulk density of the substance.

METHODS OF SIZE REDUCTION

The following are the methods of size reduction, in which different mechanisms are involved:

1. Cutting
2. Compression
3. Impact
4. Attrition
5. Combined impact and attrition

1. Cutting

The material is cut on a small scale by means of a sharp blade, knife, root cutter or any other sharp instrument. On a large scale, a cutter mill is used. Cutting of drug is usually done to hasten the drying of drugs.

CUTTER MILL

Principle The size reduction is done by cutting with the help of sharp knives.

Construction There are two types of knives which are fitted in this mill. These are stationary knives and rotating knives. The stationary knives are fixed in the casing whereas the rotating knives are attached to the rotor. The upper part of casing also contains a hopper inlet, whereas the lower part has a screen of desired aperture size.

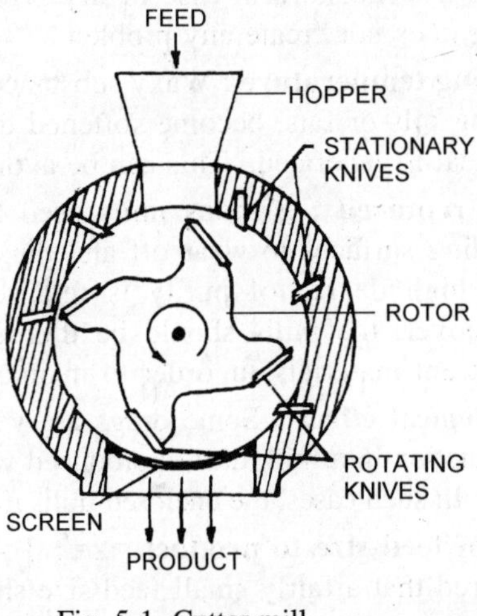

Fig. 5-1 Cutter mill

Working The material to be cut is put into the hopper of the mill. The rotor rotates at a high speed. Due to the rotation of the rotor, the material comes very close between stationary knives and rotating knives. It cuts down the material into small pieces. Screen retains the material in the mill, until the desired degree of size reduction has been affected. The product is collected which comes out of the sieve.

Uses The mill is used to obtain a coarse degree of size reduction of soft materials such as roots, peels or wood before extraction.

2. Compression ▩

In this method, the material is crushed by the application of pressure. On a small scale, size reduction is carried out by using pestle and mortar, whereas on a large scale, roller mill is used.

▩ ROLLER MILL ▩

Principle The material is crushed by the application of pressure. The mill works on the principle of compression of material by applying a pressure on it.

Construction It consists of two cylindrical rollers made of stone or metal, which are mounted horizontally. These rollers are capable of rotation on their longitudinal axis. These rollers may be from a few centimetres upto a meter in diameter. Generally, one of the roller is driven directly, while the second one runs freely.

Working The material to be crushed is fed from the hopper into the gap between the two rollers. Due to the rotation of these rollers, the material is crushed. The gap between the rollers can be adjusted to control the degree of size reduction.

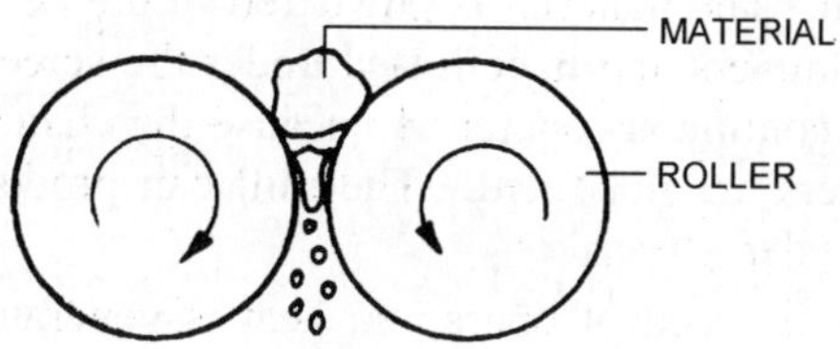

Fig. 5-2 Roller mill

Uses The roller mill is used for crushing and cracking of seeds before extraction of fixed oil from the same. It is also used to crush the soft tissues, to help in the penetration of solvent during the extraction process.

3. Impact ▩

Impact occurs when the material is more or less stationary and is hit by an object moving at high speed or when the moving particle strikes a stationary surface. In either case, the material breaks into small pieces. There is no apparatus which can be used on a small scale to affect size reduction by impact. But on a large scale, hammer mill and disintegrator are used when size reduction of material is done by impact.

▩ HAMMER MILL ▩

Principle It works on the principle of impact i.e. material is more or less stationary and is hit by an object moving at a high speed.

Construction It consists of a stout metal casing, enclosing a central shaft, to which four or more swinging hammers are attached. The lower part of the casing consists of a screen, through which material can pass and collected in a suitable receiver, when the desired degree of size reduction is reached.

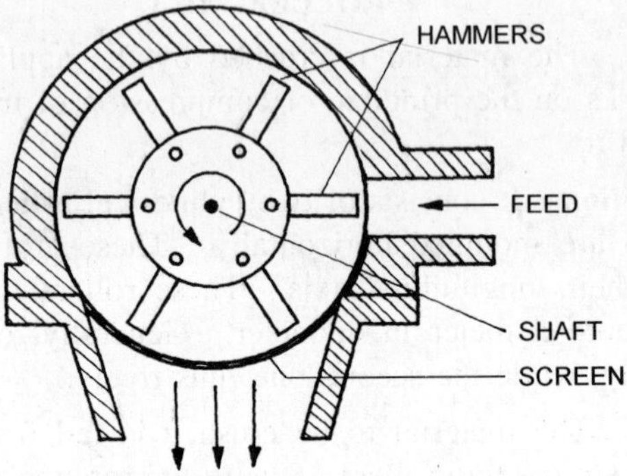

Fig. 5-3 Hammer mill

Working The material is put into the hopper which is connected with the drum. The material is powdered to the desired size, due to fast rotation of hammers and is collected under the screen. This mill has the advantage of continuous operation because the chance of jamming is less as the hammers are not fixed. The mill can produce coarse to moderately fine powder.

Due to high speed of operation, heat is generated which may affect thermolabile drugs or materials. Moreover, high speed of operation also causes damage to the mill if foreign objects such as stone or metal is present in the feed.

Uses The hammer mill is used for producing intermediate grades of powder from almost all types of substances except sticky materials that choke the screen.

▪ THE DISINTEGRATOR ▪

Principle The size reduction in disintegrator is done by impact.

Construction It consists of a steel drum having a shaft in the centre. The shaft contains a disc, on which four beaters are fixed. The shaft rotates with a speed of 5000–7000 rev./min. The side and upper inner surface of the drum is rough and undulating. The lower part of the drum has a detachable screen or sieve. The sieve has a definite pore size.

Working The beaters are mainly responsible for grinding but are helped by the undulation of the inner surface and roughness of drum.

The material is fed to beaters, through hopper which is fitted to the drum. The material is broken into small particles by impact of the beaters.

Due to high velocity of beaters the air velocity inside the chamber is increased. The air is allowed to pass through an outlet on which dust bag is tied, which retains the fine particles of powder.

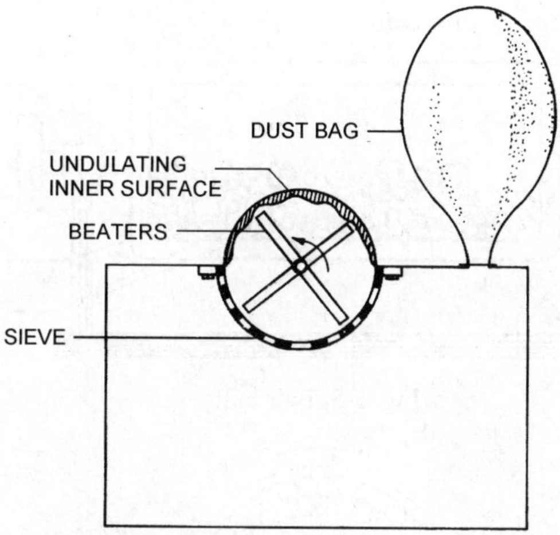

Fig. 5-4 Diagram of disintegrator in section

Uses The mill is used to powder all types of drugs including very hard drugs. The drug should be dried before feeding into the disintegrator to get fine powder. To avoid the jamming of the beaters of the disintegrator, use moderately small pieces

4. Attrition

In attrition pressure is applied on the material as in compression, but the surfaces are moving relative to each other, resulting in shear forces which break the particles. On laboratory scale, the size reduction by attrition is done by using pestle and mortar, but on a large scale roller-mill can be used.

5. Combined Impact and Attrition

The mechanism of impact and attrition can be combined in the mill to get better result. The following are the mills, in which size reduction is done by impact and attrition.

BALL MILL

Principle It works on the principle of impact and attrition.

Construction It consists of a hollow cylinder which is mounted on a metallic frame in such a way, that it can be rotated on its longitudinal axis. The cylinder contains balls that occupy 30-50% of the mill volume. The weight of the balls is kept constant. The ball size depends on the size of the feed and the diameter of the mill.

The cylinder and balls are made of metal and are usually lined with chrome. In pharmaceutical industry, sometimes the cylinder of the ball mill is lined with rubber or porcelain. The balls used in these mills are also made of rubber or porcelain.

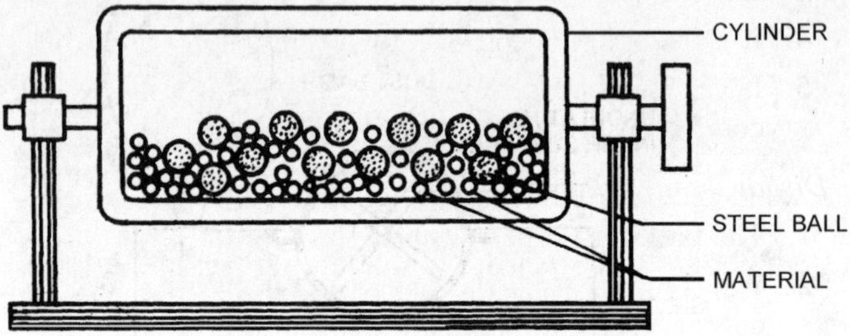

Fig. 5-5 Ball mill

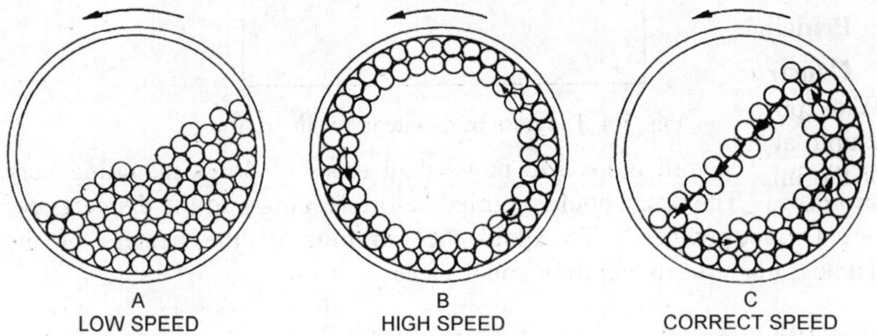

Fig. 5-6 Ball mill operation

Working The drug to be ground is put into the cylinder of the mill and is rotated. The speed of rotation is very important. At a low speed, the mass of balls will slide or roll over each other and only a negligible amount of size reduction will occur (as shown in Fig. 5-6A). At a high speed, the balls will be thrown out to the walls by centrifugal force and no grinding will occur (Fig. 5-6B). But at about 2/3rd of the speed, the centrifugal force just occurs with the result that the balls are carried almost to the top of the mill and then fall in. By this way the maximum size reduction is effected by the impact of particles between the balls and by attrition between the balls (Fig. 5-6C).

After a suitable time, the material is taken out and passed through a sieve to get powder of the required size.

Uses The mill is used to grind brittle drugs to fine powder.

Advantages of Ball Mill

1. It can produce very fine powders.
2. It can be used for continuous operation, if sieve or classifier is attached to the mill.
3. It is capable of grinding a large variety of materials of different character and of different degree of hardness.
4. It is suitable for both wet or dry grinding processes.
5. It can be used to grind toxic materials as it can be used in a completely enclosed form.

Disadvantages of Ball Mill

1. The ball mill is a very noisy machine.
2. Wear occurs from the balls as well as from the casing, which may result in contamination of the product.

▪ FLUID ENERGY MILL ▪

Principle It works on the principle of impact and attrition.

Construction It consists of a loop of pipe, which has a diameter of 20 to 200 mm, depending on the overall height of the loop, which may be upto about 2 m. There is an inlet for the feed and a series of nozzles for the inlet of air or an inert gas. It also has an outlet with a classifier

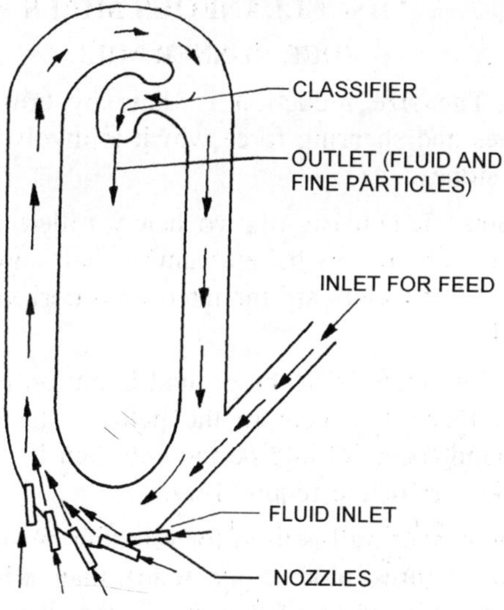

Fig. 5-7 Fluid energy mill

which allows the air to escape but prevents the particles to pass until they become sufficiently fine.

Working The air or inert gas is introduced with a very high pressure through the nozzles. Solids are introduced into air stream through inlet. Due to high degree of turbulence, impact and attritional forces occurs between the particles. The fine particles are collected through a classifier. Fluid energy mill reduces the particles to 1 to 20 micron.

To get a very fine powder, even upto five micron, the material is pretreated to reduce the particle size to the order of 100 mesh and then passed through fluid energy mill.

Uses The mill is used to grind heat sensitive material to fine powder. The mill is used to grind those drugs in which high degree of purity is required.

Advantages of Fluid Energy Mill

1. The mill is used to grind the material to fine powder.
2. The particle size of powder can be controlled due to the use of a classifier.
3. There is no wear of the mill and hence there is no contamination of the product.
4. It is useful for grinding heat sensitive substances such as sulphonamides, vitamins and antibiotics.

▩ MISCELLANEOUS MILLS ▩

▩ EDGE RUNNER MILL ▩

Principle The size reduction is done by crushing due to heavy weight of stones and shearing force which is involved during the movement of these stones.

Construction It consists of two heavy rollers and a bed made of stone or granite. The rollers have a central shaft and they revolve on its axis (Fig. 5-8). The rollers are mounted on a horizontal shaft and move around the bed.

Working The material to be ground is put on the bed and with the help of the scrapers it is kept in the path of the stone wheels. The material is ground for a definite period and then it is passed through the sieves to get powder of the required size.

Uses Edge runner mill is used for grinding most of the drugs to fine powder, but it requires more floor space than other commonly used mills. The major advantage of this mill is that it requires less attention during operation.

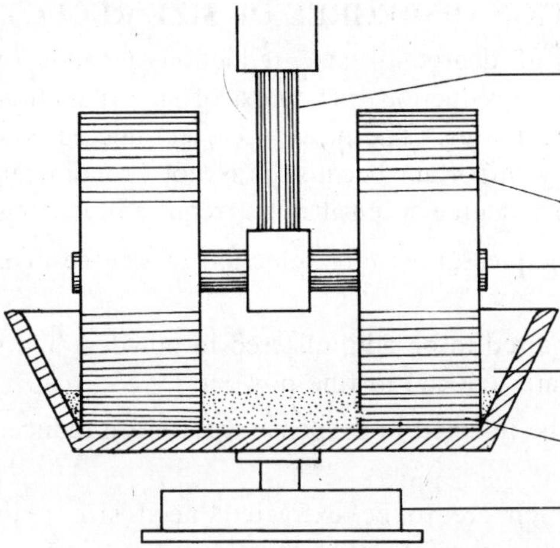

Fig. 5-8 Edge runner mill

General characteristics of various types of mills are given in Table 5-1.

TABLE 5-1

General Characteristics of Various Types of Mills

S. No.	*Name of the mill*	*Action*	*Product size*	*Uses*	*Not used for*
1.	Cutter mill	Cutting	20 to 80 mesh	Fibrous, crude (animal and vegetable drug)	Friable material
2.	Roller mill	Compression	20 to 200 mesh	Soft material	Abrasive material
3.	Hammer mill	Impact	4 to 325 mesh	Almost all drugs	Abrasive material
4.	Disintegrator	Impact	20 to 80 mesh	Almost all drugs including very hard drugs	Soft and sticky material
5.	Ball mill	Attrition and impact	20 to 200 mesh	Brittle drugs	Soft material
6.	Fluid energy mill	Attrition and impact	1 to 30 μm	Moderately hard and friable material	Soft and sticky material
7.	Edge runner mill	Crushing and shearing	20 to 80 mesh	Almost all drugs	Sticky material

SELECTION OF DEGREE OF SIZE REDUCTION

The selection of degree of size reduction depends on the use of powder after its size reduction. The cost of size reduction increases as the particle size decreases. The need of correct degree of size reduction of material is very important because it is not economical to powder a substance to a finer degree when it is not required technically.

The basic principles governing selection of degree of size reduction are as follows:

1. Drugs required to be administered in powders and suspension in mixtures are reduced to fine powder.
2. Drugs to be injected in suspension form are reduced to very fine powder.
3. Drugs which are to be extracted, need size reduction, which depends upon the following factors:
   (*a*) *Solvent or menstruum* : Water has more penetration power than other organic solvents such as alcohol (60% or more). Therefore, a higher degree of size reduction is required with alcoholic as menstruum than with water.
   (*b*) *Drug/menstruum ratio* : The rate of solution is greater in case of a larger than a small volume of solvent. Moreover, the size reduction of a solute also hastens the solution formation. Therefore, in preparing a weak preparation, the entire drug or coarse grade of drug can be used but for a stronger preparation, fine degree of size reduction is required.
   (*c*) *Physical character of the drug and localisation of the constituents* : The menstruum is slowly penetrated into hard woody drugs than into soft drugs. Therefore in the case of hard drugs it becomes necessary to reduce them to a fine powder than in the case of soft drugs for the same process of extraction and menstruum. The localisation of active principles is an important factor in deciding the degree of size reduction of drugs *e.g.* active constituents of digitalis leaves are localised chiefly in the harder tissues of leaves and hence require a fine degree of size reduction.
   (*d*) *Process* : In infusion and decoction processes the menstruum used is water and the drug/menstruum ratio is large. As such there is no need of a higher degree of size reduction. In the case of maceration and percolation processes, the drugs/menstruum ratio is comparatively smaller than for infusion and decoction. Therefore, a higher degree of size reduction is

required. The same is also very essential in case the menstruum is alcohol and extraction process is percolation.

LEVIGATION AND ELUTRIATION

Levigation Levigation is the process of wet grinding. The material is converted into paste with water and then grinding of paste is done in a mortar, using a flat headed pestle. In case of large scale grinding, it is done by using colloidal mill or a mill resembling an edge-runner mill. The process is used for the preparation of light kaolin, chalk, red and yellow mercuric oxide, calamine and camphor etc.

After the process of levigation, the paste obtained contains fine particles along with a small proportion of coarse particles. The fine particles are separated from the coarse particles by the process of elutriation.

Elutriation Elutriation is the process of separation of fine particles and coarse particles from a paste obtained after levigation. The paste is mixed with a large volume of water and the mixture is allowed to stand for a short period during which the heavy coarse particles with high density settle down on the bottom of the vessel. The fine particles with low density remain suspended in upper layers of the liquid. The upper liquid is poured off and the fine particles are allowed to settle down on the bottom. The wet paste containing fine particles is then dried.

In small scale grinding, conical flask can be used but on a large scale, elutriation tanks are used (For detail *see* chapter on size separation).

REVISION QUESTIONS

I. Very short answer type questions

Answer the following questions in brief.

1. Define the term "Comminution".
2. Name the different methods of size reduction.
3. Name the mill in which size reduction is done by cutting.
4. What are the mills in which size reduction done by compression?
5. Name the mills in which size reduction is done by attrition.
6. Write the name of the mills in which size reduction is done by impact.
7. Give the name of the milis in which size reduction is done both by attrition and impact.
8. Give the name of the mill in which size reduction is done by crushing and shearing.

9. What is the importance of particle size reduction?
10. Name the factors affecting size reduction

II. Short answer type questions

11. What are the various factors which affect the size reduction of drugs?
12. Give the advantages of a ball mill.
13. Write the advantages of a fluid energy mill.
14. Describe the process of levigation.
15. What is the elutriation process?
16. Explain the process of impact.
17. Describe the process of attrition.
18. How does stickiness affect the process of size reduction?
19. How does the presence of moisture interfere with the process of size reduction?
20. Write the importance of particle size reduction in pharmacy.

III. Long answer type questions

21. Define "Size Reduction". Explain the various factors which affect the size reduction of drugs.
22. Write in brief the different methods of size reduction of drugs.
23. Describe the construction and working of a fluid energy mill with the help of a diagram.
24. Explain with the help of a diagram the construction and working of hammer mill.
25. Write the principle, construction, working and uses of the disintegrator.
26. What are the basic principles governing selection of degree of size reduction?
27. Define "Levigation and Elutriation". Write in detail about ball mill.
28. What are the various methods of size reduction? Give the construction, working and working principle of the following mills (a) Disintegrator (b) Edge runner mill (c) Cutter mill (d) Hammer mill

IV. Objective type questions

A. Completion type questions (Fill in the blank with suitable word/words).

29. Size reduction is done by _______ in pestle and mortar.

30. In hammer mill and in disintegrator, the size reduction is done by __________.

31. Particle size reduction increases the _________ of solid substances.

32. Comminution helps to increase the _________ of drug.

33. The material having ______ moisture in dry grinding and ______ moisture in wet grinding does not produce any problem.

34. The fine particles are separated from __________ particles by the process of elutriation.

B. Matching type questions.

35. Match the items of *Column I* with appropriate items in *Column II.*

Column I Type of Mill	*Column II* Method of size reduction
(A) Cutter mill	(*i*) Combined impact and attrition
(B) Hammer mill	(*ii*) Compression
(C) Ball mill	(*iii*) Impact
(D) The disintegrator	(*iv*) Compression
(E) Roller mill	(*v*) Cutting
(F) Fluid energy mill	(*vi*) Impact
(G) Pestle and mortar	(*vii*) Combined impact and attrition

C. Multiple choice questions (*Choose the correct answer*)

36. Ball mills work on the principle of
    (1) Impact
    (2) Attrition
    (3) Crushing
    (4) Impact and attrition

37. The output of size reduction of material in a machine depends on:
    (1) Chemical nature
    (2) Physical character
    (3) Bulk density
    (4) Material structure

38. Roller mill works on the principle of:
    (1) Impact
    (2) Compression
    (3) Attrition
    (4) Compression & Attrition

39. The efficiency of a ball mill is maximum at :
    (1) Low speed
    (2) High speed
    (3) 2/3rd of speed
    (4) Very high speed

40. Give the name of the mill in which no wear occurs.
    (1) Ball mill
    (2) Edge runner mill
    (3) Fluid energy mill
    (4) Roller mill

KEY

3. cutter mill
4. Roller mill
5. Roller mill
6. Hammer mill and the disintegrator
7. Ball mill and fluid energy mill
8. Edge runner mill.
29. Compression
30. Impact
31. surface area
32. Rate of absorption
33. 5%, 50%
34. coarse
35. A (v); B(iii); C(i); D(vi); E(iv);F(vii); G(ii)
36. (4)
37. (3)
38. (4)
39. (3)
40. (3)

6

Size Separation

In normal course, the process of size reduction is followed by size separation of the powdered material. During the process of size reduction, it is not possible to obtain the particles of uniform size. Hence a special technique is used to separate particles of specified size which is known as the "process of size separation". Size separation process may be applied to the measurement of particle size, in which the proportion of each size of particle in a sample is determined and data is utilised to control raw material or to maintain the quality of manufactured product.

OFFICIAL STANDARDS FOR POWDERS

The Indian Pharmacopœia has laid down the standards for powders for pharmaceutical purposes. According to that, the degree of coarseness or fineness of a powder is expressed by reference to the nominal mesh aperture size of the sieve through which powder is able to pass.

The I.P. specifies five grades of powder which are as under:

1. Coarse powder : A powder of which all the particles pass through a sieve with nominal mesh aperture of 1.70 mm (No. 10 sieve) and not more than 40.0 per cent through a sieve with nominal mesh aperture of 355 μm (No. 44 sieve) is called coarse powder.

2. Moderately coarse powder : A powder of which all the particles pass through a sieve with nominal mesh aperture of 710 μm (No. 22 sieve) and not more than 40.0 per cent through a sieve with nominal mesh aperture of 250 μm (No. 60 sieve) is called moderately coarse powder.

3. Moderately fine powder : If all the particles of a powder pass through a sieve with nominal mesh aperture of 355 μm (No. 44 sieve) and not more than 40.0 per cent through a sieve with nominal mesh aperture of 180 μm (No. 85 sieve), it falls in this group.

4. Fine powder : In case all the particles pass through a sieve with a nominal mesh aperture of 180 μm (No. 85 sieve), it is called fine powder.

5. Very fine powder : If all the particles of the powder pass through a sieve with a nominal mesh aperture of 125 μm (No. 120 sieve), it is said to be very fine powder.

The relevant grades of powder and sieve numbers along with a nominal mesh aperture are shown in Table 6-1.

TABLE 6-1

S. No.	*Grade of powder*	*Sieve through which all particles must pass*	*Nominal mesh aperture size*	*Sieve through which 40 % of particles pass*	*Nominal mesh aperture size*
1.	Coarse powder	10	1.7 mm	44	355 μm
2.	Moderately coarse powder	22	710 μm	60	250 μm
3.	Moderately fine powder	44	355 μm	85	180 μm
4.	Fine powder	85	180 μm	—	—
5.	Very fine powder	120	125 μm	—	—

The Pharmacopœia has prescribed upper and lower limits for the three coarse grades of powder. For two fine grades of powder the pharmacopœia has prescribed only the upper limit.

When the fineness of a powder is described by means of a number, it is an indication that all the particles of the powder shall pass through the sieve of which the nominal mesh aperture in μm, is equal to that number.

SIEVES

Sieves for pharmacopœial testing are constructed from wire cloth with square meshes, woven from wires of brass, bronze, stainless steel or any other suitable material. The wires should be of uniform circular cross-section and should not be coated or plated. There should not be any reaction between the material of the sieve and the substance which is being sifted from it.

Standards for sieves Sieves used for pharmacopœial testing must specify the following:

1. *Number of sieve* : Sieve number indicates the number of meshes in a length of 2.54 cm in each transverse direction parallel to the wires.

2. *Nominal size of aperture* : Nominal size of aperture indicates the distance between the wires. It represents the length of the side of the square aperture. The I.P. has given the nominal mesh aperture size for majority of sieves in mm or in μm.

3. *Nominal diameter of the wire* : Wire mesh sieves are made from the wire having the specified diameter in order to give a suitable aperture size and sufficient strength to avoid distortion of the sieve.

4. *Approximate percentage sieving area* : This standard expresses the area of the meshes as a percentage of the total area of the sieve. It

depends on the size of the wire used for any particular sieve number. Generally the sieving area is kept within the range of 35 to 40 per cent in order to give suitable strength to the sieve.

5. *Tolerance average aperture size* : Some variation in the aperture size is unavoidable and when this variation is expressed as a percentage, it is known as the 'aperture tolerance average'. In fact, it is a limit given by pharmacopœia within which a particular dimension or average aperture size can be allowed to vary and still be acceptable for the purpose for which it is used. Fine meshes cannot be woven with the same accuracy as coarse meshes. Hence the aperture tolerance average is smaller for coarse sieves than the fine sieves.

According to I.P., a sieve must confirm to the following specifications as given in Table 6-2.

TABLE 6-2

S. No.	*Approximate sieve number*	*Approximate percentage sieving area*	*Nominal mesh aperture size (mm)*	*Tolerance average aperture size (± mm)*
1.	4	55	4.0	0.13
2.	6	51	2.8	0.09
3.	8	48	2.0	0.07
4.	10	46	1.7	0.06
5.	12	44	1.4	0.05
6.	16	41	1.0	0.03
7.	—	—	µm	± µm
8.	22	37	710	25
9.	25	36	600	21
10.	30	38	500	18
11.	36	36	425	15
12.	44	38	355	13
13.	60	37	250	13 (9.9)
14.	85	35	180	11 (7.6)
15.	100	36	150	9.4 (6.6)
16.	120	34	125	8.1 (5.8)
17.	150	36	106	7.4 (5.2)
18.	170	35	90	6.6 (4.6)
19.	200	36	75	6.1 (4.1)
20.	240	34	63	5.3 (3.7)
21.	300	35	53	4.8 (3.4)
22.	350	34	45	4.8 (3.1)

Note—Figures in brackets refer to close tolerances and those without brackets refer to full tolerance.

SIZE SEPARATION

After the drug has been subjected to size reduction, the powdered drug is separated according to its particle size. The various methods used for size separation are as under:

1. Sieving
2. Cyclone separator
3. Air separator
4. Elutriation

SIEVING

In this method, the fine powder is separated from the coarse powder by using sieves of desired number. The degree of fineness of a powder is known with the help of sieve through which the powdered material is passed. Sieves are numbered in order to distinguish them from each other.

Size separation of powder is done by passing the powdered material through a set of sieves. Sieves are arranged in descending order *i.e.* sieve of larger size is at the top and the smallest one at the bottom. The bottom sieve is attached to the receiving pan.

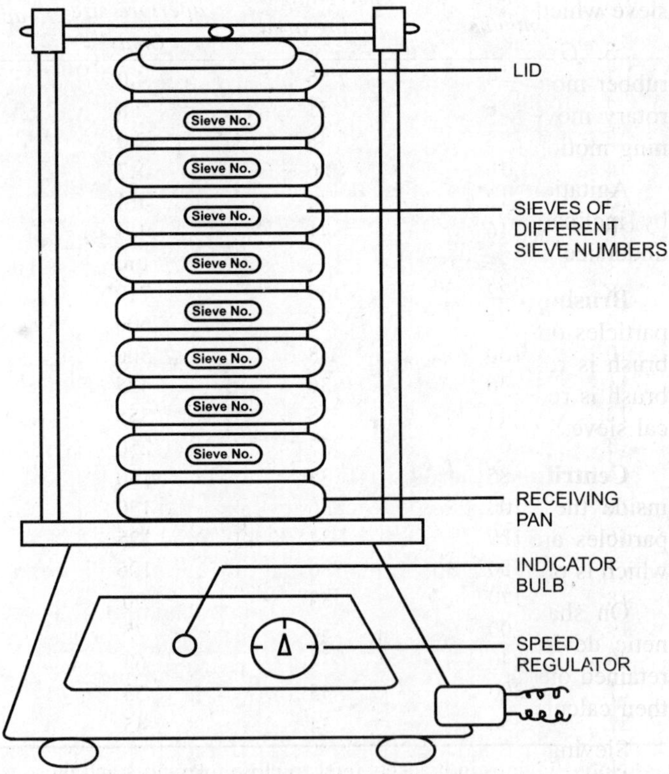

Fig. 6-1 Electromagnetic laboratory sieving machine

The material is placed in the uppermost sieve. The sieves are shaken with the help of mechanical sieve shaker or electromagnetic devices. It helps the particles to pass through the sieves.

The working of mechanical sieving devices are based on any of the following methods.

1. Agitation
2. Brushing
3. Centrifugal

Agitation methods Sieves may be agitated in a number of different ways, such as:

1. *Oscillation* : The sieve is mounted in a frame that oscillates back and forth. It is a simple method but the material may roll on the surface of the sieve.

2. *Vibration* : The sieve is vibrated at high speed by means of an electric device. The rapid vibration is imparted to the particles on the sieve which helps to pass the powdered material through it.

3. *Gyration* : In this method, a system is made so that sieve is on rubber mounting and connected to an eccentric fly wheel. This gives a rotary movement of small amplitude to sieve which in turn gives spinning motion to the particles that helps to pass them through a sieve.

Agitation methods are not continuous methods but can be made so by inclination of the sieve and the provision of separate outlets for undersize and oversize particles.

Brushing methods In this case, a brush is used to move the particles on the surface of the sieve and to keep the meshes clear. The brush is rotated in the middle in the case of a circular sieve but spiral brush is rotated on the longitudinal axis in case of a horizontal cylindrical sieve.

Centrifugal methods In this method, a high speed rotor is fixed inside the vertical cylindrical sieve, so that on rotation of rotor the particles are thrown outwards by centrifugal force. The current of air which is produced due to high speed of rotor helps in sieving the powder.

On shaking the powdered material in a mechanical or electromagnetic device using any of the above methods, the weight of powder retained on each sieve is determined. The percentage of each fraction is then calculated.

Sieving method is a rapid process and it requires very little skill. The equipment used for sieving is not expensive.

CYCLONE SEPARATOR

Principle In cyclone separator, the centrifugal force is used to separate solids from fluids. The separation depends not only on the particle size but also on density of particles. Hence depending on the fluid velocity, the cyclone separator can be used to separate all types of particles or to remove only coarse particles and allow fine particles to be carried through with the fluid.

Construction It consists of a cylindrical vessel with a conical base. In the upper part of the vessel is fitted with a tangential inlet and a fluid outlet and at the base it is fitted with solid outlet.

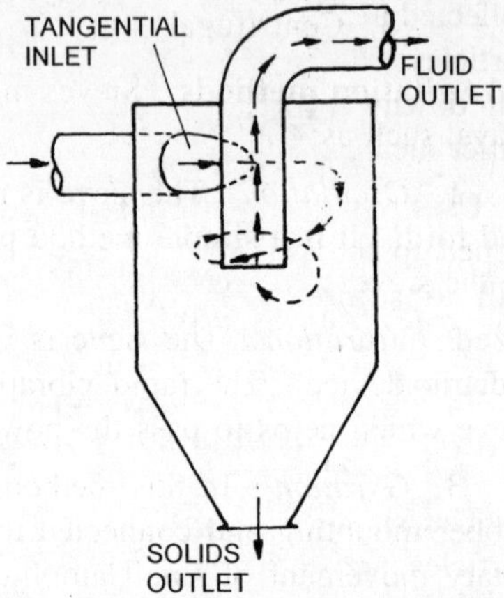

Fig. 6-2 Cyclone separator

Working The suspension of a solid in gas (usually air) is introduced tangentially at a very high velocity, so that rotary movement takes place within the vessel. The fluid is removed from a central outlet at the top. The rotatory flow within the cyclone separator causes the particles to be acted on by centrifugal force. The solids are thrown out to the walls, thereafter it falls to the conical base and discharged out through solids outlet.

Uses Cyclone separators are used to separate the suspension of a solid in a gas (air). It can be used with liquid suspensions of solids.

AIR SEPARATOR

Principle It works on the same principle as that of cyclone separator. But in this case the air movement is obtained by means of rotating disc and blades. To improve the separation, the stationary blades are used. By controlling these blades and the speed of rotation, it is possible to vary the size at which separation occurs.

Construction It consists of a cylindrical vessel with a conical base. In the upper part of the separator the vessel is fitted with feed inlet, and at the base there are two outlets, one for fine particles and other for heavy particles. The rotating disc and rotating blades are attached to the central shaft, to produce air movement.

Working As shown in the Fig. 6-3, the sample powder is passed through the feed inlet, which falls on the rotating disc. The rotating blades are attached to the same shaft. These produce a current of air as shown by the arrows. The fine particles are picked up and are carried into space, where air velocity is sufficiently reduced. The fine particles are dropped and ultimately collected at an outlet meant for fine particles. The heavy particles which fall downward are removed at an outlet meant for heavy particles.

Uses Air separator is often attached to the ball mill or hammer mill to separate and return oversized particles for further size reduction.

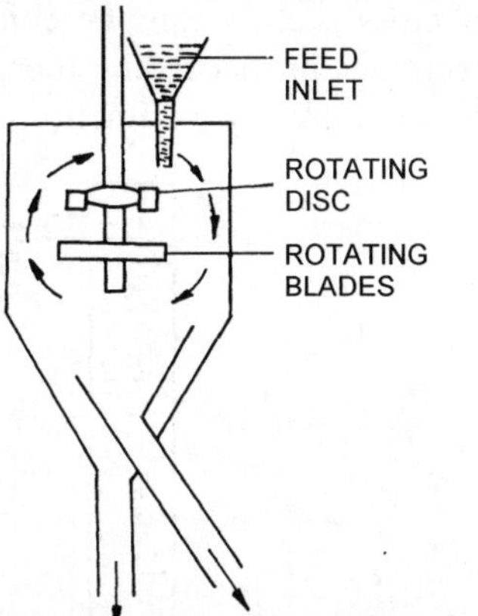

Fig. 6.3 Air separator

ELUTRIATION METHODS

The size separation of powder is based on the low density of fine particles and high density of the coarse particles. Elutriating tank is used to separate the coarse and fine particles of powder after levigation. The dry powder or paste made by levigation process is kept in an elutriating tank and mixed with a large quantity of water. The solid particles are uniformly distributed in the liquid by stirring and then it is allowed to settle down. Depending on the density of solid particles, it will either settle down or remain suspended in water. The sample is withdrawn at different heights through the outlets. These are dried and thus the powder with various size fractions are collected.

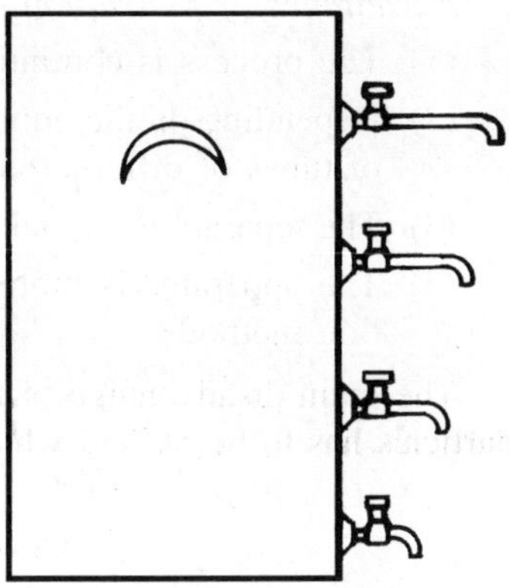

Fig. 6-4 Elutriating tank

Nowadays in elutriation process, the particles are suspended in a moving fluid, generally water or air. The apparatus consists of a vertical column with an inlet near the bottom for suspension, an outlet at the base for coarse particles and an overflow near the top for fluid and fine particles. One column will give single separation into two fractions. If more than one fraction is required a number of tubes of increasing area of cross section can be connected in series. The velocity of the fluid decreases in succeeding tubes as the area of cross section increases, thus giving a number of fractions. These fractions are separated and dried.

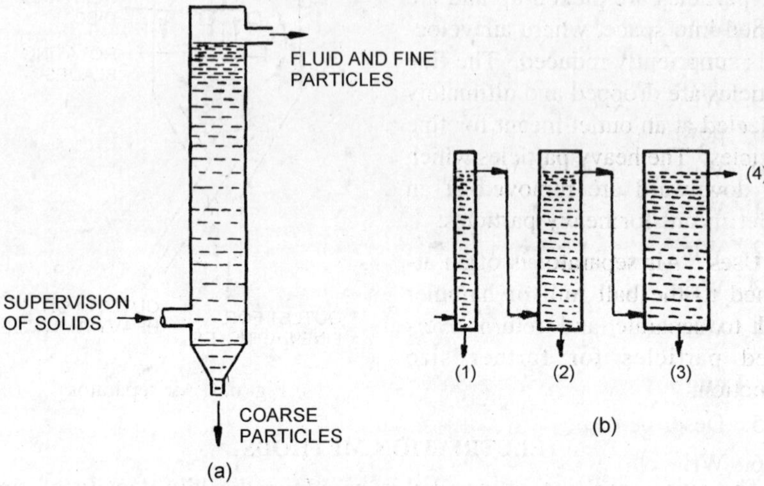

Fig. 6-5 (*a*) Elutriation (*b*) Multi-stage elutriator

Advantages of Elutriation Method

(1) The process is continuous.

(2) Depending on the number of fractions required, the same number of tubes of different area of cross section can be connected.

(3) The separation is quick as compare to other methods of separation.

(4) The apparatus is more compact than as that used in sedimentation methods.

The main disadvantage of this method is that the suspension of solid particles has to be diluted which may not be desired in certain cases.

REVISION QUESTIONS

I. Very short answer type questions

Answer the following questions in brief.

1. Define the term "Size Separation".
2. Mention the official grades of powder.
3. What do you know about elutriation?
4. Define the term "Sieve".
5. Name the various standards for sieves.

6. What are the various grades of coarse powder?
7. Write the different grades of fine powder.

II. Short answer type questions

8. What are different grades of powder specified in Indian Pharmacopoeia?
9. Why are the upper and lower limits for three coarse grades of powder prescribed by Indian Pharmacopoeia.
10. Write in brief about sieves.
11. What are the different methods used for size separation?
12. What is the importance of size separation process in Pharmacy?
13. Write the different methods of sieving.
14. What are the advantages of elutriation method?

III. Long answer type questions

15. Describe in brief, the various methods of size separation.
16. Write in detail the various grades of powder official in the pharmacopoeia.
17. Describe the construction, working and uses of air separator.
18. Describe the construction, working and uses of cyclone separator.
19. How does the elutriation method help in the size separation of powder? Write its advantages and disadvantages.
20. Explain the different methods which are generally used for sieving.
21. Write in detail about various standards fixed by the pharmacopoeia for sieves.
22. Give in detail the various grades of powder which are official in Indian Pharmacopoeia. Why pharmacopoeia has prescribed upper and lower limits for coarse grades of powder.

IV. Objective type questions

A. Completion Type Questions (Fill in the blank with suitable word/words).

23. The pharmacopœia has prescribed __________ and ________ limits for the three ______ grades of powder.
24. The pharmacopoeia has prescribed only _______ limit for the two _________ grades of powder.
25. ___________ are used to separate the suspension of a solid in a gas (air).

26. __________ is often attached to__________ mill and __________ mill to separate the oversize particles.
27. Fine powder should pass through number _________ sieve.

B. Matching type questions.

28. Match the items of *Column I* with the appropriate items in *Column II.*

Column I	*Column II*
A. Coarse powder	(*i*) only 40% passes through No. 85 sieve
B. Fine powder	(*ii*) passes through No. 120 sieve
C. Moderately coarse powder	(*iii*) passes through a sieve having nominal aperture size of 710 μm
D. Moderately fine powder	(*iv*) passes through sieve No. 10
E. Very fine powder	(*v*) passes through No. 85 sieve

C. Multiple choice questions (*Choose the correct answer*).

29. The degree of particle size of a powder is expressed in the pharmacopœia in the form of
    (1) Sieve number
    (2) Nominal mesh aperture size of sieve
    (3) Amount of powder pass through sieve
    (4) Approx. percentage sieving area
30. In the sieving method, the powder is passed through a set of sieves which are arranged
    (1) in descending order
    (2) in ascending order
    (3) at random
    (4) one's own choice
31. In cyclone separator, the powder is separated depending on its
    (1) particle size
    (2) particle size and density of particles
    (3) density of particles
    (4) shape of powder

KEY

23. upper, lower, coarse
24. upper
25. cyclone separator
26. Air separator, ball mill, hammer mill
27. 85
28. A(iv); B(v); C(iii); D(i) and E(ii)
29. (2)
30. (1)
31. (2)

7

Mixing and Homogenisation

Mixing is the most widely used operation in which two or more than two substances are combined together. Perfect mixing is that in which each particle of one material lies as nearly adjacent as possible to a particle of the other material.

The degree of mixing as defined above is not normally practicable. The desired degree of mixing depends on the purpose of the product and the objective of mixing. The main objectives of mixing may be:

1. Simple physical mixing of materials to form a uniform mixture.
2. To promote the chemical reaction to get uniform products.
3. Dispersion of solid in liquid to form suspension or paste.
4. Dispersion of two immiscible liquids to form an emulsion.

TYPES OF MIXTURES

There are three types of mixtures—(*i*) Positive mixtures, (*ii*) Negative mixtures (*iii*) Neutral mixtures.

Positive mixtures When two or more than two miscible liquids are mixed or soluble solid is dissolved in water, the mixtures are called positive mixtures. These mixtures do not present any problem in mixing. Moreover the mixture formed is irreversible.

Negative mixtures When two immiscible liquids are mixed or insoluble solids are mixed with water it forms negative mixtures. For preparing such types of mixtures a higher degree of mixing of materials is required. The mixture formed is a reversible mixture.

Neutral mixtures These mixtures are static in their behaviour. The substances do not have the tendency to mix with each other immediately, but once mixed they do not separate after mixing.

MIXING OF POWDERS

The mixing of powders is one of the common pharmaceutical operations and is used in the preparation of many types of formulations, such as, tablets, capsules and compound powders.

Mixing mechanisms The solid mixing takes place by a combination of one or more mechanisms given below:

1. *Convective mixing* : There is bulk movement of groups of particles from one part of powder bed to another. It occurs by an inversion of the powder bed by means of blades or paddles.

2. *Shear mixing* : When shear forces occur it reduces the scale of segregation by thinning of dissimilar layers of a solid material.

3. *Diffusion mixing* : It occurs when random motion of particles within a powder bed causes them to change position relative to one another. It is produced by any form of agitation of powder.

There are various physical properties which affect the perfect mixing of powders. These are discussed here under:

1. Particle size : It is easy to mix two powders having approximate the same particle sizes. The variation of particle size can lead to separation also, because the small particles move downward through the spaces between the bigger particles.

2. Particle shape : The ideal particle is spherical in shape for the purpose of uniform mixing. The irregular shapes can become interlocked and there are less chances of separation of particles once these are mixed together.

3. Particle attraction : Some particles exert attractive forces due to electrostatic charges on them. This can lead to separation.

4. Material density : It is difficult to mix two powders having different density. This is due to the fact that dense material always moves downward and settles down at the bottom. Therefore, for uniform mixing of powders, proper attention should be given to their density.

5. Proportions of materials : The best results can be achieved if two powders are mixed in equal proportions by weight or by volume. In case there is a large difference in the proportion of two powders to be mixed the mixing of powders is always done in the ascending order of their weights.

Equipment Used for Mixing of Powders

In the laboratory, the mixing of powders, is done by using pestle and mortar or with the help of a drug spatula. The method is commonly known as 'trituration'. On large scale, the following equipment are used for mixing of powders:

1. Tumbler mixer
2. Double cone mixer
3. Agitated powder mixer
4. Air mixer

Tumbler mixer It consists of a metallic vessel in which powders are mixed by slow rotation, either manually or with the help of an electric motor. Due to rotation the ingredients come over one another. For mixing of large bulk of powders, the mixing of powders is done in a vessel of a suitable design alongwith baffles which gives a thorough mixing. The tumbler mixers are generally made up of stainless steel and are of various designs, such as cubical, V shaped, Y shaped and cylindrical *etc*. These are rotated at a slow speed by using an electric motor of suitable horse power. The rotation of the vessel should be slow so that the powder does not remain stationary against the side of the vessel held by centrifugal force but lifted by baffles and fall over continuously.

Double cone blender It is developed in an attempt to overcome some of the shortcomings of rotating mixers. The mixing of powder in double cone blender is due to tumbling and shearing action with blade.

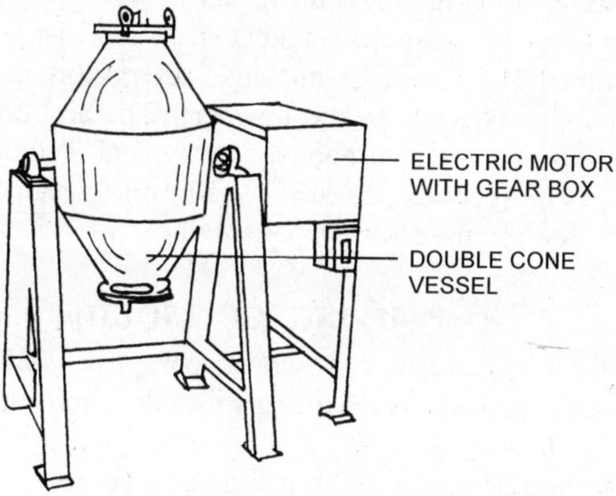

Fig. 7-1 Double cone blender

Double cone blender is made of stainless steel and is available in different capacity ranging from 5 Kg to 200 Kg or even more. The efficiency of the blender depends mainly on the speed of rotation. The rate of rotation should be optimum which depends on the size and shape of tumbler as well as nature of material to be mixed. The common range is 30-100 r.p.m.

The material to be blended is loaded approximately 50 to 60% of the total capacity of the blender. As the blender rotates the material undergoes tumbling motion and mixes the material thoroughly. Agitator blade can also be fixed in order to produce shearing action.

The double cone blender is an efficient design for mixing powders of different densities and is used mainly for small quantity of powders.

Agitated powder mixer It consists of a stationary vessel or a trough in which an arm rotates and transmits shearing action to the particles. The end-to-end movement is required for general mixing which can be achieved by fitting helical blades to the agitator. The mixer is commonly used for mixing free flowing powdered materials having uniform particle size and density.

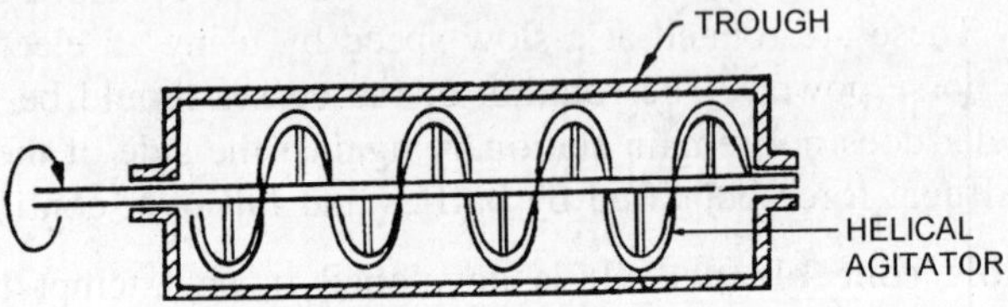

Fig. 7-2 Agitated powder mixer

Air mixer The air movement can be used for mixing of powders. The powders to be mixed are taken in a vertical cylindrical vessel and air is admitted at its base at an angle after short interval blasts. This gives a spiral movement to the powder. The air should be admitted at short intervals and not continuously. A typical method is to use eight air blasts of two seconds duration with one second interval. Thus 24 seconds are required for proper mixing.

MIXING OF LIQUIDS

Mixing of liquids is done to prepare true solution or emulsions. Mixing is required to dissolve one miscible liquid into another miscible liquid to form true solution. For making emulsion, the mixing of two immiscible liquids are done by using shear force.

Equipment Used for Mixing of Liquids

In the laboratory the emulsion is prepared by using pestle and mortar and afterward it is passed through a homogeniser to get fine emulsion. On large scale, the following equipment are used for mixing the liquids:

1. Propeller mixer
2. Turbine mixer
3. Paddle mixer

Propeller mixer It consists of a vessel and a propeller. The propeller usually operates at high speed which is upto 8000 r.p.m. which gives a satisfactory flow pattern to the liquids. During mixing of liquids, air gets entrapped in liquids or there is formation of vortex. This can be avoided by making the following changes in the position of the propeller shaft:

(*a*) Offset from the centre [Fig. 7-3(*i*)]
(*b*) Mounted at angle [Fig. 7-3(*ii*)]
(*c*) Enter the side of the vessel [Fig. 7-3(*iii*)]
(*d*) Using push pull propeller [Fig. 7-3(*iv*)]
(*e*) By the use of baffles [Fig. 7-3(*v*)]

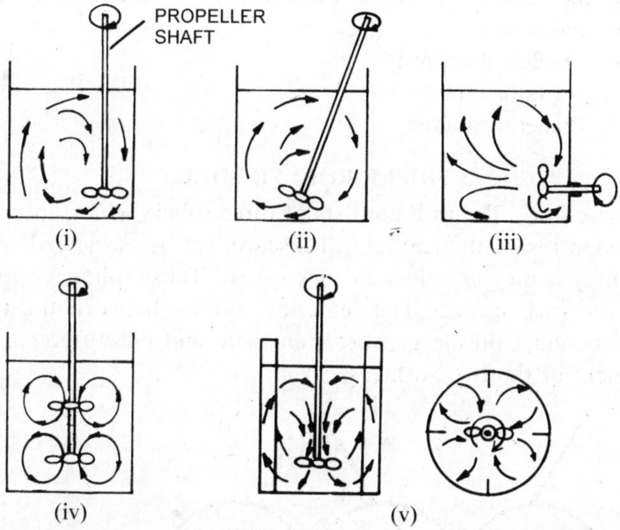

Fig.7-3 Propeller mixer showing different positions of propeller shaft

The propeller mixers are not suitable when considerable shear force is needed *e.g.* in the preparation of emulsion.

Turbine mixer It consists of a vessel and a circular disc impeller. A number of short, straight or curved blades are attached to it. The turbine impeller is usually rotated at somewhat lower speed than the propeller. The turbine mixer is used for mixing of more viscous liquids *e.g.* syrups, liquid paraffin, glycerine etc.

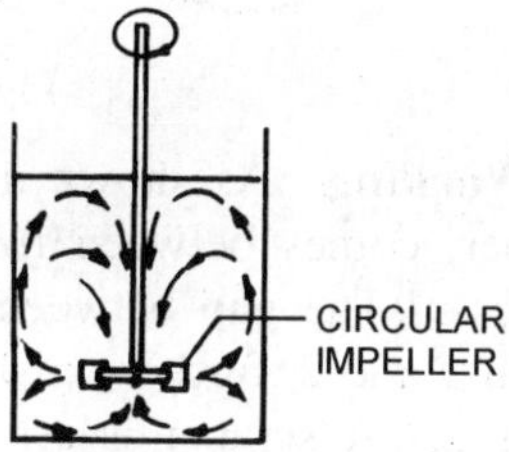

Fig. 7-4 Turbine mixers

Paddle mixer In a paddle mixer, the flat blades are attached to a vertical shaft which rotates at a low speed of 100 r.p.m. For mixing the low viscosity liquids simple flat paddles are used. But for mixing high viscosity liquids, the big paddles, often shaped to fit closely to the surface of the vessel, are used. The paddles of different sizes and shapes are used in the pharmaceutical industry according to the character and viscosity of the product.

MIXING OF SEMI-SOLIDS

The mixing of semi-solids is done for preparing ointments, creams, pill masses and wet mass for making granules etc.

Equipment Used for Mixing of Semi-solids

In case the quantity is large, the following equipment are used for mixing of semi-solids:

1. Triple roller mill
2. Agitator mixer
3. Planetary mixer

TRIPLE ROLLER MILL

Construction The mill consists of three rollers which are made of a hard abrasion-resistant material. These rollers are arranged in such a way that they come very close to each other. These rollers are rotated at different rates of speed. The material coming between the rollers is crushed depending on the gap between them and the difference in rates of movement of the two surfaces.

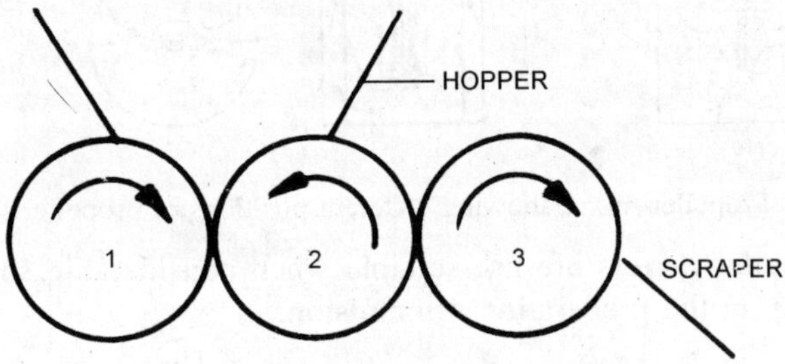

Fig. 7-5 Triple roller mill

Working As shown in Fig. 7-5, the material after passing through hopper, comes between roller 1 and 2 and is reduced in size in the process. The gap between roller 2 and 3 is usually less than that between 1 and 2, further crushes and smooths the mixture which adheres to roller 2. A scraper is arranged in such a way, that it can remove the mixed material from the roller no. 3 and does not allow the material which has not passed between both sets of the rollers to reach the scraper.

Uses The triple roller mill is very useful for the purpose of mixing of solid powder in ointment base.

AGITATOR MIXER

The semisolid mixing can be carried out in the agitator mixers meant for mixing liquids and powders. However, the mixers for semisolids are usually of heavier construction.

Sigma arm mixer is the commonly used agitator mixer for the purpose of mixing of semisolids. The mixer has two blades, the shape of which resembles the Greek letter "Sigma". The two blades move at different speeds and towards each other. The blades operate in a mixing vessel which has a double trough shape, each blade fitted into a trough. The two blades rotate at different speeds, one usually about twice the speed of the other which causes the lateral pulling of the material and is divided into two troughs. The difference in speed and shape of blades causes end-to-end movement.

Air is usually entrapped during the mixing of semisolids. This can be avoided by enclosing the sigma arm mixer and operating it under pressure.

The sigma arm mixer is commonly used for mixing of dough ingredients in the baking industry. It is used in wet granulation process in the manufacture of tablets. It is also used for mixing powdered drug with an ointment base.

▩ PLANETARY MIXER ▩

Principle In a planetary mixer, the blade tears the mass apart and shear is applied between a moving blade and a stationary wall. The mixing arm moves around its own axis and also around the central axis in order to reach every spot of the vessel. The plates in the blade are sloped, so that the powder makes an upward movement to produce tumbling motion.

Construction It consists of a stationary vessel which is made up of stainless steel. The vessel can be removed either by lowering it beneath the blade or raising the blade above the vessel. The mixing blade is mounted from the top of the vessel. . The mixing shaft is driven by planetary gear connected to an electric motor.

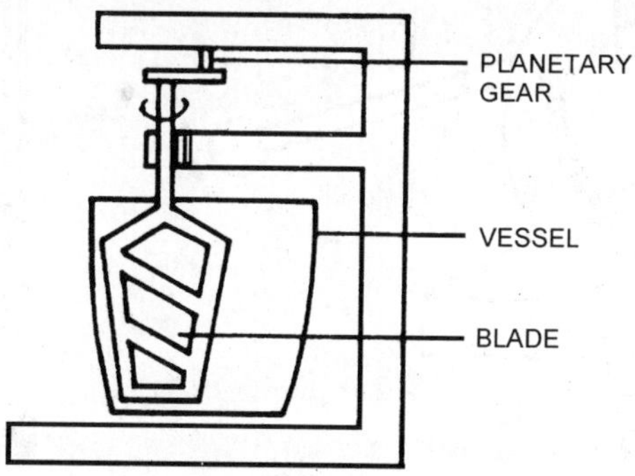

Fig 7-6 Planetary mixer

Working The blade is moved slowly at the initial stage for pre-mixing of the material and finally at increased speed for active mixing. In this way high shear can be applied for thorough mixing. The blade and the stationary vessel provide a kneading action and shear. This is due to narrow clearance between the blade and the wall of the vessel.

Uses The planetary mixer is used for its kneading action required in wet granulation. It is also used for mixing of powdered drug with an ointment base.

HOMOGENISATION

Homogenisation is the process of preparing fine emulsion from a coarse emulsion by converting the large globules to small globules. Homogenisation is done in an apparatus called 'Homogeniser'.

Principle The homogenisers are based on the principle that the large globules in a coarse emulsion are broken into smaller globules by passing them under pressure through a narrow orifice.

The commonly used homogenisers are:

1. Hand homogeniser
2. Silverson mixer homogeniser
3. Colloidal mill

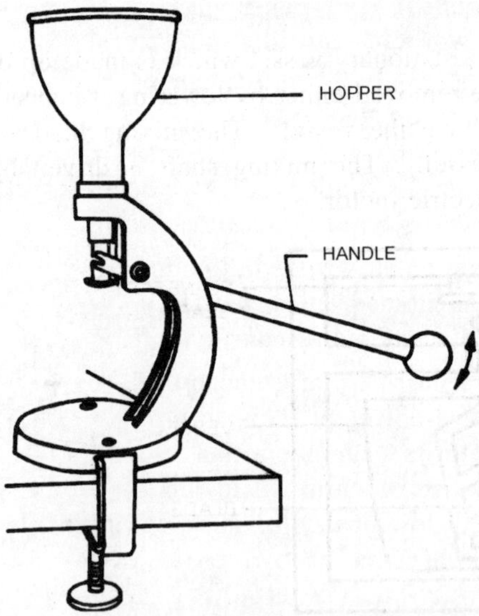

Fig. 7-7 Hand homogeniser

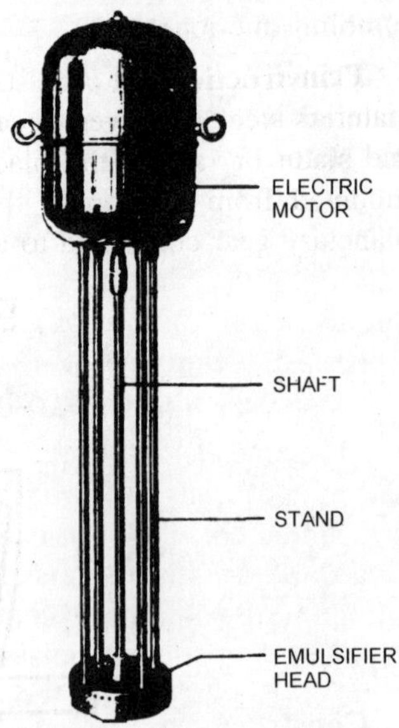

Fig. 7-8 Silverson mixer homogeniser

■ HAND HOMOGENISER ■

The homogeniser is hand-operated and the coarse emulsion is passed through a fine orifice. The emulsion is placed in the hopper of the homogeniser. The up and down movement of the handle causes coarse emulsion to draw in through inlet valve and pass through homogenising valve. In this way the emulsion is forced to pass through the fine orifice (aperture). The oil globules are broken into fine globules of uniform size.

■ SILVERSON MIXER HOMOGENISER ■

Construction It consists of an emulsifier head which is covered with fine meshed stainless steel sieve. The emulsifier head consist of a number of blades which rotate at a very high speed, in order to produce a powerful shearing action. The blades are rotated by using an electric motor fitted at the top.

Working The emulsifier head is placed in the vessel containing immiscible liquids, in such a way that it should get dipped into it. When the motor is started, the liquids are sucked through the fine holes and the oil is reduced into fine globules due to the rotation of the blades.

So a fine emulsion is produced which is then expelled out. The intake and expulsion of the mixture set up a pattern of circulation.

■ COLLOIDAL MILL ■

Principle The size reduction is affected due to shearing, when the material is passed between the narrow gap of milling surfaces of rotor and stator.

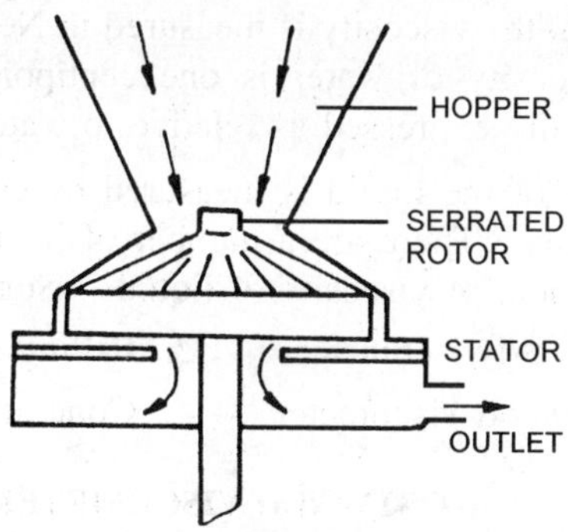

Fig.7-9 Colloidal mill

Construction Colloidal mill consists of a rotor and a stator. The rotor rotates at a speed of 3,000 to 20,000 r.p.m. The stator have conical milling surfaces between which there is an adjustable clearance between 0.002 to 0.03 inches.

Working The material *e.g.* emulsion and suspension is placed into the hopper of the mill. It is then passed through the narrow gap between the rotor and stator and thus reduced to fine particle size.

Uses Colloidal mills are capable of producing particles in micron size. These are commonly used to prepare pharmaceutical suspensions and emulsions having particle size less than one micron.

▩ VISCOSITY ▩

Every liquid has its own flow rate. Liquids like water, alcohol, chloroform and acetone move fast, whereas syrup, honey and glycerine flow slowly. This rate of flow of liquid depends on the internal resistance involved when one layer moves over another layer. In other words, the property of a liquid which gives its resistance to flow is called viscosity.

Liquids of high viscosity do not flow readily due to their high internal fractional resistance. The more the resistance to flow the more will be the viscosity of the liquid.

Viscosity of liquid decreases with rise in temperature, while it increases with fall in temperature.

Measurement of viscosity The viscosity is measured in both C.G.S. and S.I. system.

In C.G.S. system the viscosity of a liquid is measured in dyne-second per square centimetre. It is also known as "Poise". Each poise is further divided into 100 centipoise.

In S.I. system, the viscosity is measured in Newton-second per square metre. The viscosity of water is one centipoise. The viscosities of liquids are normally expressed as relative to water.

The viscosity of the liquid is measured by comparison with a liquid of known viscosity. There are a number of instruments which are used for the measurement of viscosity of liquids. Some of these are:

1. Ostwald viscometer
2. Falling sphere viscometer
3. Redwood viscometer
4. Cone and plate viscometer

▩ OSTWALD VISCOMETER ▩

Construction It consists of "U" tube having two bulbs X and Y. A capillary tube CD of a suitable bore is fitted to one arm of U tube. The viscometer is placed vertically in a thermostatically controlled bath.

Working A liquid whose viscosity is to be determined is placed in arm Y to fill the tube to mark E. It is then sucked or blown up to a point 1 cm above A. The time (t_1) for the liquid to fall from mark A to mark B is measured. The density of liquid (d_1) is determined.

The whole procedure is repeated with a liquid of known viscosity and time (t_2) is noted for the fall of liquid from mark A to B.

If η_1 is the viscosity, d_1 is the density of the liquid and t_1 is the time in second of the unknown liquid and η_2 is the viscosity, d_2 the density of the liquid and t_2 is the time in second of the known liquid, then the viscosity of the unknown liquid can be determined by:

$$\frac{\eta_1}{\eta_2} = \frac{d_1 t_1}{d_2 t_2} \quad \text{or} \quad \eta_1 = \frac{d_1 t_1}{d_2 t_2} \eta_2$$

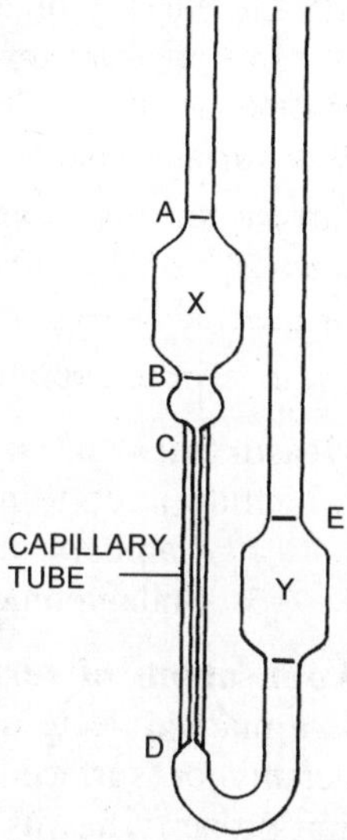

Fig.7-10 Ostwald viscometer

Applications of viscosity in pharmacy

1. Viscosity plays an important role in the stability of emulsions and suspensions.
2. Ophthalmic preparations are made viscous to prolong the contact time of the drugs *e.g.* methyl cellulose is used for this purpose.
3. Paints are made more viscous so that they may remain in contact with skin for long time *e.g.* glycerine is included in paint formulation to increase the viscosity.
4. Fats, waxes and other viscous substances are filtered at higher temperature. It is due to the fact that at higher temperature, there is decrease in viscosity and hence rate of filtration can be increased.
5. Certain pharmaceutical formulations are standardized on the basis of its viscosity *e.g.* liquid extract of liquorice.
6. The viscosity of certain liquid preparations is increased in order to improve pourability or to make the preparation more palatable.

SURFACE TENSION

The molecules of the interior of a liquid attract one another equally in all directions. At the surface of the liquid, the attraction is only in downward and sideward direction and this causes the surface layer to exist in a state of tension, which is called surface tension. Due to this tension the surface of a liquid acts like a stretched elastic membrane, which exert pressure inward on the rest of the liquid. This force, causes a liquid to assume the form of a spherical drop. In this form it has the smallest surface area for a given volume.

Surface tension is expressed in dynes/cm. The tension at liquid/gas surfaces is called surface tension and that at liquid/liquid surfaces is called interfacial tension.

The rise in temperature decreases the surface tension.

Measurement of surface tension Following are some of the methods which are used to measure the surface tension:

1. Capillary tube method
2. Drop weight method
3. Stalagmometer
4. Tensiometer method

Applications of surface tension in pharmacy The substances that cause a marked decrease in the surface tension of the solvent are called surfactants or surface active agents. The surface tension/interfacial tension property has its importance in emulsification, wetting and detergent action. The surfactants are used to increase the stability of slightly soluble materials and hence are known as "solubilising agents". Similarly a stable emulsion is produced by the use of emulsifying agent.

As surfactants decrease the surface tension between water and grease or dust, they can be used as detergent. Detergents are considered better than soaps because of their efficiency to remove dirt and grease than soaps.

▪ WETTING AGENTS ▪

Wetting agents are the substances which reduce the interfacial tension between the solid particles and liquid medium *e.g.* alcohol is added to tragacanth mucilage and glycerine is added to bentonite dispersion. Wetting agents should be used in minimum amount because excessive amount may lead to foaming or give an undesirable taste and odour to the preparation. The commonly used wetting agents are Tween 80, Sorbiton trioleate etc.

▪ REVISION QUESTIONS ▪

A. Very short answer type questions ▪

Answer the following questions in brief.

1. Define the term "Mixing"
2. What is perfect mixing?
3. What are different types of mixtures?

4. Name the different mechanisms which are applicable in mixing powders.
5. Name the various physical properties which affect the perfect mixing of powders.
6. What are the different equipments used for mixing in powders?
7. Name the different equipments which can be used for mixing of liquids.
8. Give the list of equipments used for mixing of semi-solids.
9. Define "Homogenisation".
10. Define "Viscosity".
11. What do you know about "Surface tension"?
12. What are the various units for measuring viscosity?

B. Short answer type questions ■

13. What are the main objectives of mixing?
14. Write in brief about physical properties which affect the perfect mixing of powders.
15. Draw a neat diagram of "Double Cone Blender".
16. What are the equipments used for mixing of powders? Write in brief about double cone mixer.
17. Draw the labelled diagram of "Triple Roller Mill". Write its uses.
18. What is the principle of homogenisation?
19. Define "Viscosity". Write its application in pharmacy.
20. Write in brief about "Wetting Agents".

C. Long answer type questions ■

21. Define the term "Mixing". Describe the various physical properties of solids which affect the perfect mixing of powders.
22. What are the objectives of mixing? Give a list of equipments which are used for mixing of powders. Write in detail about "Double Cone Blender".
23. What are the equipments used for mixing of liquids? Write in detail about "Propeller Mixer".
24. Write in brief about principle, construction, working and uses of "Planetary Mixer".
25. What are the preparations in which mixing of semi-solids required? Write in detail about "Triple Roller Mill".

26. Define "Homogenisation". Write the principle of homogenisation. Write in detail about "Colloidal Mill".

27. Explain with the help of a neat diagram the construction and working of any of the following mills:
    (*i*) Triple roller mill (*ii*) Colloidal mill
    (*iii*) Agitated powder mixer (*iv*) Propeller mixer
    (*v*) Double cone blender (*vi*) Planetary mixer

28. Write short notes on:
    (1) Colloidal mill (2) Silverson mixer homogeniser
    (3) Hand mill (4) Agitator mixer
    (5) Double cone blender (6) Planetary mixe

29. Define "Viscosity". What are the instruments used for measuring viscosity? Write in detail about Ostwald viscometer. Give the applications of viscosity in pharmacy.

D. Objective type questions

A. Completion type questions (Fill in the blanks with suitable word/words)

30. Mixing of powders is necessary for preparation of ________, ________ and ________ .

31. Mixing of liquids is done for preparation of ________ and ________ .

32. Mixing of semi-solids is required for preparing ________, ________ and ________ .

33. In colloidal mill the rotor rotates at a speed of ________ to ________ r.p.m.

34. In homogenisers the coarse emulsion is converted into ________ emulsion by passage under ________ through a narrow ________.

35. In C.G.S. system the viscosity of the liquid is measured in ________ which is divided into ________centipoise.

36. Surface tension is expressed in________ .

37. In agitated powder mixer, mixing of powder takes place which has ________ and ________ .

38. The rise in temperature ________ the surface tension.

39. In air mixers________ air blasts of ________ seconds duration is given after an interval of ________ seconds.

B. Matching type questions.

40. Match the items of *Column I* with appropriate items in *Column II*.

Column I	*Column II*
(A) The flat blades of paddle mixer rotate at	(*i*) produces particles in micron size
(B) Colloidal mill	(*ii*) rise in temperature
(C) Sigma arm mixer	(*iii*) 8000 r.p.m.
(D) Surface tension decreases with	(*iv*) for mixing of semisolid.
(E) The propeller of propeller mixer rotates at	(*v*) 100 r.p.m.
(F) Viscosity of liquid increases with	(*vi*) fall in temperature

KEY

30. Tablets, capsules, compound powders.
31. True solutions, emulsions
32. Ointments, creams, pill mass
33. 3000; 20,000
34. Fine, pressure, orifice
35. poise, 100
36. dynes/cm
37. Uniform particle size, density
38. Decreases
39. Eight, two, one
40. A(iv); B(i); C(iv); D(ii); E(iii);F(vi)

8

Clarification and Filtration

Filtration is the process, whereby solid particles are separated from the liquid or gas by passing it through a porous medium which retains the solid but allows the fluid to pass. When solids are present in a very small proportion *i.e.* not exceeding 1.0 per cent the process of its separation from liquid is called 'clarification'. Ultrafiltration may be defined as the separation of intermicellar liquid from solids by the use of pressure on a semipermeable membrane. The porous medium used to retain the solids is known as filter medium. The solid which gets collected on the filter is called filter cake and the clear liquid passing through the filter is known as filtrate.

When the object of filtration is to remove large visible particles by using coarse filtering medium such as muslin and cotton wool, the process is known as "straining".

Theory of Filtration The theory of filtration gives an idea about the factors influencing the rate of filtration through the filtering medium, rather than the mechanism by which the particles are retained.

The factors affecting the rate of filtration were studied by a scientist named Darcy and he expressed it in the form of an equation, which is known as "Darcy's law". The equation is:

$$V = \frac{KA\Delta P}{\eta l}$$

where V = Volume of filtrate

K = Permeability coefficient and is dependent on the nature of the precipitate to be filtered and the filter medium

A = Area of filter bed

ΔP = Pressure difference on the liquid and below the filter medium

η = Viscosity of the fluid

l = Thickness of filter cake

The above equation makes it clear that the rate of filtration depends not only on the nature of liquid undergoing filtration but also on so many other factors.

Factors Affecting the Rate of Filtration

The rate of filtration depends on the following factors:

1. Pressure : The rate of filtration of liquid is directly proportional to the pressure difference between the 'filter medium' and 'filter cake'. Thus, the rate of filtration can be increased by applying pressure on the liquid being filtered or by decreasing the pressure beneath the filter.

2. Viscosity : The rate of filtration is inversely proportional to the viscosity of the liquid undergoing filtration. Liquids which are very viscous get filtered slowly in comparison to liquids with low viscosity. Reduction of viscosity of a liquid by raising the temperature is frequently done in order to accelerate filtration *e.g.* syrups are more quickly filtered when hot than cold.

3. Surface area of filter media : The rate of filtration is directly proportional to the surface area of filter media. Pleating the filter paper or using a fluted funnel increases the effective surface area of filter paper for filtration. Filter press also works on the same principle.

4. Temperature of liquid to be filtered : Temperature plays an important role in the rate of filtration. Viscosity is reduced by a rise in temperature and the filtration of viscous oils, syrups etc. is often accelerated by filtering them while they are still hot.

5. Particle size : The rate of filtration is directly proportional to the particle size of the solid to be removed. It is easier to filter a liquid having coarse particles than that having finely divided particles because coarse filtering medium can be used to filter liquid having coarse particles and hence it increases the rate of filtration. Therefore before filtration, some method should be adopted to agglomerate the finely divided particles into coarse particles or to increase the particle size by precipitation.

6. Pore size of filter media : The rate of filtration is directly proportional to the pore size of the filter media. The liquid having coarse particles requires a coarse filtering media to remove them. So, the rate of filtration is increased when a coarse filter medium is used for filtration.

7. Thickness of cake : The rate of filtration is inversely proportional to the thickness of the filter cake formed during the process of filtration. As the filtration process proceeds, the solid particles start depositing on the filter medium, and thus, it increases the thickness of the cake and decreases the rate of filtration.

8. Nature of the solid material : The rate of filtration is directly proportional to the porosity of the filter cake. The porosity of the filter cake depends on the nature of the solid particles to be removed from the liquid. Filter aids are sometimes added to the filtering liquid to make a porous cake.

To sum up, the rate of filtration which depends on various factors can be written as:

$$\text{Rate of filtration} = \frac{\text{area of filter} \times \text{pressure difference}}{\text{Viscosity} \times \text{resistance of cake and filter}}$$

Filter Media

The surface upon, which solids are retained in the process of filtration is known as 'filter medium'. A good filter media should possess the following characteristics:

1. It should not absorb the constituents of the liquid preparation undergoing filtration.
2. It should be resistant to corrosive action of the liquid.
3. It should have smooth surface for easy discharge of cake.
4. It should allow free flow of liquid.
5. It should be resistant to chemical reaction with the contents of the liquid to be filtered.
6. It should have sufficient mechanical strength to resist the damage that occurs during filtration of liquid under pressure.

The selection of filter media depends on:

1. The quantity of the material to be filtered.
2. The nature of the product to be filtered *i.e.* its viscosity etc.
3. The size of the solid particles to be retained on the filter.
4. Purpose of filtration.

The various filtering media employed for filtration are:

1. Filter paper : Filter paper is most commonly used as filter media for general filtration. The filter papers are classified as coarse, medium and fine according to their pore size. For the filtration of pharmaceutical preparations, a fine grade of filter paper is used. The main drawback of a filter paper is that it has an absorbing property and also it sheds fine particles into the filtrate.

2. Cotton wool : Cotton wool is generally used for filtering of moderately coarse particles. The disadvantage of cotton is that, it sheds fine cotton hair in the filtrate. This problem can be solved to a large extent by using cotton wool of long staple and wetting the cotton wool plug with liquid before its use.

3. Glass wool : It consists of fine fibres of glass which are resistant to corrosive liquids. So it is used for filtering corrosive liquids, such as strong acids, alkalies and oxidising agents *e.g.* solutions of chromic acid and potassium permanganate.

4. Asbestos : It is used for the same purpose as glass wool. It is commonly used in gravimetric analysis for collecting fine precipitates which are to be subsequently ignited.

5. Fine muslin : It is used for removing very coarse particles. This is done generally before passing the liquid through a fine filter media, in order to avoid choking of the fine filter with coarse particles.

6. Filter cloth : Both synthetic and cotton cloth is used as filter media for large scale filtration *e.g.* in filter press synthetic cloth has more strength than cotton cloth. Moreover, synthetic cloth has less absorbing property than cotton cloth. Hence, synthetic clothes are preferred nowadays.

7. Membrane filters : These are made of cellulose acetate and other cellulose derivatives, nylon and polyvinyl chloride. These are mainly used to remove microorganism and very fine particles from ophthalmic solution and parenteral products.

8. Sintered glass filters : These are made from borosilicate glass. The glass is powdered and sifted to produce uniform particles. These are heated to sintered point and moulded into a flat or convex plate, which is fitted into the glass funnel of suitable shape and size. These filters are mainly used for the filtration of liquids meant for parenteral use.

Filter Aids

These are the substance which reduce the resistance of the filtrate to flow. These are added to the preparation in concentration from 0.1 to 0.5 per cent before filtration. An ideal filter aid should possess the following qualities:

1. It should be able to remain suspended in the liquid.
2. It should be free from impurities.
3. It should be inert to the liquid being filtered.
4. It should have a particle size distribution suitable for the retention of solids as required.
5. It should have a structure that permits formation of porous cake.

The object of the filter aid is to prevent the filter medium from becoming blocked and to form an open, porous cake, so reducing the resistance to flow of the filtrate. Hence filter aid must be light, porous and inert. Filter aids are mainly used in clarification process where the solids are discarded. The commonly used filter aids in pharmacy are diatomite (diatomaceous earth), perlite, asbestos, cellulose, activated charcoal, talc and kaolin etc.

The following Table 8-1 shows the advantages and disadvantages of some of the commonly used filter aid materials.

TABLE 8-1

The Advantages and Disadvantages of Filter Aid Materials

Filter aid material	*Chemical composition*	*Advantages*	*Disadvantages*
Cellulose	Cellulose	*i.* High purity *ii.* Used mainly as a coarse precoat. *iii.* Excellent chemical resistance	*i.* Expensive
Asbestos	Alumino-silicate	*i.* Good retention on coarse screens	*i.* Soluble in acids and alkalies *ii.* Give highly compressible cakes
Carbon	Carbon	*i.* May be used for filtering strong alkaline solutions	*i.* Expensive *ii.* Available in coarse grades only
Diatomaceous earth	Silica	*i.* Available in various size range *ii.* Used for fine filtration	*i.* Slightly soluble in dilute acids and alkalies
Perlite	Silica and alumino-silicate	Available in wide size range	*i.* Soluble in acids and alkalies *ii.* May give highly compressible cakes

FILTERING DEVICES USED IN PHARMACEUTICAL INDUSTRY

Various filtering devices used in pharmaceutical industry are:

1. Filter press
2. Meta filters
3. Filter leaf
4. Membrane filters
5. Filter candles
6. Sintered filters

Filter Press

There are two basic forms of the filter press but only the Plate and Frame Press has a wide application in pharmaceutical industry.

PLATE AND FRAME FILTER PRESS

Construction It consists of plates and frames. The frame is open and is used as an inlet for the material to be filtered. Plate has a grooved surface which gives support to the filter cloth. The plate and frame may be made of various metals which provide resistance to corrosion or prevent metallic contamination of the filtrate. Filter cloth is fitted on each side of the plate The plates and frames are placed alternatively and fitted in the outer frame of the press. Each plate acts as a single filtration unit. The outlet of each plate is connected to a common outlet pipe.

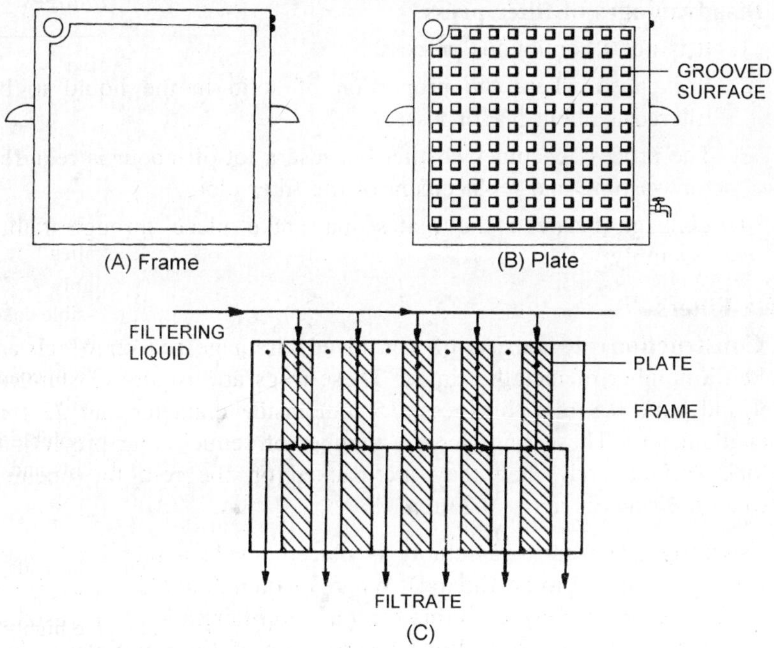

Fig. 8-1 Diagram showing principles of operation of filter press

Working As shown in the diagram (C) the filtering liquid enters the frame under pressure from the feed channel. The filtrate passes through the filter medium on to the surface of the plate.

The filtrate is collected in the plates from where it is collected through common outlet pipe. The cake is deposited in the frames. The process of filtration is continued until the frame is filled with filter cake.

When the process is stopped, the frame is emptied and the cycle is restarted.

The thickness of the cake can be varied by using frames of different thickness. The thickness of filter cake depends mainly on the solid content present in the filtering liquid and the resistance of filter cake.

Advantages of filter press

1. The filtering media can be used repeatedly.
2. Operation and maintenance is simple.
3. It requires less space.
4. It provides a large surface area for filtration.
5. Efficient washing of cake is possible.

Disadvantages of filter press

1. It is not a continuous process.
2. It is used where the proportion of solid in the liquid to be filtered is about 5% or less.
3. The process becomes costlier because a lot of labour is required for washing and replacement of the filter cloth.
4. Leakage between the plates may take place through faulty assembly.

Meta Filters ■

Construction It consists of a grooved, drainage rod on which are packed a number of metallic rings. These rings are usually of stainless steel and have 0.8 mm thickness, 15 mm inside diameter and 22 mm outer diameter. These rings have a number of semicircular projections on one surface and when they are packed on the rod, the opening between the rings is about 0.2 mm.

Working The entire assembly is placed inside a pressure vessel, containing the liquid to be filtered. When vacuum is applied, liquid will flow from outside to inside. In this form a metafilter can only be used as strainer for coarse particles. But for separation of finer particles, a bed of suitable materials such as Kieselguhr is used. In this way the pack of rings acts as a base on which the true filter medium is supported.

Uses The meta filter are mostly used for clarification of syrups, elixirs and parenteral solutions.

Advantages of meta filter

1. It possess considerable strength and hence can withstand high pressure.

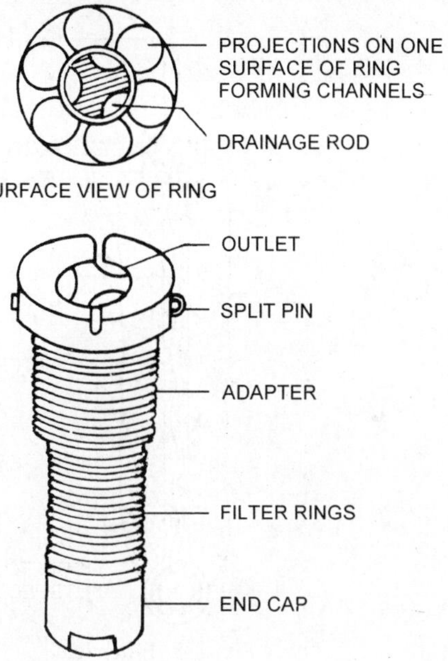

Fig. 8-2 Meta filter

2. It is an economical filter.
3. The corrosive liquids can be filtered without any problem.
4. Cake can be removed effectively without any difficulty.

Filter Leaf

Construction It is the simplest form of filter. It consists of a frame enclosing a drainage screen or a grooved plate. Filter cloth is used as the filtering medium, the whole unit being covered with filter cloth. The frame used may be of any shape *i.e.* square, rectangular or of a circular shape.

Working The filter leaf is placed in a vessel containing the liquid to be filtered. When vacuum is applied, the pressure inside the leaf is decreased. Due to the difference in external pressure and pressure inside the leaf, the liquid moves inside the filter through filter cloth. The filtrate is collected in the receiver, whereas the cake gets collected on outside of the cloth.

This method has the advantage that the liquid can be filtered from any vessel and cake can be washed simply by immersing it in a vessel containing water. The cake can be removed just by flowing air in the reverse direction.

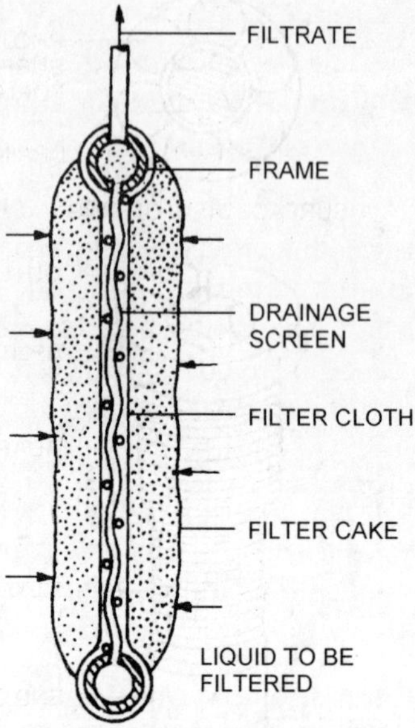

Fig. 8-3 Filter leaf

Membrane Filters

Membrane filters are made of thin and flat membranes of cellulose derivatives, such as, cellulose acetate and cellulose nitrate. These filters are brittle when in dry condition and can be stored for an indefinite period. The filters are between 50 and 150 μ thick and are available in sizes upto 60 cm^2.

A membrane filter has 400 to 500 million pores per square centimetre of filter surface. The pores are absolutely uniform in size and occupy about 80% of filter volume. To avoid rapid clogging of a membrane, pre-filtration is often required. The selection of a membrane filter for a particular application depends on the particles to be removed. Table 8-2 shows the approximate pore size required to remove specified particles.

TABLE 8.2

S. No.	*Pore size (micron)*	*Particles to be removed*
1.	0.2	All bacteria
2.	0.45	All coliform group bacteria
3.	0.8	All airborne particles
4.	1.2	All non-living particles which are dangerous in *i.v.* fluids.
5.	5	All significant cells from body fluids.

A membrane filter is fixed in a metallic holder before its use. These filters are mainly used for sterilisation of both aqueous and oily liquids. The membrane filters cannot be used for filtration of organic solvents, such as alcohols, ketones, esters and chloroform.

Filter Candles

These are ceramic filters and are made of porcelain or Kieselguhr. Kiesel-guhr filters are usually softer than the porcelain variety. These are cylindrical candles with an opening which is connected to vacuum pump for reducing the pressure under it, during the filtration process. The candles are available in a range of different pore size which is designated by a number.

The candle is placed in the solution to be filtered. When vacuum is applied, the liquid will pass through the thick wall of the candle and gets collected inside the candle from where it is removed.

The filter candle gets blocked with continuous use. This can be cleaned by scratching the external surface with a nail brush and passing water through it in the reverse direction.

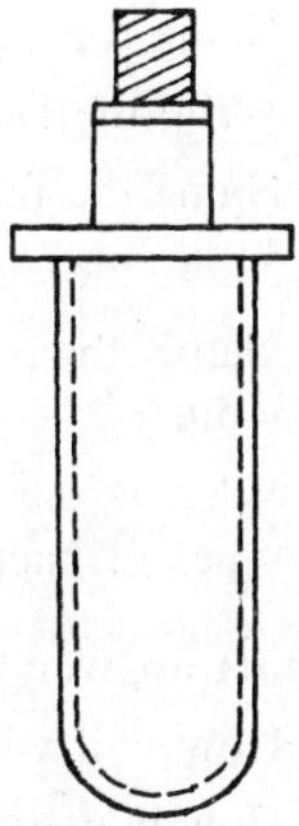

Fig. 8-4 Filter Candle

These candles are used for sterilisation of solutions. It has the tendency to absorb materials from aqueous solutions. Therefore, it is not used commonly.

Sintered Filters

These are made of borosilicate glass. Borosilicate glass is finely powdered, sieved and particle of desired size are separated. It is then packed into a disc mould and heated to a temperature at which adhesion takes place between the particles. The disc is then fused to a funnel of suitable shape and size.

The sintered glass filters are available in different pore size. Hence the funnel with a sintered filter is numbered according to the pore size. The filtration is carried out under reduced pressure. These funnels are used for bacterial filtration.

Sintered filters are also available in stainless steel which has a greater mechanical strength. However these are very much liable to attack by the solutions passing through them.

■ REVISION QUESTIONS ■

I. Very short answer type questions ■

Answer the following questions in brief.

1. Define the term "Filtration".
2. What do you know about "Clarification"?
3. Explain the term "Filter media".
4. What does the term "Ultra filtration" mean?
5. Name the commonly used filter aids.
6. Write the Darcy's law equation.
7. Name the factors which affects the rate of filtration.
8. Name the various filter media commonly used.
9. Name the commonly used filtering devices in pharmaceutical industry.
10. What is the pore size (micron) of membrane filter to remove all types of bacteria?

II. Short answer type questions ■

11. How will you clean a blocked filter candle?
12. How does rise in temperature of viscous liquid help to increase its rate of filtration?
13. Explain the factors which affect the rate of filtration.
14. Write the qualities of an ideal filter aids.
15. Mention the advantages of filter press.
16. What are the advantages of a meta filter?
17. How can you increase the surface area of filter media?
18. Write in brief about membrane filter.
19. Write short note on filter leaf.
20. What are the qualities of an ideal filter medium?

III. Long answer type questions ■

21. Define the term "Filtration". Write the theory of filtration.
22. Explain the construction and working of filter press. What are the advantages and disadvantages of filter press?
23. Explain the construction and working of the following:-
    (a) meta filter
    (b) filter leaf

24. Differentiate between filtration, clarification and straining. Describe the various filter media used in pharmacy.
25. What are the factors which affect the rate of filtration? Write in brief about membrane filter.
26. What are the qualities of a ideal filter medium? Write in brief about filter candle and sintered filters.
27. Write short notes on the following:-
    (a) Filter media
    (b) Filter aids
    (c) Sintered glass filter
    (d) Filter candle
    (e) Darcy's law
    (f) Membrane filter
28. What is "Darcy's"? Explain the various factors which affects the rate of filtration.

IV. Objective type questions

A. Completion type questions (Fill in the blanks with suitable word/words)

29. The rate of filtration is _________ proportional to the viscosity of the liquid.

30. The rate of filtration is ________ proportional to the surface area of filter media.

31. Filter candles are called ____________ filter and are made of __________ or ________.

32. Sintered filters are made of _________ glass and filtration is done________.

33. The rate of filtration is__________ proportional to the thickness of the cake formed during filtration.

34. The membrane filters are _________ and _________ thick and are available in sizes upto ______________.

35. The metallic rings of meta filter have ___________ thickness _____________ inside diameter and ________outer diameter.

36. The membrane filter has ________ to ____________ millions pores per square centimetre of filter surface.

B. Matching type questions.

37. Match the items of *Column I* with appropriate items in *Column II.*

Column I	*Column II*
A. Rise in temperature	(*i*) used as a strainer.
B. Filter aids	(*ii*) 400 to 500 millions pores per square cm.
C. Darcy	(*iii*) removes all bacteria.
D. Straining	(*iv*) accelerates the filtration rate of viscous liquid.
E. Meta filter	(*v*) used in conc. of 0.1 to 0.5 per cent.
F. A membrane filter (0.2 μ pore size)	(*vi*) studied the factors affecting the rate of filtration.
G. Membrane filter	(*vii*) removes coarse particles using coarse filter.

KEY

10. 0.2 micron
11. Scratching the external surface with nail brush.
17. Using pleated filter paper or fluted funnel.
29. Inversely
30. Directly
31. Ceramic, porcelain or Kieselguhr
32. Borosilicate, under reduced pressure
33. Inversely
34. 50 and 150 μ, 60 cm square
35. 0.8 mm, 15 mm, 22 mm.
36. 400 to 500
37. A(*iv*); B(*v*); C(*vi*); D(*vii*); E(*i*); F(*iii*) and G(*ii*).

9

Extraction Processes

'Extraction' may be defined as the treatment of the plant or animal tissues with solvent, whereby the medicinally active constituents are dissolved, and most of the inert matter remains undissolved.

The solvent used for extraction is known as "Menstruum" and the inert insoluble material that remains after extraction is called "Marc".

The various processes used for extraction are of:

1. Infusion
2. Decoction
3. Maceration
4. Percolation
5. Digestion

The various preparations prepared by using one of the above methods are Infusions, Decoctions, Spirits, Elixirs, Extracts *etc*. All these preparations are commonly known as 'Galenicals'.

SOLVENT USED IN EXTRACTION PROCESSES

In extraction process a solvent is employed which is capable of penetrating the tissues of the drug and dissolve the active principles contained in its cell. The various solvents used are as under:

1. Water : Water is a solvent for protein, colouring matter, gums, glycosides, sugars, alkaloidal salts, enzymes, many organic acids and most of the organic salts.

Waxes, fats, fixed oils and most alkaloids are insoluble in water.

Advantages of water

1. It is cheap.
2. It has a wide solvent action.
3. It is non-toxic.
4. It is non-inflammable.

Disadvantages of water

1. It dissolves a wide range of substances which are undesirable and may interfere with the clarity of the preparation or cause fermentation or decomposition of the preparation.

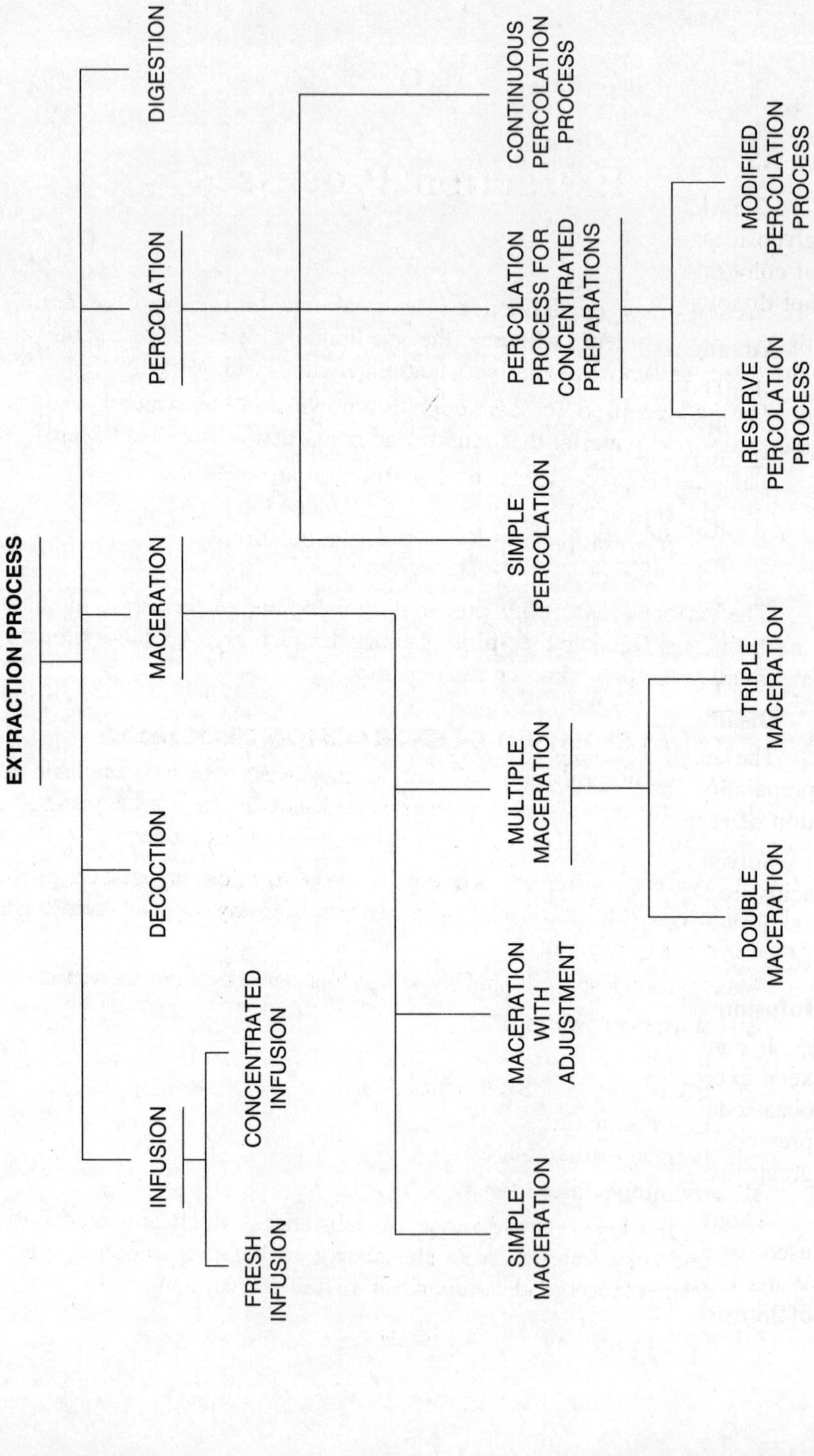
EXTRACTION PROCESS
INFUSION
DECOCTION
MACERATION
PERCOLATION
DIGESTION
FRESH INFUSION
CONCENTRATED INFUSION
SIMPLE MACERATION
MACERATION WITH ADJUSTMENT
MULTIPLE MACERATION
DOUBLE MACERATION
TRIPLE MACERATION
SIMPLE PERCOLATION
PERCOLATION PROCESS FOR CONCENTRATED PREPARATIONS
RESERVE PERCOLATION PROCESS
MODIFIED PERCOLATION PROCESS
CONTINUOUS PERCOLATION PROCESS

2. Water helps in the growth of mould and bacteria. Hence, some preservative is needed during extraction of crude drugs.
3. Water causes hydrolysis of many substances.
4. Large amount of heat is required to concentrate the aqueous preparations than the non-aqueous preparations.

2. Alcohol : Alcohol is a solvent of alkaloids, alkaloidal salts, glycosides, volatile oils and resins. Alcohol also dissolves many forms of colouring matter, tannins, many organic acids and salts. Alcohol does not dissolve albuminous matter, gums, waxes, fats, fixed oils and sugar.

Advantages of alcohol as a solvent

1. The mould and bacteria cannot grow in a solution in which alcohol concentration is 20% or more.
2. It is neutral and hence extraction products obtained from it are compatible with other products.
3. It is non-toxic in the concentration mostly present in the preparations.
4. A small amount of heat is required to concentrate the alcoholic preparations.
5. It dissolves selective active constituents of drugs.

Disadvantages of alcohol as a solvent

The main disadvantage of alcohol as a solvent is its cost. The preparation becomes costly when alcohol is used as solvent for extraction of active constituents of the drug.

Solvents such as solvent ether, chloroform, light petroleum, certain acids are used rarely for extraction of active constituents from crude drugs.

PROCESSES USED FOR EXTRACTION

Infusion

It consists of pouring water over the drugs and then allowing it to keep in contact with water for the stated period, usually 15 minutes, with occasional stirring and finally filtering off the liquid. The marc is not pressed. The boiling water is commonly used as a solvent, since it has a greater solvent action than cold water.

Apparatus Coffee pot or a teapot is the simplest form of apparatus used for preparing infusion. The drug is placed at the bottom of the pot. Water is added and it is well stirred three or four times during the period of infusion. Infusion can also be prepared by enclosing the drug in a muslin bag and then suspending it just below the level of the water in a beaker. Stirring is not required in this case because the water slowly circulates due to increase in specific gravity of water near the drug. When water comes in contact with the drug, it dissolves the active constituents and becomes heavier. The heavier layers come down and their place is taken by fresh water. As a result, there is slow circulation of water and hence stirring is not required. When hot water is used as menstruum, cooling of water occurs more rapidly at the surface than in the mass of the liquid. The lower layers of water which are hotter and contain less dissolved active constituents will rise and displace the upper layers. Hence, there is a slow circulation of water which makes stirring unnecessary.

Special pots known as 'infusion pots' are used for the preparation of infusion. It consists of a loose perforated shelf resting on a projection near the top of the pot. The drug is placed on the perforated shelf. The pot is filled with water and the perforated shelf is adjusted below the surface of water.

There are two types of infusion:

1. Fresh infusions
2. Concentrated infusions

Fresh infusions A fresh infusion is an aqueous solution of active constituents of a vegetable drug prepared by the process of infusion *e.g.* Fresh infusion of Quassia.

Coarse powder of drug is used in the preparation of infusion. Water is used as menstruum because it has more penetration power and dissolves the active constituents of the drug. Pharmacopœia states that fresh infusion should be used within 12 hours after its preparation because it gets spoiled due to fungal or bacterial growth.

Concentrated infusions Concentrated infusions are prepared by double or triple maceration process. Concentrated infusions are eight times stronger than the fresh infusion. Alcohol in the concentration of 20-25% is used as menstruum. Hence, these preparations can be stored for a longer period due to preservative action of alcohol. The dilution of 1 volume of concentrated infusion with 7 volumes of water resembles the corresponding fresh infusion in potency *e.g.* Concentrated Infusion of Quassia and Concentrated Compound Infusion of Chirata.

Decoction Process

In this process, the drug is boiled with water for a stated period usually 10 minutes. After boiling, the liquid is strained and water is passed through the content of the strainer to make the required volume.

This process is mainly used for vegetable drugs of hard and woody nature having thermostable water soluble constituents.

TABLE 9-1
Comparison Between 'Infusion' and 'Decoction'

Infusion	*Decoction*
1. Cold or boiling water is used as menstruum.	1. Drug is boiled in water.
2. Drug having soft tissue is used.	2. Drug of a hard tissue is used.
3. Drug constituents may be volatile.	3. Drug constituents should be non-volatile.
4. Final volume is not adjusted.	4. Adjustment to volume is done.
5. When boiling water is used as menstruum, precautions are taken to prevent the escape of heat by covering the vessel with a cloth.	5. No such precaution is required because the final volume is adjusted at the end.

Maceration Processes

The various types of maceration process are:

1. A process for tinctures made from organised drug *e.g.* roots, stems, leaves etc. This process is called "Simple Maceration".
2. A process for tinctures made from unorganised drugs such as oleo resins and gum resins. This process is known as "Maceration with Adjustment".
3. Process for concentrated preparations which include both "Double Maceration" and "Triple Maceration".

1. Maceration Process for Tinctures made from Organised Drugs (Simple Maceration)

Apparatus A wide mouth bottle or any other container which can be well stoppered is used for maceration process. A closed container is essential to prevent the evaporation of menstruum which is mostly concentrated alcohol. Otherwise this may lead to variation in strength as no adjustment in volume is made.

Method In this process, the drug is placed with the whole of the menstruum in a closed vessel for seven days. During this period shaking is done occasionally. After seven days, the liquid is strained and marc is pressed. The expressed liquid is mixed with strained liquid. It is then filtered to make a clear liquid. The final volume is not adjusted.

Explanation

1. Shaking of the drug during maceration is essential in order to replace the saturated layers around the drug with fresh menstruum.
2. After straining, the marc is pressed in a filter press, hydraulic press or hand press *etc*. The marc can be squeezed out in a fine muslin piece, when the quantity of the drug is very small.
3. The pressed liquid is mixed with the strained liquid and then filtered. No final adjustment in volume is made, since the volume of pressed liquid is likely to vary with the process of pressing the marc. If the final adjustment in volume is made, it will give variation in the concentration of active principles although the volume of the final preparation may be the same.
4. Filtration is necessary to remove insoluble cell contents obtained during the pressing of the marc.

Examples The tinctures made by simple maceration process are:

1. Tincture of Orange.
2. Tincture of Lemon.
3. Tincture of Squill.

2. Maceration Process for Unorganised Drugs or Maceration with Adjustment

Method In this process, the unorganised drug is placed with 4/5th of the menstruum in a closed vessel for a period of 2-7 days. During this period, shaking is done occasionally. After the stated period, the liquid is filtered and the final volume is made up by passing the remaining 1/5th of the menstruum through the filter. The marc is not pressed.

Explanation

1. The period of maceration is reduced from 7 to 2 days in some cases, because the unorganised drugs behave like simple chemicals which dissolve in the solvent very easily and quickly.
2. 4/5th of the menstruum is used to contact it with the drug in order to take into account, the increase in volume after dissolving the soluble matter of the drug. The volume is made up at the end with 1/5th of the remaining menstruum.
3. The marc left is a compact gummy matter. It does not retain the menstruum and hence it is not necessary to press the marc.
4. The final volume is made up because all the active constituents of drug get dissolved in the menstruum. Marc is not pressed.

Hence, there is no change in the concentration of the preparation in case the final volume is made up.

Examples The tinctures made by maceration with adjustment are:

1. Tincture of tolu
2. Compound tincture of benzoin

3. Maceration Process for Concentrated Preparations or Multiple Maceration process

Multiple maceration process is carried out in the same way as simple maceration process, but the menstruum used is divided into two parts in double maceration process and into three parts in triple maceration process.

Double Maceration Process In this process, the drug is macerated twice by using the menstruum which is divided into two parts in such a manner that the same volume is used for each maceration. The quantity of menstruum required for two macerations are calculated as follows:

(*i*) Volume of menstruum required for first maceration =

$$\frac{\text{Total vol. of menstruum} - \text{Vol. to be retained by the drug}}{2} + \text{Vol. to be retained by the drug}$$

(*ii*) Volume of menstruum required for second maceration = Total vol. of menstruum – Vol. of menstruum used in first maceration

The volume of menstruum to be retained by the drug is determined by experiment, in a test batch of drug by adding a known volume of menstruum to known weight of the drug. After maceration, straining and pressing of the marc, measure the volume of liquid obtained. Difference in the volume obtained and the volume used represents the volume retained by the weighable quantity of the drug used.

In double maceration process, the whole of the drug is macerated for 48 hours with the quantity of menstruum required for first maceration. Strain the liquid and press the marc. Macerate again for 24 hours with the remaining menstruum required for second maceration. Strain the liquid and press the marc. Mix the liquids obtained from the two macerations and allow it to stand for 14 days and then filter.

Examples The following concentrated infusions are prepared by double maceration process.

1. Concentrated infusion of orange
2. Concentrated compound infusion of chirata
3. Concentrated compound infusion of gentian

Triple Maceration Process In this maceration process, the drug is macerated thrice by using the menstruum which is divided into three parts in such a manner that the same volume is used for each maceration. The quantity of menstruum required for three macerations is calculated as follows:

(*i*) Volume of menstruum required for first maceration =

$$\frac{\text{Total vol. of menstruum} - \text{Vol. to be retained by the drug}}{3} + \text{Vol. to be retained by the drug}$$

(*ii*) Volume of menstruum required for 2nd and 3rd maceration =

$$\frac{\text{Total vol. of menstruum} - \text{Vol. of menstruum used in 1st maceration}}{2}$$

The whole of the drug is macerated for one hour with a part of menstruum required for first maceration and strained. Macerate again for one hour with a part of menstruum required for second maceration and strained. Macerate again for one hour with a part of menstruum required for third maceration and strained. Press the marc lightly. Then combine the liquids obtained from second and third maceration and evaporate it to a specified extent. Mix it with the liquid obtained from first maceration. Add alcohol 90% equal to 1/4th of the volume of the finished product. Adjust volume with water. Allow it to stand for 14 days and filter.

TABLE 9-2

Comparison Between 'Maceration Process' and 'Infusion Process'

Maceration process	*Infusion process*
1. Menstruum used is usually alcohol, but it may be aqueous.	1. Cold or boiling water is used as menstruum.
2. Drug is made in contact with menstruum for 2-7 days.	2. Drug is made in contact with menstruum for 15 mts.
3. The process is conducted at room temperature.	3. The process may or may not be conducted at room temperature.
4. Marc is pressed after maceration except in modified maceration process.	4. Marc is not pressed.
5. Volume is not made up in simple maceration but adjustment to volume is done in modified maceration process.	5. Volume is not made in infusion process.

TABLE 9-3

Comparison of Maceration Process for 'Organised Drugs' and 'Unorganised Drugs'

Organised drugs (*simple maceration*)	*Unorganised drugs* (*maceration with adjustment*)
1. Drug along with the whole of the menstruum is used in maceration process.	1. Drug along with 4/5th of the menstruum is used in maceration process.
2. The period of maceration is 7 days.	2. The period of maceration is 2-7 days as specified.
3. Strain off the liquid and press the marc.	3. Decant the liquid. Marc is not pressed.
4. Mix the pressed liquid with the macerate and clarify by subsidence or filtration. Filtrate is not adjusted to volume.	4. Filter the liquid and pass the remaining 1/5th of menstruum through filter to make up the final volume.
5. Examples of tinctures made by this process are: (*a*) Tincture of Orange (*b*) Tincture of Lemon (*c*) Tincture of Capsicum	5. Examples of tinctures made by this process are: (*a*) Compound Tincture of Benzoin (*b*) Tincture of Tolu (*c*) Tincture of Myrrh

Examples The following concentrated infusions are prepared by triple maceration process:

1. Concentrated Infusion of Quassia
2. Liquid Extract of Senna

Percolation Processes

The various percolation processes used for the extraction of drugs are:

1. Simple percolation or percolation process for tinctures.
2. Percolation processes for concentrated preparations such as :
   (*a*) Reserve percolation process
   (*b*) Modified percolation process
3. Continuous hot percolation or Soxhelation.

1. Simple Percolation Process

Apparatus Three types of percolators are used.

1. Conical percolator : The percolator is made of glass or of metal, usually copper, which is tinned inside. It is conical in shape having the lower diameter not less than half of the upper diameter. There are less

TABLE 9-4
Comparison Between
'Double Maceration' and 'Triple Maceration'

Double maceration	*Triple maceration*
1. Menstruum is divided into two parts.	1. Menstruum is divided into three parts.
2. The drug is macerated for 48 hours in first maceration followed by second maceration.	2. The drug is macerated thrice having each maceration of one hour duration.
3. Strain the liquid after each maceration and press the marc.	3. Strain the liquid after each maceration and press the marc after the last maceration.
4. The pressed liquid is mixed with the strained liquids of both macerations and then the volume is adjusted after adding more of menstruum.	4. Combine the strained liquid obtained from the second and the third maceration evaporate it to a specified extent. Mix it with strained liquid obtained after first maceration. Add 'alcohol 90%' equal to 1/4th of the volume of the finished product.
5. Alcohol 25% is used as menstruum.	5. Water is used as menstruum but 'alcohol 90%' is added at the end equal to 1/4th of the volume of the finished product.

chances of choking of conical percolator in case the drug swells up, because a drug can slope against the wall of the percolator. The main disadvantage of the conical type percolator is that there is undue loss of menstruum due to evaporation because of its bigger upper diameter.

2. Cylindrical percolator : The percolator is cylindrical in shape *i.e.* upper and lower diameters are same. These are used in case of those drugs which are difficult to get exhausted and there are less chances of swelling of the drug after imbibition. When a higher concentration of alcohol or any other volatile solvent is used as menstruum a cylindrical percolator is preferred.

3. Steam jacketed percolator : When percolation is carried at a higher temperature, in order to increase the solvent action of the menstruum, the percolator is heated by steam.

Method Simple percolation process is used for preparation of tinctures. There are three stages in the official method for preparation of tinctures by simple percolation process. These are:

(*a*) Imbibition
(*b*) Maceration

(*c*) Percolation

(*a*) *Imbibition* : The powdered drug is moistened with a sufficient quantity of menstruum and allowed to stand for 4 hours in a closed vessel. Pack the moistened drugs into a percolator and add sufficient quantity of menstruum to saturate the material. When liquid starts coming out from the outlet of percolator, the outlet is closed. Then a

TABLE 9-5

Comparison Between 'Simple Maceration Process' and 'Multiple Maceration Process'

Simple maceration	*Multiple maceration*
1. The drug is macerated with the whole of the menstruum.	1. The menstruum is divided into two parts in double maceration & into three parts in triple maceration process.
2. The period of maceration is 7 days.	2. In Double Maceration The drug is macerated for 48 hours in the first maceration followed by a second maceration for 24 hours. In Triple Maceration The drug is macerated thrice of one hour duration in each case.
3. After maceration, strain the liquid and press the marc.	3. In Double Maceration After each maceration, strain the liquid and press the marc. In Triple Maceration Strain the liquid after each maceration and press the marc after the last maceration.
4. Mix the pressed liquid with the strained liquid and then filter. Volume is not made up.	4. In Double Maceration Mix the pressed liquid with the liquid obtained from the two macerations and then the volume is adjusted by adding more of menstruum. In Triple Maceration Combine the strained liquid of 2nd & 3rd maceration and evaporate to a specified extent. Mix it with the liquid obtained from the first maceration. Add alcohol 90% equal to 1/4th of the volume of the finished product.
5. The final volume is not made up.	5. The final volume is made up in multiple maceration process.

sufficient quantity of menstruum is added in order to leave a layer above the drug.

(*b*) *Maceration* : The moistened drug is left in contact with menstruum for 24 hours. During this period, the menstruum dissolves the active constituents of the drug and becomes almost saturated with it.

(*c*) *Percolation* : It consists of the downward displacement of the saturated solution formed in maceration and extraction of the remaining active constituents present in the drug by the slow passage of the menstruum through the column of the drug.

After collecting 3/4th of the required volume of the finished product or when the drug is completely exhausted, the marc is pressed. Mix the expressed liquid with the percolate. Add sufficient quantity of menstruum to produce the required volume and then filter.

Explanation

1. The drug is powdered in percolation process so that it may be uniformly packed in the percolator. The powder size may vary from coarse powder to fine powder. The degree of size reduction depends on the nature of the tissues of the drug, the menstruum used and the solubility of the active constituents of the drug in the menstruum.

2. *Imbibition* : This is done in order—

(*a*) To allow the swelling of the tissues of the drug before packing it into the percolator. If the drug is packed in a dry state, it will cause blockage of the percolator.

(*b*) Imbibed drug can be uniformly packed in the percolator. When the dry powdered drug is packed in the percolator, there is a tendency of menstruum to wash the drug down toward the bottom of the percolator, where it forms an impermeable layer.

(*c*) Imbibition allows the entrapped air to escape. If a dry drug is packed in the percolator, the enclosed air will resist the flow of menstruum and it will also disturb the packing.

(*d*) The quantity of menstruum to be used for moistening of the drug depends upon the swelling power of the drug, generally, half the number of mls of menstruum as the number of grams of the drugs to be extracted. The best way to check the proper moistening of the drug is to press the drug lightly and see if it can retain the impression or not.

3. *Packing of the drug in a percolator*

(*a*) Before packing of the imbibed drug into the percolator, it is passed through a sieve to break any lump or masses.

(*b*) Glass wool, moistened with the solvent is placed at the bottom of the percolator to prevent the blockage of the outlet or tap. Cotton wool should not be used.

(*c*) The moistened drug is then added, a little at a time, into the percolator and pressed lightly after each addition, till whole of the drug is packed into the percolator . The drug should be uniformly packed upto 2/3rd or 3/4th of the percolator in order to facilitate a free flow of the menstruum through the drug.

(*d*) A piece of filter paper is placed on the packed drug. Washed sand is then placed on the filter paper. This is done to prevent disturbance of the top layers of the drug when menstruum is added into the percolator.

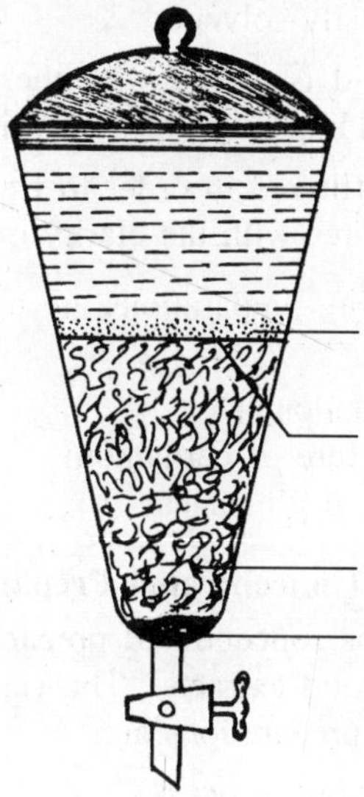

Fig. 9-1 Packing of the percolator

(*e*) A sufficient quantity of menstruum is added to saturate the material. When the liquid starts coming out from the percolator, outlet is closed. Again add a sufficient quantity of the menstruum in order to leave a layer above the drug and allow it to macerate for 24 hours. The percolator is closed to prevent evaporation of the solvent.

4. *Maceration* : During the period of 24 hours of maceration, the menstruum penetrates into the tissues of the drug and dissolves the

active constituents. A short maceration before percolation enables the extraction of active constituents of the drug with a considerably less quantity of the menstruum.

5. After 24 hours of maceration, open the outlet of the percolator and collect the percolate which measures about 3/4th of the volume required for the finished product.

During percolation, the top of the drug column should not become dry. The percolation is continued till the drug is completely exhausted. The rate of collection of percolate is generally 10-30 drops per minute.

6. The exhaustion of drug may be tested by doing the specified chemical test depending on the constituents present in the drug or absence of colour in the percolator or absence of bitter taste of percolate.

7. After exhaustion of the drug or after collecting the required quantity of the percolator, the marc is taken out from the percolator. It is pressed to recover the costly solvent.

8. The expressed liquid is mixed with the percolate and then the final volume is made by adding more of menstruum.

9. The preparation is filtered in order to free it from cell debris or other material which interferes with the clarity of the preparation.

Examples The following preparations are made by simple percolation process.

1. Tincture of belladonna
2. Compound tincture of cardamom
3. Strong tincture of ginger etc.

Percolation Processes for Concentrated Preparations

Percolation processes for concentrated preparations are used for preparing liquid extracts and solid extracts. The various processes used for the preparing concentrated preparations are:

(*a*) Reserve percolation process
(*b*) Modified percolation process

Reserve Percolation Process In this process, a part of the percolate, generally 3/4th the volume of the finished preparation, is reserved. Then the percolation process is continued till the drug is completely exhausted. The percolate is subjected to evaporation or distillation (to recover the costly menstruum) to convert it into a soft extract. This soft extract is dissolved in the reserve portion of percolate and then sufficient menstruum is added to produce the required volume.

The portion of the percolate which is reserved must be the first percolate because it is more concentrated. The portion of the percolate which is evaporated contained traces of active constituents of the drug. Hence, the major portion of the active constituents of the drug are saved from deterioration.

Modified Percolation Process In percolation process for preparation of tinctures, the drug/percolate (d/p) ratio is about 1 : 4. The d/p ratio is reduced to 1 : 3 by modifying the percolation process and hence there is a lot of saving in heat, time and menstruum.

Percolation is a displacement process. The strong solution of active constituents of drug formed during maceration is displaced by the fresh menstruum when percolation process is started. It is proved that stationary menstruum (menstruum remaining in contact with the drug) dissolves more matter than the flowing menstruum. Hence, more menstruum is required to exhaust the drug when simple percolation process is used. But if continuous percolation stage has suitable breaks by short maceration stages, the d/p ratio can be reduced to 1 : 3.

e.g. In Simple Percolation Process:

Drug (200 g) → Imbibition (for 4 hrs) → Maceration (for 24 hrs) → Percolation and collect the percolate, *i.e.* 3/4th of the volume of finished preparation.

In Modified Percolation Process:

Drug (1000 g) → Imbibition (for 4 hrs) → Maceration (for 24 hrs) → Percolation and collect 1000 ml of percolate

→ Maceration (for 12 hrs) → Percolation and collect 1000 ml of percolate

→ Maceration (for 12 hrs) → Percolation and collect 1000 ml of percolate

Drug : Percolate
1000 gm : 3000 ml
d/p = 1 : 3

Since d/p ratio is 1 : 3, test for exhaustion must be done. The process is continued in case the drug is not completely exhausted.

After exhaustion of the drug, the percolate is evaporated and then mixed with the main percolate. The final volume is made by adding more of menstruum.

Continuous Hot Percolation Process *or* Soxhlet Extraction or Soxhelation When active constituents of the drug are not freely soluble in the solvent or difficult to be displaced from the cells of the drug, then it becomes necessary to extract the crude drug by the action of hot menstruum for a considerable length of time. The fixed oils from seeds and alkaloids from the drug are extracted by continuous hot percolation process using benzene, chloroform, petroleum, ether *etc*.

Apparatus The apparatus used for continuous hot percolation process is soxhlet apparatus which consists of three parts:

A. Flask containing the boiling solvent.

B. Soxhlet Extractor in which the drug to be extracted is packed. It has a side tube which carries the vapours of the solvent from the flask to the condenser and a syphon tube which syphons over the extract from soxhlet extractor to the flask.

C. A condenser in which the vapours of the solvent are condensed again into solvent.

Procedure The drug to be extracted is packed in a paper cylinder made from a filter paper and it is placed in the body of soxhlet extractor. The solvent is placed in the flask. The apparatus is then fitted as shown in Fig. 9-2.

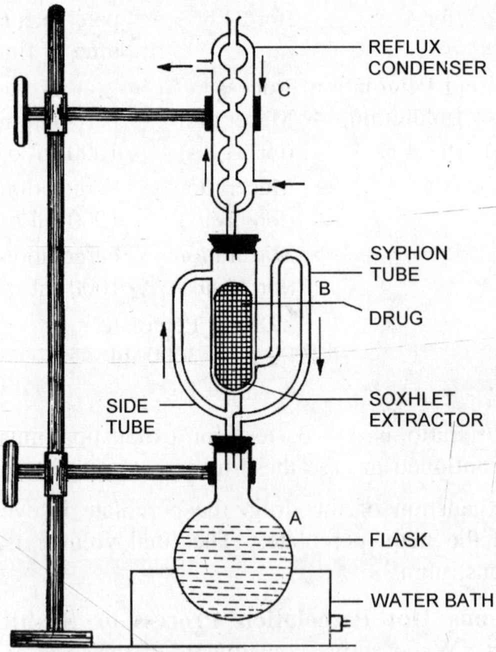

Fig. 9-2 Soxhlet apparatus

When solvent is boiled on heating the flask, it gets converted into vapours. These vapours enter into the condenser through the side tube and get condensed into hot liquid which falls on the column of the drug. When the extractor gets filled with the solvent, the level of syphon tube also raises up to its top. The solvent containing active constituents of the drug in the syphon tube syphon over and run into the flask, thus emptying the body of extractor. This alternation of filling and emptying the body of extractor goes on continuously. The soluble active constituents of the drug remain in the flask while the solvent is repeatedly volatilised. The process of filling and emptying of the extractor is repeated until the drug is exhausted. Normally the process is repeated about 15 times for complete exhaustion of the drug.

Limitation of Continuous Hot Percolation Process The continuous hot percolation process cannot be used in following cases.

1. *Physical character of the drug* : The physical character of the drug is such that it would block the soxhlet apparatus in case it is used for its extraction by this method *e.g.* opium, gum, resin, orange peel etc.
2. *Solvent* : Only pure solvents or constant boiling mixtures can be used for this process.
3. *Chemical constituents of the drug* : The process is unsuitable for drugs having thermolabile active constituents such as enzymes, alkaloids, anthraquinone derivatives, esters etc.

Digestion ▪

In digestion process, the drug is extracted by heating at a particular pressure. This will increase the penetration power of the menstruum, so that there is complete extraction of the drug. Precautions should be taken so that the increased temperature may not harm the active constituents of the drug.

The apparatus know as "Digestor" is used for extraction of the drug by this method. It is a vessel made up of metal. The whole of the drug along with the menstruum is placed in the body of the digestor. Place the cover over it and bolt it with the help of nuts. The drug is treated with menstruum for a definite period under specified conditions of temperature and pressure.

Factors Affecting Choice of Extraction Process ▪

The final choice of the process to be used for the extraction of a drug will depend on a number of factors which are as follows:

1. Character of drug : The knowledge of pharmacognosy of the drug is essential to select the right method of extraction process. The maceration process is used when the drug is soft, unorganised unpowderable and to avoid powdering of it. The percolation process is used when the drug is hard and tough.

2. Therapeutic value of the drug : When the drug has considerable therapeutic value, the maximum extraction is required, so the percolation process is used e.g. Belladonna. In case the drug has little therapeutic value, the efficiency of extraction is unimportant, and maceration process can be used to extract the drug.

3. Cost of drug : The costly drugs are extracted by using the percolation process, whereas cheap drugs are extracted by maceration process.

4. Stability of drug : Continuous hot extraction process should be avoided when the constituents of the drug are thermolabile in nature. In that case maceration or percolation process may be used to extract the active constituents of the drug.

5. Solvent : If water is used as a solvent the maceration process should be recommended. The percolation process should be preferred if non-aqueous solvents are used for extraction. If the desired active constituents of drug demand a solvent other than a pure boiling solvent or an azeotrope, continuous hot extraction process should be avoided and reserve percolation process may be used.

6. Concentration of product : The dilute products such as tinctures can be made by using maceration or percolation process, depending on the other factors. For semi-concentrated preparations, such as concentrated infusions, double or triple maceration process can be used. The liquid extracts or dry extracts which are concentrated preparations are prepared by using percolation process.

▩ INTRODUCTION TO AYURVEDIC DOSAGE FORM ▩

Ayurvedic system of medication is the most ancient method of treatment for all types of ailments. In Ayurvedic systems, the crude drugs, metals, minerals, ghee, oil and stones *etc*. are used as medicine in various forms. The following are some of the common ayurvedic dosage forms which are used in this system.

I. Liquid Dosage Forms

1. Kwaths (क्वाथ) : It is also a decoction and is generally prepared by boiling one part of vegetable substance or drug (roots, woods, barks and leaves of fresh plant) in coarse powder or cut or sliced into small pieces with 8 or 16 parts of water in earthen pot till the whole is reduced to 1/4th or 1/8th or 1/16th quantity of water. Kwath should be prepared a fresh every day.

2. Araks (अर्क) : These are distilled essences or liquors made by soaking drugs in water for 24-48 hours and then distilling the same. The distillate collected is called 'Araks'. Arkas are just like aromatic waters prepared by distillation used in allopathic system of medicine. Araks are used in fever, dyspepsia and as cooling lotion when it is applied externally.

3. Arishtas (आरिष्ट) : These are weak alcoholic preparations prepared by making a decoction of the drugs and then allowing them to undergo fermentation by the help of raw sugar or honey. The fermentation is done for a period of 7-10 days in hot weather and for 15-30 days in cold weather. e.g. Dashmularishta, Ashokarishta

4. Asavas (आसव) : These are medicated alcoholic liquors prepared by the fermentation of raw vegetable juices with honey or jaggery or treacle. The various parts of the plant such as roots, leaves and barks etc. are cut into pieces and infusion is prepared in water in air-tight earthen jars. Honey or treacle is mixed in it. The fermentation is done for at least six months.

The asavas are prepared by the fermentation of infusion of the drugs, whereas aristas are prepared by the fermentation of decoction of the drugs. Asāvas are used as stomachic, stimulants, tonics and astringents etc. e.g. Kumariasva, Chandanasva, Madhukasava.

5. Kanjika (काञ्जिका) : It is a sour liquid produced from the fermentation of powdered paddy (*Brassica juncea*) and other grains. It is a clear transparent fluid with an acid taste and vinous smell. It is cooling, useful as a drink in fever and burning of the body *etc*.

6. Kshirpaka (क्षीरपाक) : It is a decoction in milk which is prepared by boiling one part of drug in 8 parts of milk and 32 parts of water till the milk alone remains. The decoction is then strained.

7. Swarasas (स्वरस) : These are fresh expressed juices prepared by crushing green fresh medicinal plants in a mortar and expressed. Strained through a clean muslin cloth. eg. Tulsi swarasa

8. Hima (हिमा) : It is a cold infusion. One part of the drug is put in 6 part of cold water and kept overnight in an earthern pot. Next day the drug is taken and macerated well and filtered through a clean cloth. The preparation thus prepared is called hima kalpana.

9. Phanta (फन्टा) : It is hot infusion. The coarse powder of a drug is put into hot water, rubbed and filtered with a cloth. The preparation is not very potent.

10. Paniyas (पानीय) : These are weak forms of decoction prepared by boiling one part of medicinal substances in 32 or 64 parts of water, till water is reduced to half the quantity, strained and given to appease thirst.

11. Peya (पेया) : It is a decoction which is prepared by boiling one part of a cereal in 14 parts of water till it becomes thicker than that of Manda.

12. Manda (मण्ड) : It is a decoction which is prepared in 14 parts of water and one part of cereal, usually rice.

13. Tailas (तैल) : These are medicated oils which are prepared by boiling drugs in water, milk or other liquid substances mixed with oil until water content is evaporated. The oils thus prepared are generally meant for local applications. In some cases, the oils are used internally. e.g. Bhringaraja Tailas, Maha Naryan Tailas, Dhanvantra Tailas

II. Semisolid Dosage Forms

1. Avalehas (अव्हेल) : These are thick extracts of the drugs. The decoction of the drug is prepared and after straining it is again boiled down to a thick soft consistency with sugar or honey. In case sugar is used in the preparation, the quantity used should be four times that of the drugs, whereas in case of jaggery, its quantity should be twice that of the drugs. Avalehas are used for digestive troubles, respiratory problems and as a general tonic. e.g. Kushmanda Avaleha, Draksavaleha, chyavanprasha

2. Kalkas (कल्क) : It is a paste which is prepared by grinding dry or fresh whole vegetable substances, moistened with water on a flat stone or slab with a muller. It is then mixed with honey, ghee or oil which should be double the quantity of the drug. In case sugar or jaggery is to be mixed, its proportion should be the same as that of the drug. e.g. Nimba Kalka.

3. Ghan (घन) : It is a semi-solid preparation, prepared by evaporation of the quaths to semisolid consistency. Ghans are meant for converting quaths to tablets or pills.

4. Ghritas (घृता) : These are medicated ghees or clarified butter. The ghrita or clarified butter is heated on a fire to remove water. A little turmeric juice is then added to purify it. The purified ghrita is melted with a gentle heat in earthen pot, copper or iron pan and then mixed with the medicinal paste and decoctions of medicines to be used. It is then boiled with gritas till the water content gets evaporated and it is free from the froth. It is then strained through cloth and preserved for use. It is meant for internal use.

5. Pakas (पाक) : These are jelly like soft preparations of drugs for internal use, made into paste or solid mass with sugar, milk or honey. The thin paste is also called Avaleha (linctus) and the semi-solid mass is called Paka. So pakas are of two kinds, liquids and solids.

6. Murambas (मुरब्बा) : These are preparations of drugs or fruits made by soaking them in syrup or honey.

7. Malamas (मलहम) : These are called ointments. These are semi-solid or soft preparations meant for local application for various lesions. Malamas are prepared by mixing drugs with ghee, vaseline, bees wax and coconut oil etc.

8. Rasakriya (रसकृया) : In this semi sold preparation, the swarasa is extracted, boiled down to thick consistency so as to obtain semisolid preparation known as Rasakriya. It is used mainly for the bitter drugs, so it will be easier for consumption and the dosage of the drug can be minimized e.g. Daruharidra Rasakriya.

III. Solid Dosage Forms

1. Anjan (अंजन) : These are medicated fine powder intended to be used in eyes for their local effect. To relieve pain, especially in the head, 'anjans' are recommended in Ayurveda.

2. Bhasmas (भस्म) : These are ashes which are prepared from vegetable and mineral substances. The vegetable drugs are cut into a coarse powder or pieces and then burnt till they are completely reduced to ashes. The mineral ashes are prepared from metals. The metals are first subjected to purification by treatment with oil, fat free curd and cow's urine. The purified mass is oxidised and then subjected to a process of roasting. The roasted mass is reduced to a fine powder. Ashes are also prepared from various animal products such as hart's horn, pearls and cowries etc. e.g. Swaran Bhasma, Shnakha Bhasma, Loha Bhasma

3. Churnas (चुर्ण) : These are powdered mixtures prepared by mixing dry mineral, animal or vegetable substances in a pestle mortar. The powdered mixture is then passed through cloth, linen or fine sieve. In case jaggery is to be mixed with powder, it should be equal to the quantity of churan and in case of sugar, it should be double the quantity of churan. Churnas are usually taken with milk, hot water and cow's urine. Churnas are usually given in bulk. Its action is quick but its effect is only temporary. e.g. Triphala Churna, Sudarshan Churna and Ashwagandhadi Churna.

4. Rasas (रस) : These are preparations of metals containing mercury in any form. These preparations contain various kinds of poisons. They are made into pills and tablets so as to fix the proportion of the dose. Rasas are generally taken with kvath, milk or water and sometimes with honey, ghee or both. These are prepared either by Kharleya or Kupi pakva method.

5. Gutikas (गुटिका) : These are large pills. These are prepared from the pill mass. The pill mass is prepared by reducing a decoction of vegetable substances to a thick consistency and then mixed with powdered medicines, raw sugar, honey, gum, guggal *etc.* The pill mass is then converted into pill pipes and finally converted into gutikas. e.g. Bilvadi Gutikas

6. Pisty (पिष्टी) : It is prepared by mixing various stones with the rose arak or kavera arak till it is converted into a fine powder. It is considered to be better than Bhasams of stones.

7. Vatikas (वटी) : These are small pills which are prepared in the same way as gutikas. e.g. Triphalavati.

8. Varti (वर्टि) : These are called suppositories. These are meant for rectal use. Anjan varti are used for application of drug in the eye. Vaginal varti are also prepared for vagina. e.g. Gudavarti.

9. Ksharas (क्षार) : Medicinal plants or herbs or specified parts of them are wholly or completely burnt and their ashes are allowed to dissolve or mix in water. It is filtered and then evaporated to a fine white residue, which is called Kshar. This is very effective preparation used in liver and spleen ailments.

Note : Asavas, Aristas, Avalehas, Kvaths, Ghirtas, Tailas are regular preparations of crude drugs containing a different strength of active principles of the drug.

▪ REVISION QUESTIONS ▪

I. Very short answer type questions ▪

Answer the following in brief.

1. Define the term "Extraction".
2. Name the various processes used in the extraction of crude drugs.

3. Give a list of galenicals which are prepared by extraction.
4. What are the different types of maceration process?
5. Why is stirring of the drug required during maceration and infusion processes?
6. Why is the marc pressed in certain extraction processes?
7. Why is the marc not pressed in the maceration process for unorganised drugs?
8. Name the various steps of simple percolation process.
9. What are the drugs which cannot be extracted by soxhelation process?
10. What are the advantages of water as a solvent?

II. Short answer type questions

11. Give the advantages and disadvantages of alcohol as a menstruum.
12. Why water is preferred as a menstruum in various extraction processes?
13. Why is a short period of maceration required before the actual percolation
14. Which type of drugs cannot be extracted by soxhelation process?
15. Why is boiling water commonly used as a solvent in infusion process?
16. What are the advantages and disadvantages of water as a solvent?
17. Give the advantages and disadvantages of alcohol as a solvent.
18. How will you test the exhaustion of the drug in the percolation process?
19. Why imbibition is necessary before packing of the drug into the percolator?
20. What are the various steps in packing of a drug in a percolator?
21. Why volume is not made up in simple maceration process?
22. Why multiple maceration process is needed in certain preparations?
23. Why is maceration done in a covered vessel?
24. Mention the various limitations of continuous hot percolation process.
25. Write in brief about modified percolation process.
26. Describe briefly the "Reserve percolation process" of extraction.

III. Long answer type questions

27. Describe in detail the simple maceration process for extraction.
28. What is "Multiple Maceration"? Write its merits and demerits.
29. Explain in detail about maceration with adjustment. How does it differ from simple maceration process?
30. Describe the simple percolation process which is used in the preparation of tinctures.
31. Explain in detail about continuous hot percolation process with a neat diagram of soxhlet apparatus. What are the limitations of this process?
32. Write in detail about modified percolation process.
33. Define the term "Extraction". What are the factors which affects the choice of extraction process?
34. Why imbibition is necessary before packing of the drug in a percolation? Write in brief about percolation processes for concentrated preparations.
35. Write in brief about common ayurvedic dosage forms.
36. Differentiate between the following:
    (*a*) Infusion and Decoction
    (*b*) Infusion and Maceration
    (*c*) Double Maceration and Triple Maceration
    (*d*) Simple Maceration and Multiple Maceration
    (*e*) Maceration process for organised drugs and unorganised drugs.
37. Write short notes on:
    (*a*) Infusion (*b*) Decoction
    (*c*) Maceration (*d*) Percolation
    (*e*) Reserve percolation process (*f*) Soxhelation
    (*g*) Multiple Maceration process (*h*) Digestion
38. Describe in brief:
    (*a*) Asavasa (*b*) Avalehas
    (*c*) Bhasmas (*d*) Kvaths
    (*e*) Rasas (*f*) Gutikas
    (*g*) Aristas

IV. Objective type questions

A. Completion type questions (Fill in the blanks with suitable word/words)

39. Alcohol in the conc. of __________ is used as ________ in multiple maceration process.

40. One volume of conc. infusion when diluted with ________ volume of water resembles the corresponding fresh infusion in __________.

41. The process of extraction in which the drug is kept in contact with menstruum for 15 minutes is called ________.

42. Simple maceration is done in a covered vessel for _____ days to prevent _________ of menstruum which is mostly _________ in nature.

43. In double maceration process, the whole of the drug is macerated for ________ with a part of menstruum and then it is macerated again for _________ with the remaining menstruum.

44. In soxhelation process _______ solvent or ____________ mixtures are used.

45. When a drug is extracted by heating at a particular pressure the process is called _________.

B. Matching type questions.

46. Match the items of *Column I* with appropriate terms in *Column II.*

Column I	*Column II*
A. Concentrated infusions	(*i*) unsuitable for drugs having thermolabile active constituents.
B. Multiple maceration process	(*ii*) for preparation of tinctures from organised drugs.
C. Soxhelation process	(*iii*) the drug is boiled with solvent.
D. Decoction	(*iv*) prepared by double or triple maceration
E. Simple maceration process	(*v*) used for preparation of conc. preparation
F. Compound tincture of benzoin	(*vi*) prepared by simple maceration
G. Tincture of orange	(*vii*) conc. of alcohol is 20-25%
H. Double maceration	(*viii*) prepared by maceration process for unorganised drug

KEY

39. 20-25%, menstruum.
40. Seven, potency.
41. Infusion.
42. Seven, evaporation, volatile.
43. 48 hours, 24 hours.
44. pure, constant boiling mixtures.
45. Digestion.
46. *A*(*iv*); *B*(*v*); *C*(*i*); *D*(*iii*); *E*(*ii*); *F*(*viii*); *G*(*vi*); *H*(*vii*).

10

Heat Processes

Heat is the form of energy which is used in processes like fusion, ignition, boiling, desiccation, exsiccation, evaporation, distillation, sublimation, freeze drying etc.

Heat may be generated by burning of solids, liquids, gaseous substances, fuels or by using the heating effect of an electric current.

Heat may be transferred from the source of heat to the articles or from one place to another place by any one of the following methods:

(*i*) *Conduction* : In this method, the heat energy transfer takes place by transmission of momentum of individual molecules. Heat transfer in solids and liquids takes place by this method.

(*ii*) *Convection* : In this method, the heat transfer takes place by the actual motion of the particles *i.e.* during the process of mixing. Heat transfer in liquids takes places by this method.

(*iii*) *Radiation* : In this method, the energy transfer takes place through space *i.e.* without using any medium. The heat of the sun reaches the earth by this method.

Heating is done either by direct heating or by indirect heating. In direct heating the material is placed in a vessel and heated by the direct source of heat. In case of indirect heating the apparatus like water bath, steam bath sand bath, acid bath and glycerin bath are used to heat the vessel containing the material.

DESICCATION

Desiccation is the process of complete removal of mechanically admixed water from substances.

Apparatus used for laboratory scale Desiccator is used for this purpose. It is a closed glass vessel. A suitable dehydrating agent, such as concentrated sulphuric acid, phosphorous trioxide, phosphorous pentaoxide, anhydrous calcium chloride, anhydrous lime or dried silica gel is placed at the lower part of the desiccator. The china-dish having the material to be desiccated is placed on the perforated plate which is held in place by its projected arms. The desiccator is closed with a cover which has ground edges and is usually greased to ensure an air tight joint. Some desiccators are provided with a ground glass stopcock in an outlet which may be attached to the vacuum pump to evacuate the air. This results in acceleration of the process of desiccation.

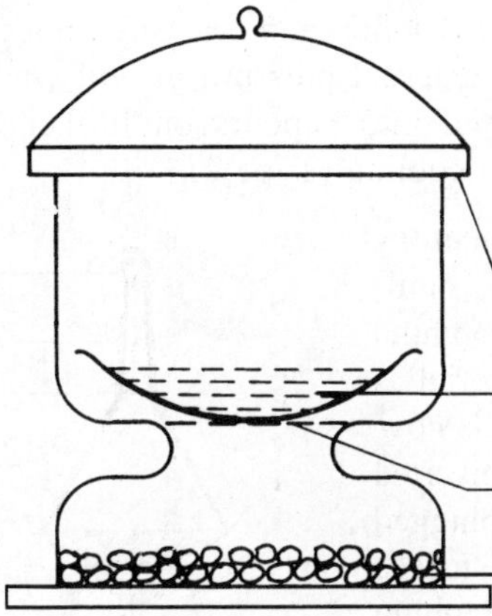

Fig. 10-1 Desiccator

Applications

1. It helps in the size reduction of crude drugs. The presence of water in the crude drugs has a greater elasticity and cannot be powdered properly. As such, for powdering the drug it is first dried.
2. It reduces bulk and weight of drugs and hence increases the potency of a medicinal substance. Moreover, it reduces the cost of transportation and storage.
3. It helps in the preservation of vegetable and animal drugs. Presence of moisture causes decomposition of drugs due to bacterial growth and hence desiccation helps in its preservation.

SUBLIMATION

It is the process in which a solid gets converted into vapours without the formation of a liquid and on cooling, the vapours get converted into solid. The product obtained after sublimation is called "Sublimate".

Theory When a solid is heated it is converted either directly into vapours or first gets converted into liquid and then on further heating it form vapours.

Solid ⟶ Vapour ⟶ Solid (Type 1)

Solid ⟶ Liquid ⟶ Vapour ⟶ Liquid ⟶ Solid (Type 2)

The difference between the above two types is due to pressure. If a solid can at some temperature exert a vapour pressure equal to the external pressure, it will on heating to this point pass direct to vapour and reverse changes will occur on cooling the vapour *i.e.* "True Sublimation" (Type 1) will occur. If a solid cannot at any temperature exert a vapour pressure equal to the external pressure, it will when heated first liquefy and then get converted into vapours on further heating. The reverse changes will occur on cooling (Type 2).

Apparatus used for laboratory scale On a laboratory scale, sublimation can be done by using a china dish and a funnel. The material is placed in a china dish which is covered with a funnel, placed in inverted position. The funnel stem is plugged with cotton-wool. The outer surface of the funnel is cooled by wrapping it with cotton wool soaked in cold water. The china dish is heated over a sand bath and the vapours are condensed in a funnel.

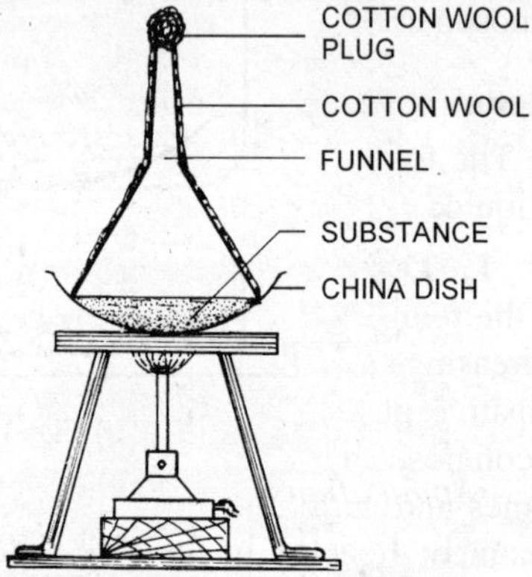

Fig. 10-2 Sublimation process

Applications

1. Various chemicals are purified by sublimation in pharmacy *e.g.* iodine sublimed sulphur, menthol, mercuric chloride, camphor, benzoic acid, ammonium chloride naphthalene etc.
2. It is also used for separating sublimating substances from non-sublimating substances.

Types of Sublimates ■

Depending upon the physical character, there are three types of sublimed substances which are as under:

1. Cake sublimate : This occurs when there is a very little difference in the condensing surface and the sublimating point of the volatile substance *e.g.* mercuric chloride and ammonium carbonate.

2. Powder sublimate : This occurs when there is much difference in the heating and cooling chamber and the sublimate will condense more rapidly in the form of small particles *e.g.* sulphur.

3. Crystalline sublimate : Some substances sublime in crystalline form and the size of crystal depends upon the condition of condensation *e.g.* benzoic acid, iodine, naphthalene, menthol etc.

EVAPORATION

Evaporation means a free escape of vapour from the surface of a liquid below its boiling point *i.e.* evaporation can take place even at room temperature. The vapours formed exert a pressure known as vapour pressure which varies with the temperature. The vapour pressure is maximum at the boiling point of liquid because vapours are formed throughout the liquid. The vapour pressure of a liquid is equal to the atmospheric pressure at its boiling point.

Factors Affecting Evaporation

The following are the factors which affect the rate of evaporation of a liquid:

1. Temperature : The rate of evaporation is directly proportional to the temperature of the liquid. The evaporation can be accelerated by increasing the temperature but it will cause decomposition of heat sensitive principles of many drugs. Many glycosides and alkaloids are decomposed at a temperature below 100°C. Hormones, vitamins, enzymes and antibiotics being more heat-sensitive materials, needs special treatment in order to avoid decomposition *e.g.* Malt extract is concentrated by evaporation under their reduced pressure to avoid loss of enzyme.

2. Temperature and time of evaporation : It has been observed that exposure to a relatively high temperature for a short period of time may be less harmful to the active principles of a drug than a lower temperature with exposure for a longer period. On the basis of this fact, liquid is exposed to high temperature for a short period in film evaporator.

3. Temperature and moisture content : Some drug constituents decompose more readily in the presence of moisture if heated at a high temperature. This is due to the hydrolysis of the active constituents.

To avoid decomposition of the active principles of such materials the evaporation is done at a low temperature and then the final drying is done at a high temperature when only little moisture remains in it.

4. Types of product required : On evaporation of the liquid the concentrated liquid, semisolid and solid are formed. The selection of the method and the equipment required for evaporation depends upon the type of the product required.

5. Effect of concentration : During evaporation the upper layer of the liquid under evaporation has a tendency to form a film and formation of precipitate in the product which results in lowering down of the rate of evaporation. Therefore, efficient stirring is required in order to prevent degradation of the product at the bottom due to excessive heat and it will also prevent deposition of solids.

6. Surface area : The rate of evaporation is directly proportional to the surface area of the evaporator, in which the liquid is evaporated. The larger the surface area of the evaporator, the shorter is the time it takes to evaporate the liquid.

7. Vapour pressure of the liquid to be evaporated : The rate of evaporation is directly proportional to the vapour pressure of the evaporating liquid. The liquid has the maximum vapour pressure at its boiling point. As such the rate of evaporation can be increased by raising the temperature of the evaporating liquid. The rate of evaporation of liquid is the maximum at its boiling point.

EVAPORATORS

The equipment used in the process of evaporation are called evaporators. The evaporators are divided into three groups.

1. Natural circulation evaporators
2. Forced circulation evaporators
3. Film evaporators

Natural Circulation Evaporators

The evaporators in which the movement of the liquid takes places as a result of convection current set up by the heating process, are called natural circulation evaporators *e.g.* evaporating pans, evaporating still and short tube evaporators.

Evaporating pans It consists of a hemispherical pan made from copper or stainless steel and surrounded by steam jacket. The hemispherical shape provides a large surface area for evaporation. The evaporating pans may be fixed or made to tilt.

In case the evaporating pan is fixed, the emptying of the pan is done from the product outlet. In other cases the evaporators are mounted in such a way that they can be tilted to remove the product. The evaporating pans are heated by steam which passes through a steam jacket.

Advantages

1. It is the simplest equipment for the purpose of evaporation of the liquid.

2. It is an economical evaporator.
3. It is easy to clean, use and maintain.

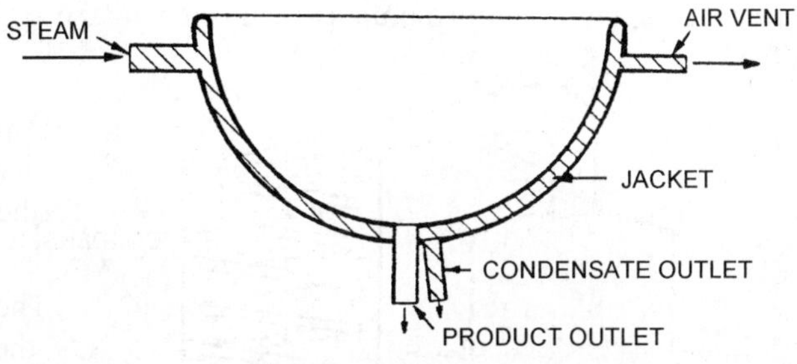

Fig. 10-3 Evaporating pan

Disadvantages

1. Due to natural circulation of the product, the coefficient of the heat transfer is poor and solids get deposited which causes the decomposition of the product.
2. The heating surface is limited and decreases proportionally to increase in size of the pan.
3. It is not suitable for concentration of thermolabile materials because the liquid is heated all throughout in an open atmosphere. Further there is no provision to evaporate under a reduced pressure.
4. The evaporating pan cannot be used for the evaporation of thermolabile pharmaceutical materials which are dissolved in an organic solvent, such as, ethyl alcohol, as there is no provision to recollect the costly organic solvent.
5. The evaporating pan is an open one and the vapours can pass direct to the atmosphere which may lead to saturation of the atmosphere with vapours. This in turn may cause discomfort to the worker. It may also slow down the process of evaporation.

Evaporating still This type of evaporator is commonly known as a "Still" because the evaporating pan is covered and is connected to a condenser so that the vapours are condensed into the liquid. As shown in Fig. 10-4 there is a vessel similar to the evaporating pan with a cover that connects it to the condenser, so that the liquid is distilled off.

Advantages

1. It is simple in construction.
2. It is easy to clean and maintain.

3. The vapours are condensed in it. It increases the speed of evaporation and the costly solvent can be recovered *e.g.* ethyl alcohol.
4. There can be a provision for evaporation under a reduced pressure in case the vacuum pump is connected to the evaporating still.

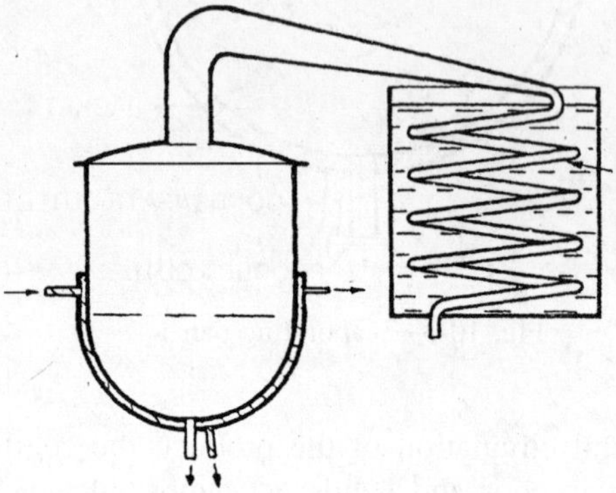

Fig. 10-4 Evaporating still

Disadvantages

1. The heating surface is limited.
2. The evaporating still is not suitable for the thermolabile materials as the liquor is heated all the time in it.
3. Due to natural circulation, the coefficient of the heat transfer is poor.

Short tube evaporator It consists of a number of tubes which are from 1 to 2 metres in length and from 40-80 mm in diameter. About 1000 tubes are fitted in a vessel upto 2.5 metres or more in diameter. This part of the evaporator is called "Calandria". The tubes are filled with liquid and surrounded by steam. The level of the liquid is maintained slightly above the top of the tubes so that the space which is left in the evaporator can be used for the purpose of separation of vapour from the boiling liquid.

The liquid in the tubes is heated by steam and it begins to boil. The mixture of the liquid and vapour will come out of the tube which sets up a circulation with boiling liquid rising up in the smaller tubes of calandria and returning down the large central down take.

Advantages

1. The heating area is increased by using a tubular calandria.
2. The coefficient of the heat transfer is 3-5 times more as compared to the evaporating pan.

3. The condenser and receiver can be attached to the evaporator in order to recover the costly solvent.

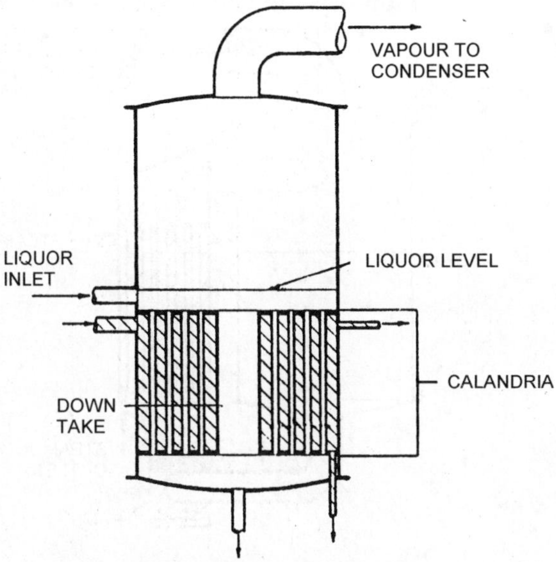

Fig. 10-5 Short tube evaporator

Disadvantages

1. It is quite complicated and hence it is expensive to construct it.
2. It is difficult to clean it.
3. The maintenance of the evaporator is quite costly.

Forced Circulation Evaporators

In these types of evaporators, some mechanical device is fitted to circulate the contents heating in it *e.g.* an evaporating pan in which the material is agitated by a stirring rod or by a mechanical propeller.

As shown in Fig. 10-6, the liquid is circulated by means of a pump and as it is under pressure in the tubes the boiling point is raised and no boiling takes places. As the liquid leaves the tubes and enters the body of the evaporator, there is a drop in pressure and vapour gets removed from the super heated liquid.

Advantages

1. The rapid liquid movement improves heat transfer.
2. The evaporator is useful for the evaporation of the viscous liquids or materials that deposit solids or foam readily.

3. The rapid evaporation rate makes this evaporator useful for concentration of thermolabile materials under a reduced pressure *e.g.* concentration of insulin and liver extract.

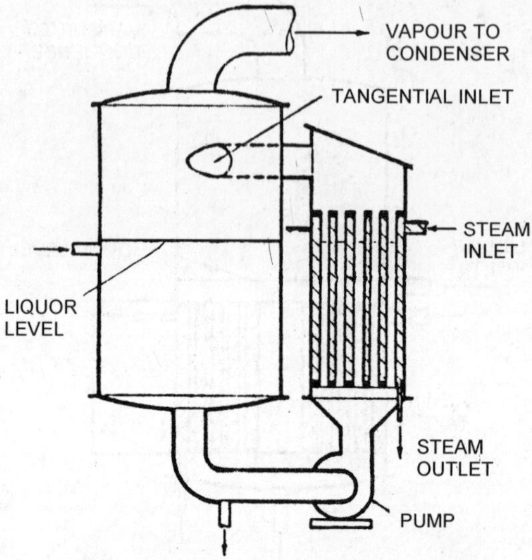

Fig. 10-6 Forced circulation evaporator

Film Evaporators

In film evaporators, the material is spread as a film on the heated surface to provide a large evaporated surface. There are two types of film evaporators.

1. Climbing film evaporators
2. Horizontal film evaporators

Climbing film evaporators In these evaporators, a large number of vertical tubes about 7 metres in length and 50 mm in diameter are enclosed in an outer jacket to which steam is supplied. Thus the tubes are heated externally. The pre-heated feed liquid is admitted at the base. Here it boils and the vapours formed take the liquid up the tube at a velocity of about 6-7 metres/second. At the top the mixed vapour and the concentrated liquid are ejected at a considerable speed into a separator. The separator allows the vapour to escape from the top and the concentrated liquid is collected at the bottom. The liquid takes only a few seconds to travel the length of the tube, so the evaporator is very suitable for heat-sensitive substances. Sometimes a number of units are fitted in a group to effect fuel economy by using the hot vapours produced in one unit to heat the subsequent unit and so on.

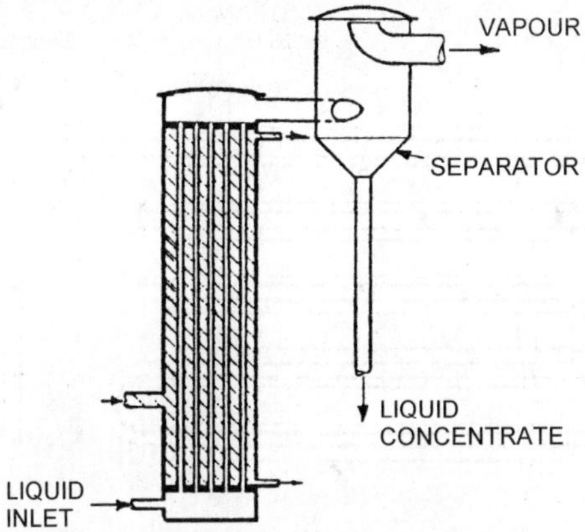

Fig. 10-7 Climbing film evaporator

Advantages

1. The use of long narrow tubes provides a large area for heat transfer.
2. The time of the contact between the liquid and the heating surface is very short. So, it is most suitable for the concentration of a liquid containing the thermolabile materials.
3. The evaporation rate is very high inspite of a short heating time.
4. There is no elevation of boiling point, although the tubes are very long.
5. The method is suitable for materials which produce foam.

Disadvantages

1. It is quite an expensive evaporator.
2. It is difficult to clean and maintain it.
3. It is difficult to maintain at proper feed rate. If it is too high, the proper concentration will not be made, on the other hand if the feed rate is too low, the film cannot be maintained.

Horizontal film evaporator In this type of evaporator, several parallel 8 feet long tubes are joined together in series. Each tube is enclosed in the opposite direction to the feed liquid in the inner tube. The liquid passes through the tubes, gets evaporated as it moves along the tube and finally passes to a separator. The concentrated liquid is collected at the bottom while the vapour is led off to the atmosphere or used for some heating purpose. It is usually employed in a single unit, so that it can be operated under a reduced pressure.

The viscosity, density and surface tension of the liquid being evaporated influences its viscosity through the tube. So it is not practicable to

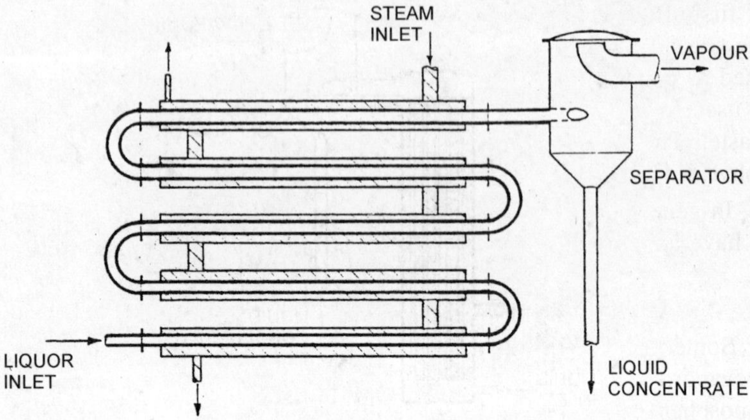

Fig. 10-8 Horizontal film evaporator

concentrate liquid with a high viscosity by using a climbing film evaporator. In such cases a "Falling film evaporator" may be used. It resembles the climbing film evaporator but is inverted so that the feed liquid enters the top of the tubes and the concentrate as well as vapour leave from the bottom.

MULTIPLE EFFECT EVAPORATION

In single effect evaporators, steam is used to heat the liquid which provides the latent heat of vaporisation. The vapours are condensed in the condenser, where the latent heat is given up to the cooling water and it goes to waste. To avoid this wastage, two evaporators are connected together with a piping arrangement so that the vapour from the calandria

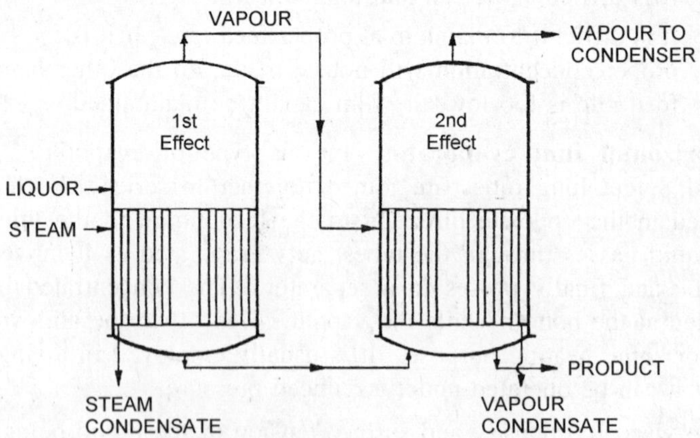

Fig. 10-9 Multiple effect evaporation

of first effect (which is heated by steam) is used to heat the calandria of the second effect. This means that the calandria of the second effect is used as condenser for the first effect, so that latent heat of vaporisation is used to evaporate more quantity of the liquid instead of its going as waste. The vapour from the second effect then taken to a condenser and converted into liquid.

In general, not more than two or three effects are combined together to have an economical and efficient evaporation of liquids.

EVAPORATION UNDER REDUCED PRESSURE

Sometimes the solutions containing heat-sensitive drugs get destroyed if evaporation is done at the boiling point of the solution under normal atmospheric pressure. The liquid boils when its vapour pressure is equal to the pressure of the surrounding atmosphere. If the pressure in an evaporator is reduced the aqueous liquid will boil at a temperature below 100°C. Table 10-1 indicates the relationship between pressure and boiling point of water.

TABLE 10-1

S.No.	*Pressure (bars)*	*Boiling point of water (°C)*
1.	1	100
2.	0.7	90
3.	0.47	80
4.	0.31	70
5.	0.12	50
6.	0.10	45
7.	0.07	40
8.	0.03	25

The evaporation under a reduced pressure should be done with care because there is a danger of overheating of the liquid. There is an increase in the viscosity of the liquid as the external pressure is reduced. The boundary layer thickness will increase which causes difficulties in heat transfer and hence there is a risk of overheating.

Advantages of evaporation under reduced pressure

1. The evaporation occurs at a low temperature which prevents damage to heat-sensitive materials.
2. The evaporation occurs at a low temperature which gives a higher temperature gradients without the need for excessive steam pressures.

REVISION QUESTIONS

I. Very short answer type questions

Answer the following questions in brief.

1. Define the term "heat".
2. How the heat is transferred?
3. What does the term "desiccation mean"?
4. Define the term "sublimation".
5. What are different types of sublimates?
6. Define the term "evaporation".
7. What are the different types of evaporators used in pharmacy?
8. Name the factors which affect the rate of evaporation of a liquid.

II. Short answer type questions

9. Explain how heat is transferred from the source to the articles.
10. Write the applications of desiccation in pharmacy.
11. What are the various types of sublimates prepared by sublimation?
12. What are the applications of sublimation process in pharmacy?
13. Write the advantages of multiple effect evaporators.
14. Write the advantages and disadvantages of an evaporating pan.
15. How will you differentiate between natural circulation evaporators and forced circulation evaporators?

III. Long answer type questions

16. Define the term "Evaporation". Describe the various factors which affect the rate of evaporation of liquid.
17. Explain the term "Sublimation". How sublimation is done in laboratory? What are different types of sublimates? Write its application in pharmacy.
18. Classify the different types of evaporators. Explain with the help of a neat sketch the working of a film evaporator.
19. Explain with the help of a neat sketch one of the evaporators covered under the group of natural circulation evaporators.
20. What are the different types of film evaporators? What are the advantages and disadvantages of climbing film evaporators?
21. Write Short notes on:
    (a) Sublimation (b) Desiccation
    (c) Evaporating pan (d) Climbing film evaporator
    (e) Horizontal film evaporator (f) Multiple effect evaporation

IV. Objective type questions

A. Completion type questions (Fill in the blanks with suitable word/words).

22. The sublimation process reduces _______ and _______ of the drugs and hence increases the potency.
23. The transfer of heat in a solid and a liquid takes place by __________method.
24. Desiccation is the process of complete removal of ________ water from substances.
25. The liquid boils when its __________is equal to to the atmospheric pressure.
26. The rate of evaporation is ________ to the surface area of the evaporator.
27. In film evaporators the material is spread as _______ on the heating surface to provide a large ___________.

B. Matching type questions.

28. Match the items of *Column I* with appropriate items in *Column II*

Column I	Column II
A. Heat of the sun reaches the earth	(*i*) convection
B. The rate of evaporation is directly proportional	(*ii*) increase in surface area
C. The efficiency of film evaporators	(*iii*) use of a tubular calandria
D. Heat transfer in liquid takes place by	(*iv*) radiation
E. The heating area is increased	(*v*) temperature
F. In forced circulation evaporators	(*vi*) mechanical device is fitted to circulate the heating liquid

KEY

22. Bulk, weight
23. Conduction
24. Mechanically admixed
25. Vapour pressure
26. Directly proportional
27. Film; evaporated surface
28. *A*(*iv*); *B*(*v*); *C*(*ii*); *D*(*i*); *E*(*iii*); *F*(*vi*).

11

Distillation

Distillation is the process of converting liquid into its vapours by heating and reconverting it again into liquid by condensing the vapours. It is a method of separating substances which differ in their vapour pressures.

The distillation process is carried out in an apparatus which consists of:

(*a*) Still, in which volatile material is boiled.

(*b*) Condenser, in which vapours are condensed.

(*c*) Receiver, in which distillate is collected.

TYPES OF DISTILLATION PROCESSES

The following are the various types of distillations:

1. Simple distillation
2. Distillation under reduced pressure
3. Fractional distillation
4. Steam distillation
5. Destructive distillation

1. Simple Distillation

It is a process of converting a liquid into its vapour in a distillation still, transferring the vapour to another place and condensing it again into liquid.

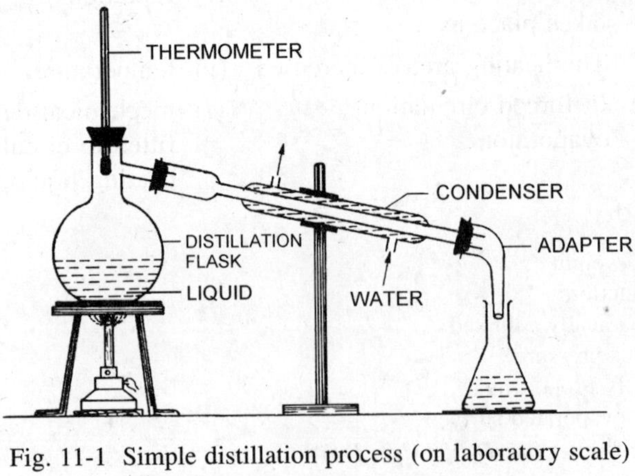

Fig. 11-1 Simple distillation process (on laboratory scale)

Apparatus used for laboratory scale It consists of a distillation flask with a side arm sloping downward which is connected to a condenser. The condensed vapours are collected in a flask called 'receiver'. The whole apparatus is made of glass (*see* Fig. 11-1).

The distillation flask should be of such a size that it can contain half to two-thirds of the liquid to be distilled. The thermometer is fitted in the distillation flask to note down the temperature, at which the vapours are distilled. Bumping is avoided by adding small pieces of porcelain or porous pot before distillation.

Applications of simple distillation in pharmacy

1. It is used for the preparation of distilled water and water for injection.
2. Many volatile oils and aromatic waters are prepared by simple distillation.
3. Organic solvents are purified by distillation.
4. Many official compounds are prepared by distillation *e.g.* Spirit of nitrous ether and Aromatic spirit of ammonia.
5. Concentration of liquid and to separate non-volatile solid from volatile liquids such as alcohol and ether.

2. Distillation Under Reduced Pressure ▪

Theory Liquid boils when its vapour pressure is equal to the atmospheric pressure. The boiling point of the liquid may be lowered to the desired temperature by reducing the pressure on its surface.

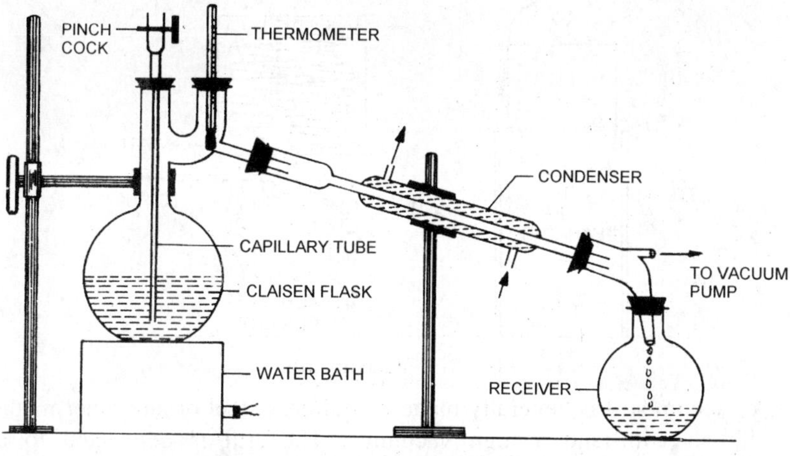

Fig. 11-2 Distillation under reduced pressure (on laboratory scale)

Apparatus used for laboratory scale It consists of a double-neck distillation flask known as "claisen flask". In one of its necks a thermometer is fitted and in the second neck a capillary tube is fitted which prevents bumping of the heated liquid. The capillary tube should be so fine as to permit only a slow stream of bubble which can be controlled with a pinch cock. Thick walled glass apparatus with inter-changeable standard glass joints are used for vacuum distillation. The claisen flask is connected to a receiver through condenser. Vacuum pump is attached to the receiver to attain the desired degree of vacuum. Heating of claisen flask is not started until the desired vacuum has been attained.

Applications in pharmacy

1. It is used for the concentration of extracts containing thermolabile (constituents which are sensitive to heat) in order to prevent their destruction.
2. It is used for separating substances which undergo decomposition when heated under normal atmospheric pressure.
3. It is used for obtaining a light porous mass on distillation of the liquid extract.

▪ VACUUM STILL ▪

The vacuum stills are employed for distilling substances under reduced pressure on a large scale. A typical vacuum still is shown in Fig. 11-3.

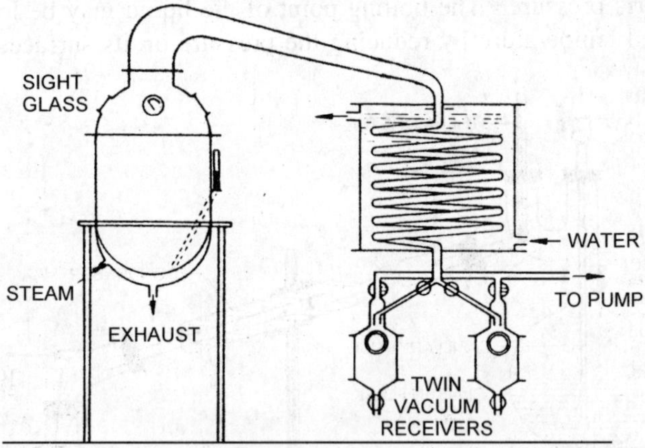

Fig. 11-3 Vacuum still

A vacuum still is generally made of stainless steel or any other metal which can withstand a high vacuum. The still is connected to a condenser. The vacuum is created by means of a vacuum pump. The vacuum still is filled by attaching a pipe to a tap in the lower part of the hood and the pump is started. The other end of the pipe dips into the liquid to be distilled so that it can be drawn into the still. An observation window in the hood is very helpful to the operator to see the progress of distillation and also the level of the content of the liquid to be distilled. Two receivers are generally attached to the condenser in order to collect the distillate without stopping distillation. However, they may be used alternately by a suitable arrangement of the cocks.

Applications in pharmacy

1. Distillation of substances that have a high boiling point at atmospheric pressure.
2. Distillation of thermolabile substances that get damaged by a high temperature.
3. Removal of the last traces of a volatile solvent.

3. Fractional Distillation (Distillation of miscible liquids)

Theory When a substance is dissolved in a liquid, the vapour pressure of the liquid is lowered. When two miscible liquids are mixed together, each will act as solute or solvent for the other. So, when a mixture of two such liquids is heated, the vapour pressure of each is lowered. The pressure exerted by each liquid in the mixture is known as "partial pressure". The liquid boils when the sum of the partial pressures is equal to the atmospheric pressure. The vapours arising from two miscible liquids at boiling point is richer in the component exerting the greater partial pressure.

Apparatus used for laboratory scale The apparatus used for laboratory scale is as shown in Fig. 11-4. Fractionating column is fitted between the distillation flask and the condenser. Fractionating column is used for continuous separation of two miscible liquids. Long fractionating column is used in the mixture where the boiling point is quite close to each other and short fractionating column is used in those cases where there is a considerable difference in the boiling point of the mixture of miscible liquids.

In fractional distillation, the mixture of miscible liquids is heated in the still. The vapours formed are allowed to pass through the fractionating column, where a part of the vapour is condensed and while returning to the still comes into an intimate contact with the rising vapour resulting in further fractionation of the liquid being distilled. The liquid with higher boiling point is condensed first and vapour becomes richer with the liquid having the lower boiling point which gets condensed in a condenser.

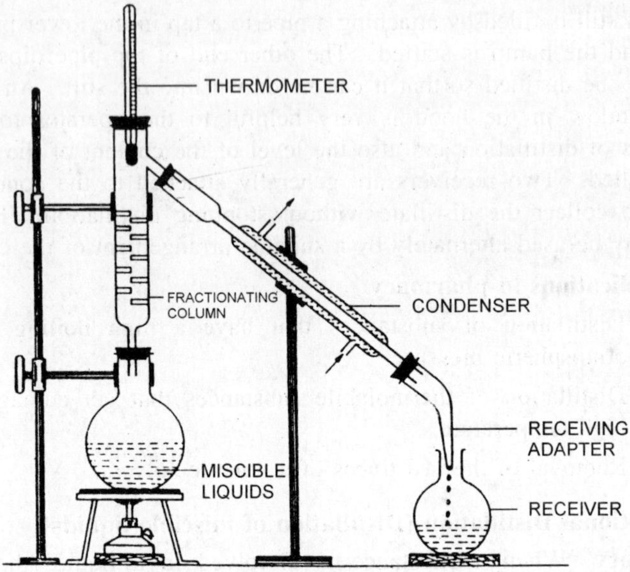

Fig.11-4 Fractional distillation (on laboratory scale)

Applications in pharmacy

1. Alcohol is purified from the mixture of alcohol and water obtained from fermentation tank.
2. It is used for the separation of miscible liquids, such as, alcohol and water, acetone and water, chloroform and benzene.

4. Steam Distillation (Distillation of two immiscible liquids)

Theory When two immiscible liquids are heated together, then the mixture boils when the sum of the vapour pressure equals to the atmospheric pressure. The temperature at which mixture boils is lower than that of either of the liquids *i.e.* the boiling point of the mixture is lower than that of the liquid with the lower boiling point. The temperature at which the mixture boils remains stationary until one of the liquids has been completely removed from the still.

Apparatus used for laboratory scale It consists of a "Steam Can" fitted with a cork having two holes. Through one of the holes passes a bent tube leading the steam to the flask containing the non-aqueous liquid. This tube should reach almost to the bottom of the flask. Another long tube which passes through the other hole reaches almost to the bottom of the steam can. This tube acts as a safety tube, so that in case the pressure inside the steam can becomes too much, it is relieved by forcing water out of it. Moreover, when steam starts coming out from the safety tube, it indicates that the steam can is almost empty. The delivery tube carrying vapours from the flask is connected to the condenser to convert it into liquid which gets collected in the receiver.

The non-aqueous liquid is placed in the flask. A small quantity of water is added to it. The steam can and the flask are heated simultaneously, so that a uniform flow of steam passes through the boiling mixture.

Distillation is continued until all the non-aqueous liquid has distilled over. The distillate is then collected in florentine receiver where oil is completely separated from water.

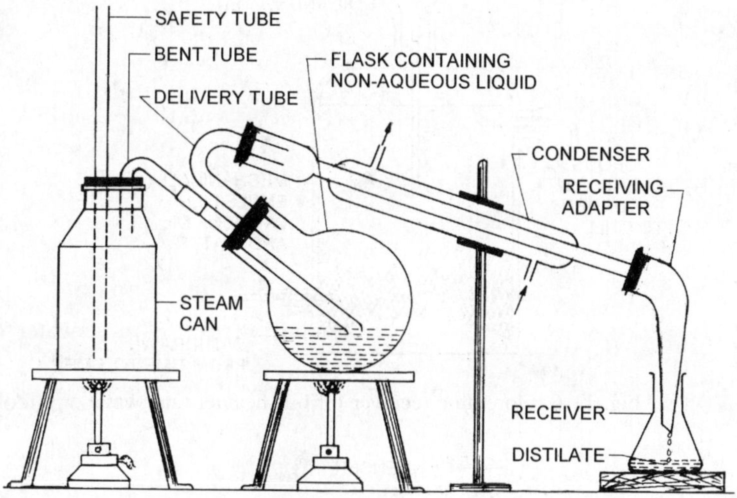

Fig. 11-5 Steam distillation (on laboratory scale)

Applications in pharmacy

1. It is used for the preparation of volatile oils.
2. It is used to determine the percentage of volatile oil in the drug.
3. It is used for the distillation of volatile oil for its purification without any decomposition.

FLORENTINE RECEIVERS

It is used for the separation of oil and water. Florentine receivers are of two types:

Type I : used for separation of oil heavier than water.

Type II : used for separation of oil lighter than water.

The receiver used for oil heavier than water has two taps (Fig. 11-6). The tap fitted near the bottom of vessel is used for collecting oil, whereas the tap fitted near the top of the vessel is used for water to overflow.

The receiver used for oil lighter than water is fitted with syphon at the bottom which works when it gets filled with water (Fig. 11-7) whereas the tap fitted near the top is an outlet for the flow of oil.

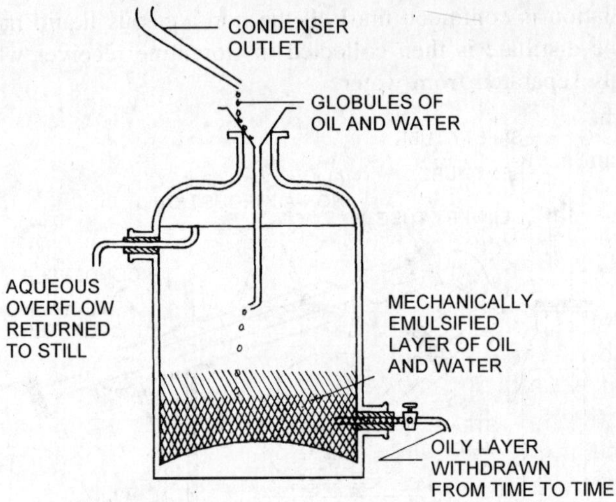

Fig. 11-6 Florentine receiver for oils heavier than water

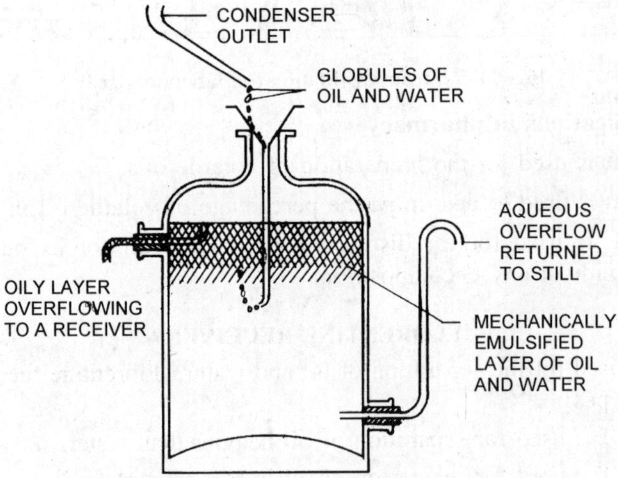

Fig. 11-7 Florentine receiver for oils lighter than water

5. Destructive Distillation

This is also known as Dry Distillation. The dried organic matter is heated in the absence of air, in a suitable apparatus, until all the volatile substances are driven off and the residue is left behind. The residue is subjected to carbonisation. Destructive distillation is mainly used in industry for obtaining many valuable products from wood and coal.

Destructive distillation of wood gives acetone, menthol, cresol, wood tar etc. while charcoal remains in the still. Destructive distillation of coal gives burning gases the ammonia, and the coke remains in the still. Destructive distillation of animal bones gives ammonia, amines and hydrocarbons.

Ichthammol is prepared by the destructive distillation of fish fossils.

PURIFIED WATER I.P.

Water which is free from volatile and non-volatile impurities is called purified water. It is prepared by distillation, ion-exchange treatment, reverse osmosis or any other suitable process. It contains no added substances and meets the requirements for chemical purity specified for it. It is liable to get contaminated by micro-organisms, hence purified water should not be used in preparations meant for parenteral administration. It should be stored in tightly closed containers.

WATER FOR INJECTION I.P.

Water which is free from volatile and non-volatile impurities, micro-organisms and pyrogens is called "Water for Injection". It is obtained by distilling potable water, purified water or distilled water from a neutral glass or suitable metal still fitted with an efficient device for preventing the water drops to go along with water vapours into the condenser. The first portion of the distillate is rejected which contains volatile impurities. The remainder is collected in suitable containers, previously rinsed with freshly distilled water and closed so as to avoid contamination. It contains no added substances. Water for injection must meet the purity requirements stated under purified water. It need not be sterile but it should comply with the test for pyrogen. Water for injection is stored in tightly-closed neutral glass containers.

STERILE WATER FOR INJECTION I.P.

It is water for injection which is sterilised and suitably packed. It contains no anti-microbial agent or other added substances. It has pH between 4.5 and 7.5. It must comply with the tests for sterility. It should also comply with the requirements of the tests for carbon dioxide, chloride, sulphate, nitrates and nitrites, ammonium, calcium and heavy metals. It must comply with the test for pyrogens.

Sterile water for injection should be stored in single-dose containers not larger than of one litre in size.

Preparation of Purified Water I.P. and Water for Injections I.P. by Distillation The potable water is used for the preparation of purified water. It contains—

(*i*) Dissolved gases such as carbon-dioxide and ammonia
(*ii*) Dissolved salts and solids

This can be avoid by taking the following precautions:

1. By heating the feed water. This removes the dissolved gases. The solubility of gases decreases as the temperature is raised. For the purpose of economy the water feeding the boiler should be passed through the condenser jacket for heating the water.

2. A constant level device is attached to the boiler to avoid excessive concentration of salts. Inspite of this, some of the solids will be deposited and it becomes necessary to de-scale the boiler after a certain period.

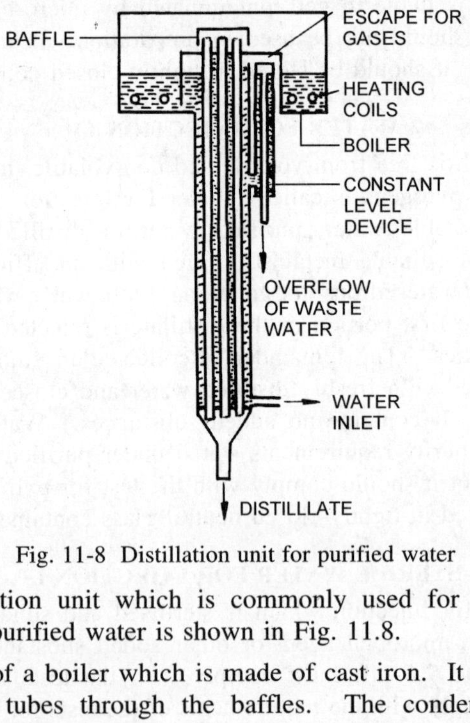

Fig. 11-8 Distillation unit for purified water

The distillation unit which is commonly used for the continuous production of purified water is shown in Fig. 11.8.

It consists of a boiler which is made of cast iron. It is connected to the condenser tubes through the baffles. The condenser tubes and baffles are made of stainless steel. Baffles are provided over the top of the condenser tubes to avoid water drops getting mixed with the vapours. It is done to avoid carry-over of pyrogen and other water soluble materials in the droplet. The cooling water enters at the bottom of the condenser and is heated by the condensing vapours. The flow rate is adjusted in such a way that water gets heated at 90°-95°C before it enters the boiler. The top of the condenser jacket is open, so that gases from the water can escape into the atmosphere.

A constant level device is fitted in such a way that only the heated water free from gases enters the boiler.

■ REVISION QUESTIONS ■

I. Very short answer type questions ■

Answer the following questions briefly.

1. Define the term "Distillation".
2. What are the different types of distillation?
3. How will you separate two immiscible liquids?
4. How is bumping avoided in distillation process?
5. How is oil and water separated?
6. Define the term "Fractional distillation".
7. What is purified water?
8. Why purified water is not used in preparing parenteral products?
9. What is "Water for Injection"?
10. Name the dissolved gases which is present in water.

II. Short answer type questions ■

11. Write the applications of simple distillation in pharmacy.
12. What is theory of distillation under reduced pressure?
13. Differentiate between purified water and water for injection.
14. Explain the theory of fractional distillation.
15. Explain the theory of steam distillation
16. Write the applications of steam distillation
17. Write in brief about florentine receiver.
18. Give a brief account of destructive distillation.
19. Write the applications of fractional distillation.

III. Long answer type questions

20. Define "distillation". What are different types of distillation? Write in detail about distillation under reduced pressure.
21. What do you mean by steam distillation? Explain with a neat sketch the working of the apparatus used for the distillation on a laboratory scale. Mention its applications in pharmacy.
22. How will you separate two immiscible liquids in pharmacy? Draw a labelled sketch of the apparatus used in the laboratory. Give its applications in pharmacy.
23. Differentiate between purified water and water for injection. How purified water is prepared in the laboratory?
24. Write short notes on the following:-
    (a) Fractional distillation
    (b) Steam distillation
    (c) Vacuum still
    (d) Florentine receiver
    (e) Destructive distillation

IV. Objective type questions

A. Completion type questions

25. Liquids which decompose at or below their boiling point are purified by__________.
26. Fractional distillation is used for the separation of two ______________liquids.
27. Long fractionating column is used in separating miscible liquids where the __________ to each other.
28. Steam distillation is used for the separation of two __________ liquids.
29. Sterile water for injection has pH between ______________ to ________________ and must comply with the test for ________________.
30. The ______________ of the liquid may be __________ to desired _________ by reducing the pressure on its surface.
31. When a substance is dissolved in a liquid, the vapour pressure of the liquid is _________.
32. The vacuum still is used or distilling substances __________ on a large scale.

KEY

3. Steam distillation
4. Small pieces of porcelain
8. contaminated by micro-organism
10. carbondioxide and Ammonia
25. Distillation under reduced pressure.
26. Miscible
27. Boiling point is very close.
28. Miscible
29. 4.5 to 7.5, sterility
30. Boiling point, lowered, temperature
31. Lowered
32. under reduced pressure.

12

Introduction to Drying Processes

"Drying" is an important technique used in the pharmaceutical industry. Proper drying can prevent deterioration of the product and it also improves the solubility of the product. In majority of the cases, drying operations are used to remove liquid or moisture from the solid substances. Thus "drying is defined as the final removal of liquid from solids by vaporisation with the aid of heat." The equipment used for drying is called a "dryer".

There are various nonthermal methods which also help in drying. For example, the expression of a solid to remove liquid, the extraction of liquid from a solid by the use of a solvent, the adsorption of water from a solvent with the help of desiccants such as, anhydrous calcium chloride, the absorption of moisture from gases by passage through a sulphuric acid column and by the process of desiccation.

Theory of drying Drying involves both heat and mass transfer operations. To dry a material, two steps are needed *viz.*:

(*a*) Heat must be supplied to provide latent heat of vaporisation.
(*b*) The liberated vapour must be removed by moving an air stream.

The theory of drying can be understood more easily by keeping in mind the fact that a film of liquid is formed at the surface of the material being dried. The rate of evaporation of this film is related to the rate of heat transfer, as per the equation (1) given below:

$$\frac{dw}{d\theta} = \frac{q}{\lambda} \tag{1}$$

where $dw/d\theta$ = the rate of evaporation pounds of water per hour
q = overall rate of heat transfer (BTU per hour)
λ = latent heat of vaporisation of water (BTU per hour)

The rate of diffusion of moisture into the air stream is expressed by the rate equations, similar to those for heat transfer. The driving force is a humidity differential, whereas heat transfer is a temperature differential. Thus equation (1) can be written as:

$$\frac{dw}{d\theta} = K'A(H_s - H_g) \qquad (2)$$

where $dw/d\theta$ = the rate of diffusion expressed as pounds of water per hour

K' = the coefficient of mass transfer [pounds of water/(hour) (square foot) (absolute humidity difference)]

A = area of the evaporating surface in square feet

H_s = the absolute humidity at the evaporating surface (pounds of water per pound of dry air)

H_g = the absolute humidity in the passing air stream (pounds of water per pound of dry air)

The coefficient of mass transfer K' is not a constant but it varies with the velocity of the air stream passing over the evaporating surface, thus:

$$K' = cG^n \qquad (3)$$

where c = a proportionality constant

G = the rate of flow of air [pounds of dry air/(hour) (square foot)]

n = a fractional exponent usually about 0.8[2]

After a certain period, the rate of evaporation is equal to the rate of diffusion of vapour. The rate of heat transfer can be equated with the rate of mass transfer *i.e.* equation (1) can be equated with equation (2) *i.e.*

$$\frac{dw}{d\theta} = \frac{q}{\lambda}$$

$$= K'.A.(H_s - H_g) \qquad (4).$$

If the overall rate of heat transfer (q) is expressed as the sum of the rates of heat transfer by convection, radiation and conduction, then equation (4) can be written as:

$$\frac{dw}{d\theta} = \frac{(q_c + q_r + q_k)}{\lambda}$$

$$= K'.A.(H_s - H_g) \qquad (5)$$

where q_c = the rate of heat transfer by convection

q_r = the rate of heat transfer by radiation

q_k = the rate of heat transfer by conduction

The rate of drying may be accelerated by increasing any of the individual terms in equation (5).

The rate of convection heat transfer (q_c) can be increased by increasing the air flow rate and by raising the inlet air flow rate. The rate of radiation heat transfer (q_r) can be increased by introducing a high temperature radiating heat source into the drying chamber. The rate of conduction heat transfer (q_k) can also be speeded up by reducing the thickness of the material being dried and by allowing it to come in contact with raised-temperature surfaces. The rate of drying can be increased by increasing the coefficient of mass transfer (K'). This is done by increasing the air velocity. By dehumidifying the inlet air, there is an increase in humidity differential ($H_s - H_g$) which speeds up the rate of drying.

Applications of Drying

1. In the pharmaceutical industry it is used as a unit process in the manufacture of granules which can be dispensed in bulk or converted into tablets or capsules.
2. Drying can also be used to reduce the bulk and weight of the material, thereby lowering the cost of transportation and storage.
3. It helps in the preservation of crude drugs of plant from mould growth, which occurs due to presence of moisture.
4. It helps in the size reduction of crude drugs. The presence of moisture in the crude drug does not allow it to get powdered easily.
5. Drying is also used in the processing of materials *e.g.* the preparation of dried aluminium hydroxide, the spray drying of lactose and in the preparation of solid extracts.

■ EQUIPMENT USED IN DRYING PROCESSES ■

The equipment used for drying are known as "Dryers". The following are some of the different types of dryers in common use in the pharmaceutical industry:

1. Tray dryers
2. Tunnel dryers
3. Rotary dryers
4. Fluidised-bed dryers
5. Vacuum dryers
6. Freeze dryers.

Tray Dryer ■

The simplest form of dryer in this category is a cabinet with a heater at the bottom *e.g.* "Laboratory Oven". These ovens are of very little value because there is no control of heat transfer or humidity. If a fan is fitted to the oven, the forced hot air is circulated which helps in increasing the heat transfer and also in reducing the local vapour concentrations. Despite this there is no adequate control.

The best type of a tray dryer is that of the directed circulation form, in which air is heated and is directed across the material in a controlled flow. The material to be dried is spread on tiers of the trays. The trays used have solid, perforated, or wire mesh bottoms. The screen trays are lined with paper so that air circulates across rather than through the drying material. The paper is used as a disposable tray liner to reduce cleaning time and also to prevent contamination of the product.

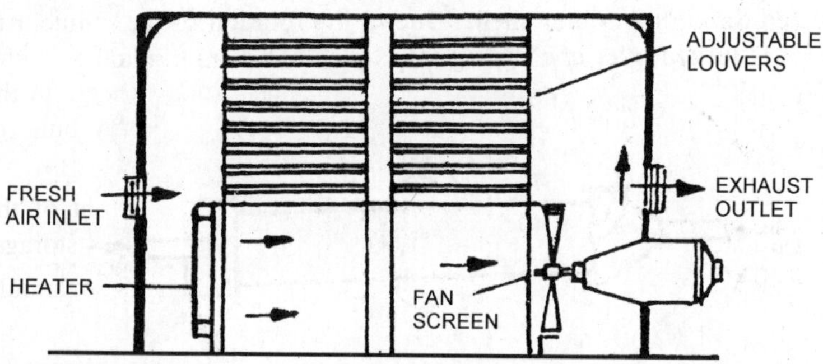

Fig. 12-1 Tray dryer

In modern tray dryers, a uniform temperature and air flow is maintained by the use of a well-insulated cabinet with strategically placed fans and heating coils. As shown in Fig. 12-1, there is an alternate arrangement of the shelves so that air can flow uniformly without any obstruction (as indicated by the arrows). Heater is fixed in such a way that the air is re-heated before passing over each shelf. When the air passes over each shelf a certain amount of heat is given up to provide latent heat of vaporisation. In such type of dryers there can be a good control of heat and humidity provided it is designed correctly.

Uses Tray dryers are used for drying of crude drugs, chemicals, powders and granules used in tablet manufacturing.

Tunnel Dryer

A tunnel dryer is a modification of the tray dryer in which the oven is replaced by a tunnel which receives damp material at one end and discharges the dried product at the other end. It may be operated batchwise or continuously. The tunnel dryers can be of any size and the movement of solid material can be effected by placing it on trays on rails and at suitable intervals a tray may be pushed into the inlet which displaces the tray from the dry end. The conveyor belt system can also be used to pass the material through the tunnel.

Rotary Dryer ■

Rotary dryer is a modified form of the tunnel dryer in which the material is passed through a rotating cylinder, counter current to the stream of heated air. It consists of a cylindrical shell (about 10 m in length) which is mounted with a slight slope, so that the material fed in at one end will move through it on its slow rotation at about 10 revolutions per minute. Heating of the cylindrical shell is done directly by passing hot air current or indirectly by steam tubes or heated gases circulated through an outer shell. Due to the rotation of the cylinder the material is turned over and drying takes place from individual particles.

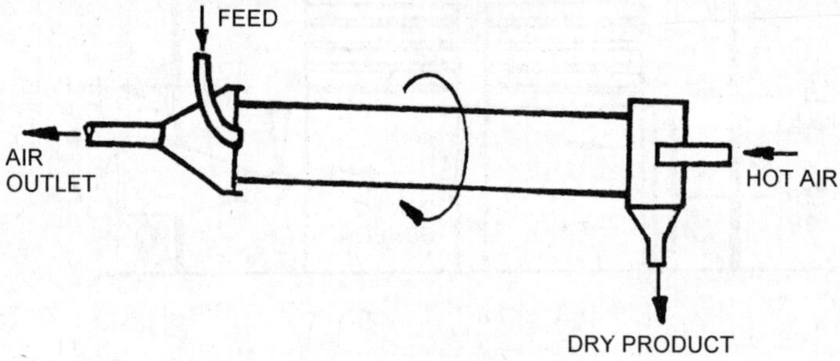

Fig. 12-2 Rotary dryer

Uses The rotary dryer is used for the purpose of drying any powdered or granular solid. On a large scale operation, rotary dryers are used for continuous drying.

Fluidised Bed Dryer ■

In a fluidised bed dryer, good contact between hot air and particles to be dried is obtained which causes rapid drying.

Theory If a gas is allowed to flow upward through a bed of solid particles at a velocity greater than the settling velocity of the particles, the particles are partially suspended in the gas stream. The resultant mixture of solids and gas behaves like a liquid and the solids are said to be fluidised. Each individual solid particle is surrounded by the drying gas with the result that drying takes place in a much shorter period. Moreover the intense mixing between the solids and hot gas provides a uniform condition of temperature, composition and particle size distribution.

Two types of fluidised bed dryers are used in the pharmaceutical industry. There are:

1. Vertical fluidised bed dryers
2. Horizontal fluidised bed dryers

A typical vertical fluidised bed dryer is shown in Fig. 12-3. The fluidising air stream is induced by a fan which is mounted in the upper part of the dryer. The air is heated to the required temperature in air heaters and passed through the wet material contained in a drying chamber fitted with a wire mesh support at the bottom. The air flow rate is adjusted by means of re-circulation control and fabric filter bags are provided to prevent the passage of fine particles. This type of fluidised bed dryer is a batch type dryer and the drying chamber is removed from the unit for charging and dumping. The fluidised bed dryers are available in different capacities ranging from 5 kg to 200 kg with an average drying time of about 20-40 minutes.

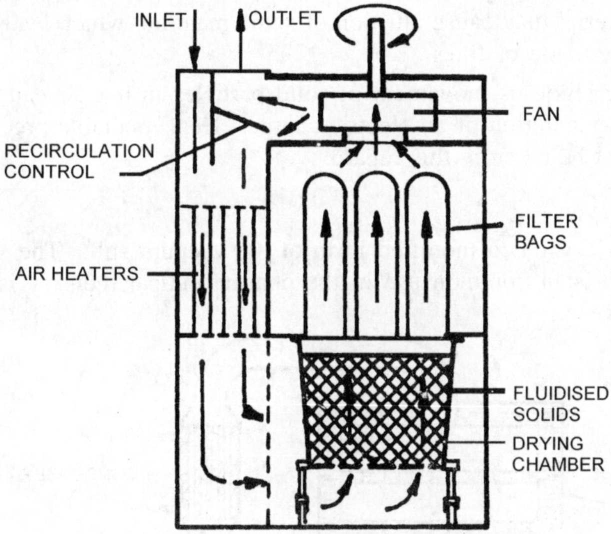

Fig. 12-3 Fluidised bed dryer

Horizontal vibrating conveyer fluidised bed dryers are used for continuous drying of a large volume of the material.

Advantages of Fluidised Bed Dryer

1. It gives a high drying rate. The fluidised bed dryer method is 15 times faster than the routine method of a tray dryer.
2. The method is suitable for drying of thermolabile materials because heating time is minimised.
3. In a fluidised bed dryer, drying takes place from individual particles and not from the entire bed. As such most of the

drying takes place at a constant rate and there is less danger of overheating.

4. The temperature inside the fluidised bed dryer can be controlled. Moreover the temperature is uniform.
5. The free movement of individual particles prevents the risk of soluble materials migrating which may occurs in static beds.
6. The fluidised bed dryer has a high output and occupies a small floor space.
7. It can be used for drying any powdered material but it is mostly used for drying of granules meant for the manufacture of tablets.

Disadvantages of Fluidised Bed Dryers

1. The turbulence produced when hot air is passed through the material may cause attrition of some material, which leads to the production of fines.
2. The vigorous movement of solid particles in hot air can lead to the generation of an electric charge. Hence suitable precautions must be taken in this regard.

Vacuum Dryer

Vacuum dryer is a modified form of the vacuum still. The vacuum dryer which is in common use in the pharmaceutical industry is called "vacuum oven".

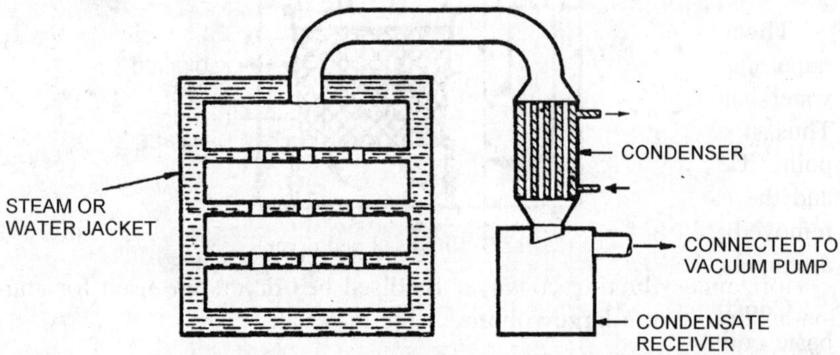

Fig. 12-4 Vacuum dryer

It consists of a jacketed vessel made of a material which can withstand vacuum within the oven and steam pressure in the jacket. The oven can be closed by a door that can be locked tightly to provide an air-tight seal. The oven is connected to a vacuum pump through a condenser and a receiver. Generally, vacuum oven is operated at the pressure of about 0.03 to 0.06 bar. At this pressure water boils at 25-35°C. In the pharmaceutical industry an oven of the size of about 1.5 m cubes having 20 shelves is commonly used.

Nowadays, the vacuum ovens with a number of small compartments with small doors are available rather than one big compartment with a heavy door.

Advantages of Vacuum Dryer

1. The dryer is useful for drying of heat sensitive materials because drying takes place at a low temperature.
2. A porous and soft dry extract is produced when a liquid extract is dried in a vacuum dryer.
3. The valuable solvent can be recovered from the extract, when it is dried in a vacuum dryer as solvent vapours are condensed in the condenser.

Disadvantages of Vacuum Dryers

1. The labour and running costs are rather high.
2. The vacuum dryer is of limited capacity.
3. Heat transfer coefficients are low.

Freeze Dryer ■

In the freeze drying process, there is removal of water vapours from a frozen solution by sublimation. Therefore it is also called sublimation drying process or lyophilisation.

Theory In this process, the material is frozen in a suitable container connected to a high vacuum system, so that the vapour pressure of water vapours is reduced to less than that of the material being dried. Thus, it reduces the temperature and pressure to values below the triple point. Under these conditions, any heat transferred is used as latent heat and the ice sublimes directly to the vapour state. The water vapour is removed from the system by condensation in a condenser maintained at a temperature lower than a frozen material.

Construction Freeze dryers are composed of the following four basic components:

1. A chamber for vacuum drying
2. A vacuum source
3. A heat source
4. A vapour-removal system as vacuum pump or steam ejector or both

The chamber of vacuum drying is generally designed for batch operation but by using special inlet and outlet mechanisms, continuous drying operation can be achieved. It consists of shelves for keeping the material.

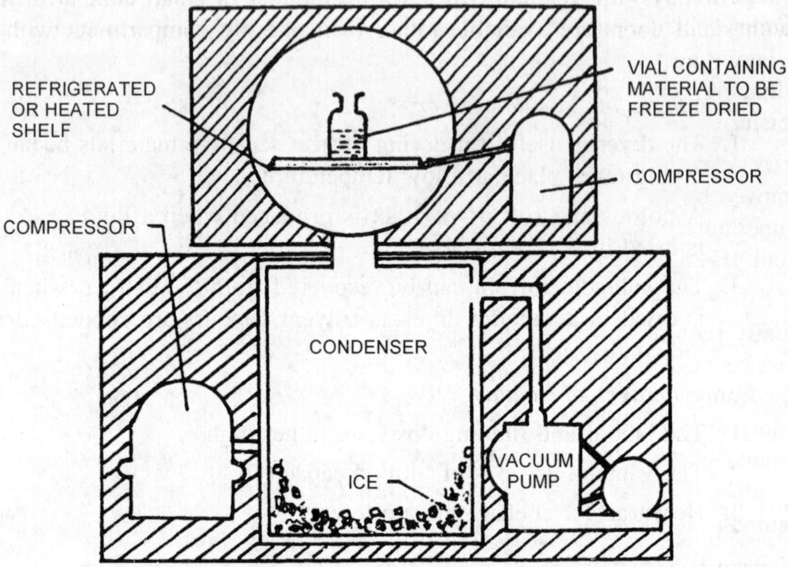

Fig. 12-5 Essential components of a freeze-drying system

The rate of drying is increased by keeping the distance between subliming surface and condenser much less than the mean path of molecules. The condenser consists of a relatively large surface cooled by solid carbon dioxide mixed with acetone or ethanol. The temperature of the condenser must be much lower than the evaporated surface of freezed substance. This condition can be maintained by cleaning the condenser surface repeatedly.

Heat is provided by conduction or radiation or both. Vacuum is achieved by vacuum pump or steam ejector or a combination of the two.

Working The working of freeze dryer involves the following steps:

(i) *Pre-treatment* : This step is done to reduce the volume of the solution to be introduced into the container which has limited capacity. The solution is pre-concentraed under normal vacuum tray drying. Sometimes solid or liquid desiccants are also used for this purpose. This reduces the actual drying by 8-10 times.

(ii) *Pre-freezing* : This is done to solidify water. The ampoules, vials and bottles in which aqueous solution is packed, are frozen in cold shelves at a temperature below –50°C.

(iii) *Primary drying* : The material to be dried is spread in order to increase the surface area for sublimation. The temperature and pressure is kept below the triple point of water (0.0098 °C and 4.58 mm of mercury) for the sublimation of water. Heat is supplied which transfers as latent heat and ice sublimes directly into vapour state which are ultimately removed. Primary drying help to remove about 98-99 % moisture.

(iv) *Secondary drying* : The moisture left in the primary drying is removed by an ordinary vacuum drying. The vacuum drying is done at a temperature of 50°-60°C. The rate of drying is very slow and its takes about 10-20 hours.

(v) *Packing* : The biological products dried by freeze drying are usually required to be in a sterile condition for injection. So attention must be paid to packaging of freeze dried products to ensure protection from moisture. The containers should be closed under the controlled atmospheric condition and also observing aseptic conditions. The ampoules are sealed immediately after drying, whereas the vials and bottles are closed as such or after replacement of vacuum by inert gas, if required. The containers are labelled and packed in card-board boxes.

Advantage of Freeze Drying Process

1. The product obtained is light and porous having excellent solubility.
2. The chances of hydrolysis is minimised as drying takes place at a very low temperature.
3. Drying takes place under vacuum; hence, oxidation is minimised as there is no contact with air.
4. The heat sensitive materials can be dried.
5. The loss of volatile material is minimum.
6. The freeze dried material can be stored at room temperature if properly sealed in an inert atmosphere.
7. The sterility of the product can be maintained.

Disadvantages of Freeze Drying Process

1. The process is very expensive because a complicated plant is used.
2. The product obtained by freeze drying process is very hygroscopic. So packaging requires special precautions.
3. The period of drying is quite long. It is usually not less than 10 hours.

Uses of freeze drying process The process is mainly used for drying of biological products such as antibiotics, blood products, vaccines, enzyme preparations, microbiological cultures and other thermolabile pharmaceutical substances.

DRYERS USED FOR SOLUTIONS AND SUSPENSIONS

Sometimes solutions and suspensions are required to be converted into solids. This is done by using special types of dryers. The main purpose of these dryers is to spread the liquid to a large surface area so that drying can occur rapidly. Two types of dryers are used for this purpose:

1. The dryers in which there is spreading of the liquid in the form of a thin film *e.g.* Drum Dryer.
2. The dryers in which there is dispersing of the liquid as a spray of small droplets *e.g.* Spray Dryer.

Drum Dryer

The drum dryer consists of a hollow roller with a smoothly polished external surface heated internally by steam. It rotates on its longitudinal axis. The liquid to be dried is placed in a trough known as a "feed pan". The liquid is picked up by the roller as it rotates, covering the surface in a thin film which gets dry during the revolution of the roller. On the completion of one revolution, the dried film is removed mechanically by a scraper known as a "doctor knife".

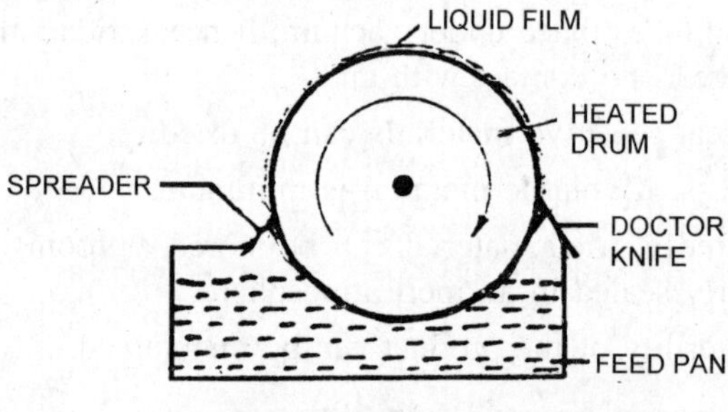

Fig. 12-6 Drum dryer

Advanatages of Drum Dryer

1. The dryer is compact. It occupies much less space as compared to a spray dryer.
2. The product obtained in the drum dryer is in the form of flakes which are used conveniently for many purposes.

3. The liquid is exposed to heat for a few seconds.
4. In order to reduce the temperature of drying, the drum can be enclosed in a vacuum chamber.
5. There is rapid drying because the liquid gets spread in the form of thin film over a large area resulting in rapid heat and mass transfer.

Disadvantages of Drum Dryer

1. Technical skill is required to operate a drum dryer. A careful control on feed rate, film thickness, speed of rotation and temperature is necessary.

Applications A drum dryer is used for drying of solution or suspension *e.g.* drying of milk products, starch products, ferrous salts and suspension of Zinc oxide or Kaolin.

Spray Dryer

In a spray dryer the liquid to be dried is sprayed in the form of mist. The minute droplets are readily evaporated and get converted into solid particles, which fall to the bottom of the chamber. The vapours are transferred into a separator where the fine dry particles which are carried along with vapours are separated and collected.

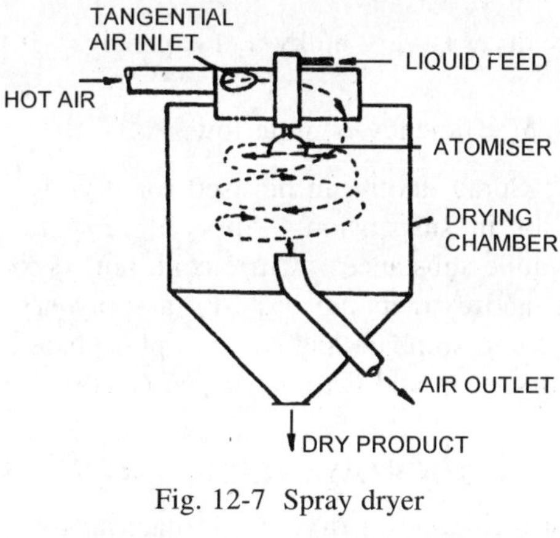

Fig. 12-7 Spray dryer

Spray dryers are available in many forms and designs. A typical spray dryer is shown in Fig. 12-7 The drying chamber is just like the cyclone separator, so as to ensure good circulation of air to facilitate heat and mass transfer and also to ensure that the dried particles are separated by the centrifugal action.

The character of the particles depends on the liquid to be converted in the form of droplets. As such it is important to use the right type of atomiser. Two types of atomisers are used:

1. Jet atomiser
2. Rotary atomiser

Jet atomisers are easily blocked resulting in variation of the droplet size. Rotary atomisers are preferred to avoid this problem.

Advantages of Spray Dryer

1. The liquid when sprayed through an atomiser gets converted into small droplets and it also provides a large surface area for heat and mass transfer so that evaporation is rapid.
2. Due to rapid evaporation, the droplets do not attain a high temperature so that most of the heat used is in the form of latent heat of vaporisation.
3. The dry product obtained has a high density, hence it has an excellent solubility.
4. Labour costs are low.
5. The product obtained is free flowing having almost spherical particles which is quite helpful in the tablet manufacturing.

Disadvantages of Spray Dryer

1. The spray dryer is very bulky and expensive. It occupies a large space.
2. The thermal efficiency is quite low.

Applications Spray dryer can be used for drying of any substance both in solution or in suspension. Spray dryers are very useful for drying of thermolabile substances. Citric acid, borax, sodium phosphate, hexamine, gelatin and extracts are dried by a spray dryer. The suspensions of starch, barium sulphate and calcium phosphate are also dried by a spray dryer. Milk, soap and detergents, too are dried by a spray dryer.

MICROWAVE DRYING

It is a modern technique of drying the material by using microwave energy. The energy in the form of microwaves is converted into internal heat by interaction with the material itself. This allows rapid heat transfer throughout the material which in turn can lead to rapid drying.

The heating effect is produced by the interaction of a rapidly oscillating electric field (915 or 2450 megahertz) with the polarised molecules and ions in the material. As the field reverses polarity, it relaxes and allows the molecules to return to their random orientation, giving up stored potential energy as random kinetic energy or heat. The interaction of the alternating field with ions causes billiard-ball-like collisions with unionised molecules and the impact energy is converted into heat.

Industrial microwave dryers are usually of static bed continuous type. Material to be dried are placed on conveyer belts and conveyed through the microwave applicator. Generally, heating is done by a stream of hot air followed by microwave treatment to remove last traces of moisture.

Microwave drying is useful for drying of thermolabile pharmaceutical materials such as, vitamins, enzymes, proteins and flavours.

▪ REVISION QUESTIONS ▪

I. Very short answer type questions ▪

Answer the following questions in brief.

1. Define the term "drying".
2. Name the various equipments used for drying of solid materials?
3. What are the dryers used for dying of solutions and suspensions?
4. What is "freeze drying"?
5. What are the various non-thermal methods for drying?
6. How do the solution and suspensions converted into solids?

II. Short answer type questions ▪

7. What are the two main steps in drying a material?
8. Write the applications of drying.
9. Explain the theory of fluidised bed dryer.
10. Discuss the theory of freeze drying process.
11. Write the advantages and disadvantages of fluidised bed dryer.
12. Give the advantages and disadvantages of drum dryer.
13. Write the applications of spray dryer.
14. Write the theory of microwave drying.
15. What types of dryer is appropriate for drying of powders and granules?

III. Long answer type questions ▪

16. Explain in detail the theory of drying. What are its applications in pharmacy?

17 Discuss the theory, construction, working of freeze drying apparatus. Write the advantages and disadvantages of freeze drying process.

18. Discuss the theory, construction and working of a fluidised bed dryer.

19. What are the dryers used for drying of solutions and suspensions? Describe the construction and working of a drum dryer.

20. Describe in brief about spray dryer. Write its advantages and disadvantages. Why spray dryer method is preferred over drum dryer method for drying of solutions and suspensions?

21. Define the term "drying". How are solid materials dried? Write in brief on any two of the following:
    (a) Tray dryer
    (b) Fluidised bed dryer
    (c) Rotary dryer
    (d) Vacuum dryer

22. Write short notes on:
    (a) Tray dryer
    (b) Rotary dryer
    (c) Fluidised bed dryer
    (d) Freeze drying
    (e) Spray drying.

IV. Objective type questions

Completion type questions (*Fill in the blanks with suitable word/words*).

23. Fluidised bed dryer method is ____________times faster than that of a tray dryer.

24. Fluidised bed dryers are available in different capacities ranging from ______________ to ______________ with an average drying time of about ______________ minutes

25. Proper drying prevents the ________________ of the product.

26. Drying is used to remove ________________ and ______________ from the solid substances.

27. Vacuum oven is operated at the pressure of about ____________ to ____________ bar.

28. Vertical fluidised bed dryer is __________ dryer whereas horizontal fluidised bed dryer is used for __________ drying of the material.

29. Vacuum dryer is modified form of ______________ still.

30. Rotary dryer is modified form of __________ dryer.

KEY

23. 15
24. 5 Kg to 200 Kg, 20-40 times
25. Deterioration
26. Liquid, moisture
27. 0.03 to 0.06
28. Batch type, continuous
29. Vacuum
30. Tunnel

13

Sterilisation

Sterilisation is the process of complete destruction of all microorganisms present in a system. The products free from living microorganisms are called "Sterile Products". Terms related to sterility are:

1. Antiseptic : The term antiseptic is often wrongly used as a synonym for disinfectant. A substance that prevents the growth of microorganisms by inhibiting their activity without destroying them is called antiseptic. A substance may be a good antiseptic but a poor disinfectant.

2. Bactericide : The substance that kills bacteria is called bactericide.

3. Bacteriostatic : The substance that arrests or retards the growth of bacteria is known as bacteriostatic.

4. Disinfection : A process that removes the infection potential by destroying microorganisms but not generally bacterial spores.

5. Germicide : A substance that kills pathogenic bacteria (bacteria producing disease) but not necessarily bacterial spores.

6. Viricidie : A substance that kills viruses.

7. Sterility : The absence of viable microorganisms is called "sterility" and preparations free from viable microorganisms are called "Sterile".

Disinfectant, bactericide and germicide are synonymous terms for a substance that kills microorganisms.

TABLE 13-1

Difference between Sterilisation and Disinfection

Sterilisation	*Disinfection*
1. It is a process by which all viable forms of microorganisms are removed or destroyed.	1. It is a process that removes infection potential by destroying microorganisms.
2. The bacterial spores are also destroyed.	2. The bacterial spores are not destroyed.
3. Sterilisation is done by any of the physical, chemical and mechanical methods.	3. Disinfection is done by using any one of the disinfectants.

Thermal Resistance of Microorganisms

The microorganisms show varying resistance to different methods of sterilisation. The degree of resistance varies with the specific microorganism, especially with the spores of microorganisms which are more resistant than the vegetative forms of the organism. Therefore, before selecting any method of sterilisation, it must be kept in mind that the method and its conditions must be lethal to the resistant spores and for that the following points should be taken into consideration.

1. Thermal death time : It may be defined as the time required to kill a specific type of microorganisms at a given temperature under specific conditions. It depends on factors like temperature, pH, presence of bactericide, number of contaminating microorganisms and their resistance to heat. There is a considerable variation in thermal death time between different types of bacterial spores. Therefore, an adequate margin of safety should be kept to kill the most resistant species of microorganisms and spores expected to be present by exceeding temperature and time for which it is applied than the known thermal death times of most of the spores.

2. Death rate of microorganisms : There is no direct method to determine when the sterility will be achieved. This is due to the reason that shortly before sterility is reached, the number of living microorganisms is so small that accurate determination of it becomes impossible due to very high errors in taking the samples. The reliable approach is to plot a graph between survivors against time of exposure.

3. Decimal reduction time (D value) : It is defined as the time in minutes required to reduce the number of viable organisms by 90%. It is one of the functions to indicate the efficiency of sterilization process. The order of death of microorganisms can be calculated from the equation.

$$K = 1/t\ (\log No - \log N) \qquad (1)$$

where K = constant which depends on organism, temperature and medium.

t = time of exposure in minutes.

No = Number of organisms viable at the beginning of time interval

N = Number of organisms viable at the end of the time interval

It was noted that after 90% reduction in microorganisms the equation (1) can be written as

$$K = 1/t$$

$$\text{or} \quad t = 1/K$$

Time t is defined as the decimal reduction time which is called the D value.

$$D = 1/K$$

The value of D can be found out by calculating the value of K from the graph of logarithm of the number of surviving organisms against time of exposure.

Factors Affecting the Thermal Destruction of Microorganisms

The following factors affect the thermal destruction of microorganisms.

1. ph : The majority of microorganisms are resistant to heat at a pH of 6 to 8. So acidic or alkaline solutions are easier to sterilise. There are certain substances like alkaloidal salts which act as buffers for acidic or alkaline pH may be used for maintaining stability. Such conditions help in the sterilisation of an injection.

2. Protective substances : In media containing high concentrations of organic substances such as proteins and carbohydrates, the microorganisms are not easily killed. The reasons are not clearly known but it is believed that protein forms a protective coat on the cells.

The most of the injections containing protein are thermolabile. Therefore they cannot be sterilised by heat. Hence they do not create much problem but this effect is found in injections containing thermostable carbohydrates such as dextrose which is used in high concentrations. But it has been observed that any increase in resistance of organisms is overcome by normal sterilising conditions.

This problem is more important in the sterilisation of glass wares and equipment such as tubes, syringes, containers etc. which are not thoroughly cleaned after use for proteins like blood or blood products and carbohydrates like dextrose because some of the microorganisms may remain hidden inside the equipment and protected from steam. Therefore, it is desirable that the glass wares and equipment should be thoroughly cleaned before sterilisation.

3. Antibacterial agents : The addition of antibacterial agent in injections can reduce the sterilisation temperature from 115°C to 100°C. This is very useful for the sterilisation of thermolabile substances. This method of sterilisation is commonly called it as sterilisation by heating with bactericide.

4. Inhibitory medicaments : There are certain medicaments which when converted into solution are harmful to microorganisms. This is due to pH in certain cases or it may be due to the toxic effect of the medicaments itself. Although some of the non-sporing microorganisms, for example *Staphylococcus aureous* are killed with in 24 hours at room temperature by a number of medicaments in their usual strength, but their spores are not killed unless they are heated to sterilising conditions of time and temperature. Therefore, there are only very few injections which can be safely regarded as self-sterilising.

5. The Inactivation factor of the process : The inactivation factor means the degree to which the viable population of organism is reduced and it is obtained by dividing the initial viable count by the final viable count.

$$\text{Inactivation factor} = 10t/D$$

where t = Exposure time in minutes, and
D = Decimal reduction time for the same temperature and conditions.

6. Initial number of organisms : When a certain number of organisms are heated at a lethal temperature, the organisms are not killed at once, but they are killed gradually as the exposure is prolonged. If certain fraction of initial number is destroyed in a particular time interval then the same fraction will be destroyed in the succeeding interval of time and will continue till all the organisms are killed and the preparation is sterilised. If the initial number of organisms is less, then the time required for sterilisation will be less. Therefore, while preparing the solutions every precautions should be taken to eliminate the entry of microorganisms and as far as possible thoroughly cleaned containers and equipment should be used.

METHODS OF STERILISATION

The methods of sterilisation can be divided into three main groups:

(A) Physical Methods:

1. Dry heat sterilisation
2. Moist heat sterilisation
3. Radiation Sterilisation
   (*a*) Use of ultra violet rays
   (*b*) Ionising radiation

(B) Chemical Methods:

1. Sterilisation by heating with bactericide.
2. Gaseous sterilisation.

(C) Mechanical Methods : Sterilisation involves the filtration of parenteral preparations through the following bacteria proof filters:

1. Ceramic filters
2. Seitz filter
3. Sintered glass filters
4. Sintered metal filters
5. Membrane filters

(A) Sterilisation by Physical Methods

(1) Dry Heat Sterilisation : All microorganisms including bacterial spores can be destroyed by heat. This is due to the oxidation of essential cell constituents. Dry heating at 100°C kills all vegetative bacteria in one hour but it does not kill spores. According to the pharmacopœia, sterilisation by dry heating is effected by heating at a temperature of 160°C for two hours. The products are heated in a hot air oven to maintain a temperature of 160°C.

Hot air oven It is used for sterilisation of pharmaceutical products and other materials. It is a double walled chamber made of steel. Insulation material, such as, glass fibres or asbestos is filled between the two walls of the oven to avoid heat loss. The door is also double-walled having asbestos gasket on its inner side. Two or three perforated shelves are fixed inside the oven to place the material for sterilisation. An electric fan is also fitted to ensure the uniform circulation of hot air in the oven in order to maintain the required temperature in all the shelves. Heating elements are fitted on the bottom of the oven and it is thermostatically controlled. A thermometer is fitted in the oven to note down the temperature inside the oven.

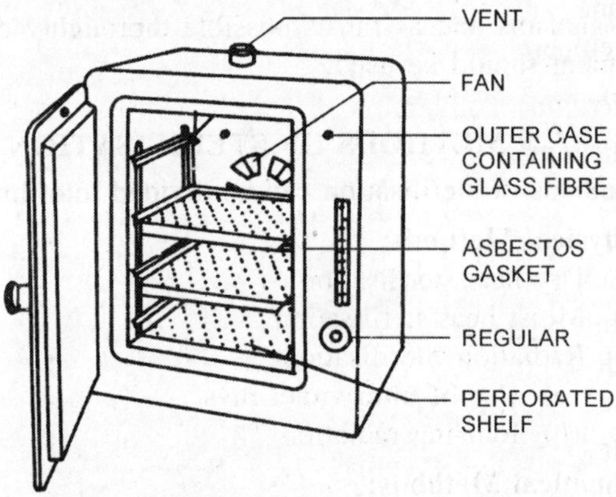

Fig. 13-1 Hot air oven

The materials to be sterilised are placed on the perforated shelves of the oven. The following precautions are to be taken while placing the material meant for sterilisation:

1. Glass apparatus must be wrapped with clean cloth or filter paper and containers must be plugged with non-absorbent cotton wool.
2. The articles and substances which are to be sterilised should not be placed at the floor of the oven as it receives direct heat and becomes much hotter.

3. The oven should not be overloaded with the materials meant for sterilisation.
4. There should be sufficient space in between the articles, so that there is uniform distribution of heat.

After heating the contents of the oven for two hours at 160°C, the articles are allowed to remain there, till the temperature comes down to 40°C. The sterilised material is then removed from the oven.

Advantages of Dry Heat Sterilisation

1. It is used for sterilisation of those substances which get spoiled during moist heat sterilisation, *e.g.* oily materials and powders.
2. The method is suitable for sterilisation of assembled equipment such as all glass syringes due to exposure to high temperature for a long time.
3. It is not so damaging to glass and metal equipment as moist heat.

Disadvantages of Dry Heat Sterilisation

1. This method is not suitable for surgical dressings.
2. This method is not suitable for most of the medicaments, rubber and plastic goods because the articles are exposed to a very high temperature for a long period.

Applications

1. It is mainly used for sterilisation of glass wares, such as, pestle and mortar, petridishes, flasks, pipettes, bottles, test tubes *etc.*
2. It is used for sterilisation of powders, such as, sulphacetamides, sulphadiazenes, kaolin, talc, zinc oxide, starch *etc.*
3. Injections where fixed oil is used as vehicle are sterilised by the dry heat method *e.g.* injection of progesterone, injection of testosterone propionate and injection of oestradiol dipropionate.
4. It is also used for sterilisation of scalpels, scissors, spatula, blades and glass syringes.

(2) Moist Heat Sterilisation : Moist heat sterilisation is more effective than the dry heat method. This is due to the fact that steam has more penetration power than dry heat and the thermal capacity of steam is more than thermal capacity of dry heat. The method is very useful for the killing of bacterial spores. The moist steam penetrates the spores and capsules of bacteria, rupture it and escaping protoplasm is coagulated.

The following combinations of temperature and time are normally employed for sterilising by heating in an autoclave:

TABLE 13.2

S.No.	*Holding temperature*	*Minimum holding time in minutes*
1.	115° to 118°	30
2.	121° to 124°	15
3.	126° to 129°	10
4.	134° to 138°	5

The condition prescribed above are to be maintained throughout the load, during the holding period of sterilisation.

Autoclave Moist heating is done in an "Autoclave". It consists of a strong metallic chamber usually made of stainless steel. It has a cover fitted with a steam vent, a pressure gauze and a safety valve. Rubber gasket is fitted on the inner side of the lid, in order to make autoclave air tight. The cover is closed with wing nuts and bolts. The electrically heated element is fitted at the bottom to heat the water to convert into steam. The perforated inner chamber is placed on the stand. The material to be sterilised is loosely packed into it.

A sufficient quantity of water is poured into the chamber after removing the perforated chamber. The level of the water is adjusted in such a way that it does not touch the bottom of the perforated chamber. The material is packed in the perforated chamber. The lid is then closed with wing nuts and bolts.

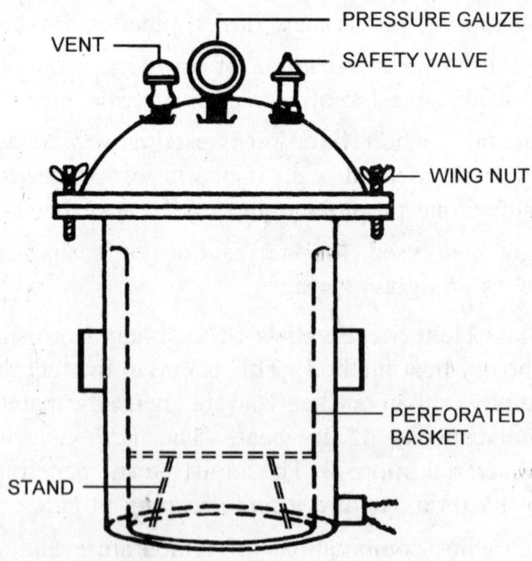

Fig. 13-2 Autoclave

The autoclave is switched on to heat the water. The vent is opened and safety valve is set at the required pressure. When steam starts coming out from the vent and it continues for 5 minutes, it is then closed. It indicates that air has been removed. The steam pressure starts raising and it comes to the desired pressure *i.e.* 10 lbs/square inch with corresponding temperature 115°C or 15 lbs/Sq.inch with corresponding temperature 121°C. After the stated period, switch off the autoclave. Allow it to cool to about 40°C before opening the vent. When whole of the steam inside the autoclave is removed, the lid is opened and the sterilised material is taken out. In industry, large size autoclaves of both horizontal and vertical position are used. They are heated directly by introducing steam prepared in a centralised boiler.

Advantages of autoclaving

1. Autoclaving destroys microorganisms more efficiently than dry heat and hence the material is exposed to a lower temperature for a shorter period.
2. It is used for sterilisation of a large number of official injections.
3. Equipment or parts of rubber and plastic, such as, Nylon and PVC can withstand the temperature and the pressure required for sterilisation.
4. A large quantity of material can be sterilised in one batch using a big autoclave.

Disadvantages of autoclaving

1. It is unsuitable for sterilisation of powders and oils.
2. It cannot be used for sterilisation of injections and articles, such as, plastics which get spoiled at 115-116°C for 30 minutes.

Applications

1. The method is used for sterilisation of surgical dressings and surgical instruments.
2. The containers and closures are sterilised by autoclaving.
3. It is used for the sterilisation of a majority of official injections which can withstand the pressure of 15 lbs/sq.inch for 30 minutes.

Other Methods of Sterilisation by Moist Heat

The following are some of the other methods besides autoclaving which are used for sterilisation by moist heat:

1. Tyndallisation
2. Pasteurisation
3. Sterilisation of vaccines

Tyndallisation method This is a fractional sterilisation method. The method was official in B.P. 1932, for sterilisation of medicaments unstable at 115°C but able to withstand low temperature heating. The method was used for sterilisation of culture media.

In this method, the solution to be sterilised is packed and sealed in its final container and heated at 80°C for one hour on each of three successive days. The first heating destroys the vegetative cells but not the bacterial spores. These bacterial spores germinate into the vegetative forms in the interval between the first and the second heating and are killed in the second heating. The third heating provides a safeguard against any spores which may not germinate until the second interval.

The method was deleted from the B.P. 1932 by the 4th Addendum (1941) and replaced by "Heating with a Bactericide".

Pasteurisation It is a partial sterilisation method which is used to make milk safe and also to improve its keeping properties. The process kills only 97 to 99 per cent microorganism, but it does not kill bacterial spores. The methods used for pasteurisation of milk are as under:

(*i*) *Holder method* : The milk is heated at 62.8°C for 30 minutes in a steam jacketed stainless steel tank containing agitators. This provides correct exposure throughout the milk and prevents skin formation. Clean dry steams is blown to the space above the liquid to prevent the formation of skin and foam. The method kills all types of bacteria including *mycobacterium tuberculosis*.

(*ii*) *Flash method* : The milk is heated to 71.6°C for 15 seconds and then quickly cooled. The milk is heated by passing through narrow horizontal pipes inside large ones through which water passes in the opposite direction. The method is commonly used by most of the firms because it is a less time consuming process. It also needs less floor space and it is a continuous process.

Sterilisation of Vaccines In case of vaccine which is a suspension of dead bacteria, the organisms are killed in such a manner that its antigenic power is preserved. The suspension of microorganism is prepared in normal saline solution and transferred into a sealed container. Sterilisation is carried out by immersing the container in a thermostatically controlled water bath at a temperature between 55° to 60°C for one hour. The strick aseptic precautions are observed to exclude any possibility of contamination. The vaccine is tested for sterility to confirm the proper sterilisation of vaccine.

(3) Radiation Sterilisation : This is of two types:

1. Sterilisation by ultra violet light
2. Sterilisation by ionising radiation

Sterilisation by ultra violet light Direct sunlight can destroy microorganism on account of its ultra violet rays of long wavelength. The sun emits both ultra violet rays of longer as well as shorter wavelength. The ultra violet rays of shorter wave length are absorbed by the earth's atmosphere. The antimicrobial activity of U.V. light depends on its wave length. It is maximum at 265 nm wave length.

Ultra violet rays for sterilisation is produced by passing a low current at high voltage through mercury vapour in an evacuated glass tube.

Applications

1. It is used for sterilisation of air to prevent cross infection in hospitals.
2. It is used for sterilisation and maintenance of aseptic area in the pharmaceutical industry.
3. It is used for sterilisation of thermolabile substances before packing *e.g.*, destruction of the virus of homologous serum jaundice in blood plasma and inactivation of viruses and bacteria in vaccine production.
4. It is also used for sterilisation of surfaces of working tables and rooms where aseptic technique is to be performed. The U.V. lamps should be installed in the ceiling and it should be shielded, in order to protect the worker from the harmful effects of U.V. radiation.

Disadvantages

1. Ultra violet rays have a low penetration power, so it is not applicable to the sterilisation of packed pharmaceuticals.
2. U.V. rays are less effective against organisms in the atmosphere or on surfaces if the relative humidity is high.
3. The radiation is partially screened by dust or grease on the U.V. lamp. So regular cleaning of lamp is necessary.
4. U.V. light is harmful for worker. The eyes and skin should be protected from direct ultra violet rays.

Sterilisation by ionising radiations The ionising radiations are X-rays and Gamma rays. These are lethal to bacterial cell and destroy the nuclei of the cell. Gamma rays are produced from radio-isotonic source such as cobalt-60 or cesium-137 or of electrons energised by a suitable electron accelerator. A dose of 2.5 Mrads is generally accepted as adequate although other dosage levels may also be employed.

The material to be sterilised is packed in the final container and then exposed to ionising radiation. Ionising radiations are much more efficient as a sterilising agent than ultra violet rays.

Advantages

1. Gamma rays have a high penetration power and, so, materials can be sterilised after filling them in the final container.
2. No aseptic precautions are required.
3. The temperature rise is negligible.
4. The method is suitable for all types of materials such as dry, moist and frozen.
5. The method is reliable and can be accurately controlled.
6. Some bacterial and viral vaccines can be sterilised without any loss of its antigenic power.
7. A large quantity of material can be sterilised because the exposure time is very short.

Disadvantages

1. The plant used is very costly. A lot of capital is required in setting up the plant.
2. The process cannot be stopped once it is started because the radiation cannot be switched off.
3. The radiations are harmful to workers.
4. It produces undesirable changes in many medicaments, such as, colour, solubility and texture of the product.

Applications

1. The method is mainly used for sterilisation of plastic syringes, hypodermic needles, scalpels, surgical blades and adhesive dressings.
2. It is also used for sterilisation of bone and tissue transplant, plastic tubing, catheters and sutures.
3. It is used for sterilisation of thermolabile medicaments.

(B) Chemical Methods of Sterilisation ■

These are of two types:

1. Sterilisation by heating with a bactericide
2. Gaseous sterilisation

1. Sterilisation by heating with a bactericide : This method may be used for sterilising aqueous preparations which are unstable at higher temperatures attained in the moist heat sterilisation processes. The method has a lower margin of safety and should be used only when moist heat sterilisation is not applicable.

In this process the medicament is dissolved or suspended in a suitable solution of the following bactericide so as to achieve the concentration of bactericides given in Table 13-3.

TABLE 13.3

S.No.	Name of the bactericide	Concentration of bactericide in per cent w/v
	For injections	
1.	Chlorocresol	0.2
2.	Phenylmercuric acetate or Phenylmercuric nitrate	0.002
	For eye drops	
1.	Benzalkonium chloride	0.01
2.	Phenylmercuric acetate or Phenylmercuric nitrate	0.002
3.	Thiomersal	0.01
4.	Chlorohexidine acetate	0.01

The preparation is then transferred into the final container which is then sealed so as to exclude microorganisms and heated at 98-100°C for 30 minutes by heating it in boiling water.

The bactericide used should possess the following properties:

1. It should be non toxic.
2. Compatible with medicaments.
3. Stable and active at various pH.
4. Stable during heating and storage.

The lethal effect of bactericide increases with the rise of temperature.

Applications The method is used for the sterilisation of injections which though reasonably thermostable do show some evidence of deterioration when heated at 115-116°C for 30 minutes (Autoclaving).

The method cannot be used for the sterilisation of injections meant for intrathecal or peridural administration. Similarly this method is not suitable for intravenous injections when a single dose exceeds 15 ml.

2. Gaseous sterilisation : In this case sterilisation is done with a chemical in gaseous state. In olden days, formaldehyde was very commonly used, but now it has been replaced by ethylene oxide. Beta propiolactone is a new chemical which is also used as a sterilising agent.

(*a*) Formaldehyde : It is an alkylating agent. In olden days, it was used in special chambers to sterilise catheters, syringes and other thermolabile hospital equipment. However nowadays, it is used for the fumigation of empty rooms after infectious diseases. Formaldehyde is inferior to ethylene oxide due to the following reasons:

1. It has a weak penetration power.
2. It is difficult to maintain a high concentration in the atmosphere.
3. It requires a high humidity to be an effective sterilising agent.
4. It is readily inactivated *e.g.* by proteins and other organic matter.
5. It is irritating to the respiratory tract.
6. It is difficult to remove the adsorbed gas.

(*b*) **Ethylene oxide** (C_2H_4O) **:** It is a colourless gas at room temperature. It can be liquefied easily and the liquid boils at approximately 10.8°C. It is readily dissolved in water and organic solvents. It is highly inflammable so it is used by:

1. *Mixing ethylene oxide with some inert gas in a fixed ratio*

   These mixtures are:

   (*i*) Ethylene oxide = 1 part
   Carbon dioxide = 9 parts

   (*ii*) Ethylene oxide = 11% *w/v*
   Trichlorofluoromethane = 79% *w/w*
   Dichlorodifluromethane = 10% *w/w*

   (*iii*) Ethylene oxide = 12% *w/w*
   Dichlorodifluromethane = 88% *w/w*

   Carbon dioxide is not so popular because it has a very high vapour pressure.

   The sterilisation is done in a chamber which can be heated to the desired degree of temperature. The material to be sterilised is packed in the chamber and is treated with a sterilising mixture for the stated time.

2. *Using ethylene oxide in the absence of air*

   The exposure is carried out in an evacuated steriliser at subatmospheric pressure. Pure ethylene oxide or a mixture containing 90% ethylene oxide and 10% carbon dioxide is used as sterilising agent.

   Ethylene oxide kills microorganisms by alkylation of protein molecules. It is active against all types of microorganisms.

Factors influencing efficiency of ethylene oxide These factors are as follows.

1. **Temperature :** Sterilisation can be done at room temperature but it takes a long time. It is very effective at the temperature of 40°C.
2. **Concentration :** It is very effective in concentration between 200 mg to 1 g/litre.

3. **Relative humidity :** Some moisture is necessary to sterilise the material by ethylene oxide. Sufficient moisture is needed during exposure to ethylene oxide in order to provide the optimum humidity in the micro-environment of the organisms. Generally 40-50% moisture is necessary to have the maximum efficiency of ethylene oxide as a sterilising agent.
4. **Power of penetration :** Ethylene oxide has a high penetration power. It can penetrate through paper, fabrics and a number of plastics and rubbers. Ethylene oxide is a very superior sterilising agent because of the said factor.
5. **Absorption :** Many materials absorb ethylene oxide, and, so it causes reduction of the gas concentration in the chamber atmosphere. The sterilised articles cannot be used until the absorbed gas has escaped. The amount and the rate of absorption depend on the nature, thickness, surface area of the articles and their wrapping and the size of the load.

Advantages

1. It is suitable for heat sensitive substances because sterilisation is effective at room temperature.
2. It is a very reactive compound, but it causes damage to only a few materials.
3. Ethylene oxide has a good penetration power; hence it can be used to sterilise the pre-packed articles.
4. The method is very reliable.
5. The method is useful for sterilisation of moist-sensitive substances and equipment because only a low humidity is required.

Disadvantages

1. The method is very slow.
2. The apparatus used for sterilisation on a large scale is very expensive.
3. The running costs are high.
4. A lot of precautions are required to be taken to use ethylene oxide as it is highly inflammable and toxic.
5. Certain toxic substances, such as, ethylene chlorhydrin are produced in certain materials.

Applications

1. The method is used for sterilisation of thermolabile materials, such as, rubber and plastic items.

2. It is also used for sterilisation of delicate instruments or electric diagnostic instruments which are used in an operation theatre.
3. The method is applicable for sterilisation of powders packed in plastic or cellophane envelopes which are permeable to gases.
4. The method is suitable for sterilisation of instruments, metallic equipment, syringes and needles.

(*c*) **Beta-propiolactone** [$(CH_2)_2OCO$] **:** It is the latest sterilising agent. It has low vapour pressure and is a liquid at room temperature. Its boiling point is 160°C hence it is non-flammable. It has less penetration power than ethylene oxide. So it is mainly used for sterilisation of operation theatres and aseptic rooms etc. It is generally used in the concentration of 2-4 mg per litre of space at 25°C. It causes irritation, blisters and burns on contact with skin. Moreover it is carcinogenic

(C) Sterilisation by Mechanical Methods

The solutions containing thermolabile medicament can be sterilised by filtration through bacteria proof filters. These filters retain the bacteria and the sterile filtrate is collected in sterilised receiver. To obtain a sterile filtrate it is necessary that the filter, receiver and all connecting parts likely to come into contact with the filtrate must be sterile. For successful sterilisation by filtration, the following points should be observed:

1. The whole of the apparatus must be sterile.
2. An aseptic technique should be followed in order to minimise the risk of contamination.
3. The assembly of filtration unit should be so adjusted that there is minimum exposure of filtrate to the atmosphere.
4. The filter selected must be fine enough to obstruct the passage of all bacteria.

The various types of bacteria proof filters used are:

1. Ceramic filters : These are also called filter candles. These are made of porcelain or kieselguhr and are available in a range of pore size. These candles are numbered according to its pore size. Kieselguhr filters are usually softer than the porcelain type.

The candle is placed in the solution to be sterilised and its opening is attached to the vacuum system. When vacuum is applied the pressure inside the candle is decreased. Due to the difference in pressure between the outside and inside of the candle, the solution moves into the candle. The filtrate is collected in sterile container. The filter becomes somewhat blocked with continuous use. This can be cleaned by scratching the outlet surface with a nail brush and passing water through it in the reverse direction.

The main disadvantage of ceramic filter is its tendency to absorb materials from aqueous solutions.

2. Seitz filter : It consists of two parts. The lower part holds a perforated disc, on it a compressed asbestos sheet is placed. Two parts are joined together with the help of nuts. As shown in Fig. 13-3, there is a valve on the upper part through which vacuum is applied. The asbestos sheet is made up of asbestos fibres but may also contain cellulose and alkaline earth such as magnesium compounds. The asbestos pads are used once only and then discarded.

Asbestos pads may yield alkali and cause precipitation of alkaloids from aqueous solutions of their salts. Due to the fibrous nature of asbestos pads, it may shed fibres into the filtrate and also absorb drugs from solution. Hence, a few millilitres of filtrate should always be rejected and sintered glass disc may also be fixed in the filtration unit immediately after seitz filter.

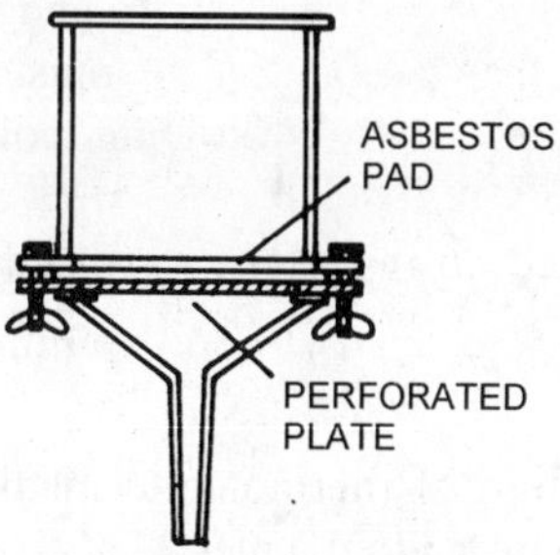

Fig. 13-3 Seitz filter

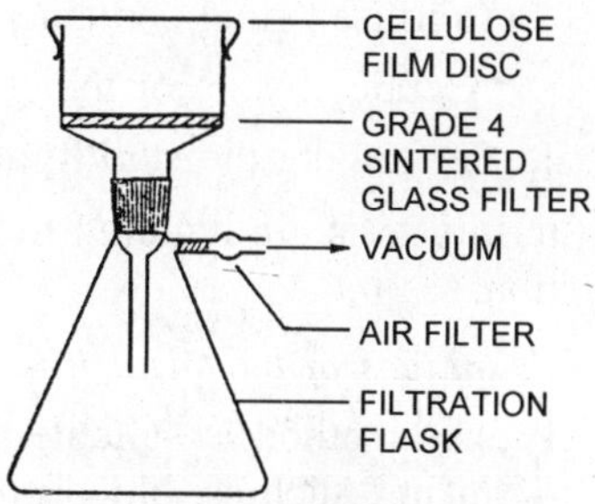

Fig. 13-4 Simple filtration unit

3. Sintered glass filters : These are made from borosilicate glass. The glass is finely powdered and particles of the required size are separated and is then packed into disc moulds. These moulds are heated until a suitable adhesion has taken place between the granules. These discs are fused to funnels of suitable shape and size. Sintered glass filters are available in different pore size and are numbered accordingly. For bacteria proof filtration number 5 or 3 must be used. The filtration is carried out under a reduced pressure as shown in Fig. 13-4.

Sintered glass filter do not absorb the medicaments from the solution. These filters are made from borosilicate glass, so it does not change the pH of the solution and also does not shed fibres.

Sintered glass filters are cleaned after use by passing water in the reverse direction. Organic matter may be removed by passing strong sulphuric acid with 1% sodium nitrate through the filter.

4. Sintered metal filters : These are the metallic counter part of sintered glass filters. These are usually made from stainless steel. They have the advantage of having greater mechanical strength, but are liable to attack by the solutions passing through them.

5. Membrane filters : These are made of cellulose acetate or cellulose nitrate. These are fixed in metallic holders similar to those used with asbestos pads. The pore size in the membranes lies in the range of 100-150μ. They are also called millipore filters.

Membrane filters are suitable for sterilising aqueous and oily solutions but are not suitable for organic solvents, such as, alcohols, ketones, esters or chloroform.

Sterilisation by filtration involves four basic steps:

1. Filtration of the solution through one of the bacteria-proof filters which have been described above.
2. Aseptic distribution of the filtered solution into the previously strerilised final containers.
3. Aseptic closure of the containers.
4. Performing the sterility test.

Sterility tests are required to be performed on injections sterilised by filtration.

Advantages of bacterial filtration

1. The method is suitable for sterilisation of thermolabile medicaments, such as, blood products, insulin and enzymes.
2. All types of bacteria *i.e.*, living as well as dead, are removed from the preparation.
3. Both clarification and sterilisation are done side by side.
4. It is an excellent method for the rapid supply of a small volume of a parenteral solution in an emergency.

Disadvantages

1. The method is not a reliable one and therefore a sterility test is necessary.
2. The suspensions and oily preparations cannot be sterilised by this method.

3. There are chances of absorption of medicaments from a solution by the filter.
4. Some filter media, such as, asbestos pads may shed fibres in the filtered product.
5. Units may leak if carelessly handled.
6. Defects in the media are not immediately detectable.
7. Aseptic technique is necessary.
8. Highly trained staff is required.
9. The process is only suitable for medicaments which are in solution form.

Applications

The method is useful for sterilisation of parenteral solutions containing thermolabile medicaments without any decomposition *e.g.* insulin, blood serum and other products containing protein matter which get coagulated upon heating.

▪ TESTS FOR STERILITY ▪

These tests are based upon the principle that if bacteria or fungi are placed in a medium which provides nutritive material, moisture, the desired pH and are kept at a favourable temperature, the organisms will grow and their presence can be indicated by the turbidity in the originally clear medium.

The tests for sterility are done by detecting the presence of viable forms of bacteria, fungi and yeast in or on pharmacopœial preparations. The tests must be carried out under strict aseptic techniques in order to avoid accidental contamination of the product during the test. All glass apparatus required for the test must be sterile.

Culture media Culture media used for test may be prepared as described in I.P. Culture media is required for aerobic and anaerobic bacteria and for fungi. The media used should comply with the tests, such as, sterility, nutritive properties, effectiveness of media as per details given in I.P.

Methods of testing Tests for sterility may be carried out by :

1. Membrane filtration method
2. Direct inoculation method

1. Membrane filtration method : The method is preferred in the following cases.

(*i*) An oil or oily preparation.

(*ii*) An ointment that can be put into solution.

(*iii*) A non-bacteriostatic solid not readily soluble in culture medium.

(*iv*) A soluble powder or a liquid that possesses bacteriostatic and fungistatic properties.

(*v*) Liquid products where the volume in a container is 100 ml or more.

The method involves the filtration of the sample under test through a membrane filter having normal porosity of 0.45 μ, and a diameter of approximately 47 mm. After the filtration, the membrane is removed aseptically from the metallic holder and divided into two halves. The first half is transferred into 100 ml of culture media meant for fungi and incubated at 20° to 25°C for not less than seven days. The other half is transferred into 100 ml of fluid thioglycollate medium and incubated at 30° to 35°C for not less than 7 days. Observe the growth in the media.

2. Direct inoculation method : In this method the specified quantity of sample under test is drawn aseptically from the container (The quantity of the substance or preparation to be used for the inoculation varies and is given in I.P.) and transferred into a vessel of culture medium. Mix the liquid with the medium and incubate for not less than 14 days. Observe the growth of microorganisms in the medium.

Observation and Results The culture medium is examined during and at the end of incubation to find out if there is any microbial growth. The following observations are possible:

1. No evidence of growth; hence the preparation being examined passes the test for sterility.

2. There is evidence of growth. So, re-testing is performed using the same number of samples, volumes to be tested and media as in the original test. If no evidence of microbial growth is then found, the preparation being examined passes the tests for sterility.

3. There is evidence of microbial growth. So, isolate and identify the organism. If they are not readily distinguishable from those growing in the containers reserved in the first test, the preparation being examined fails the test for sterility. They are readily distinguishable from those growing in the containers reserved in the first test. The second re-test is performed using twice the number of samples. The preparation being examined passes the tests for sterility in case there is no evidence of microbial growth. In case there is evidence of growth of any microorganisms in the second re-test, the preparation being examined fails the tests for sterility.

ASEPTIC TECHNIQUES

During the preparation of sterile pharmaceutical products, the sterilisation is done either before filling the product into the final container or after filling and sealing the product into its final container. In the first case, it is desirable that the area where such preparations are prepared, must be free from microorganism so as to maintain the sterility of the product. But in the second case it not necessary to follow the aseptic techniques because the products get sterilised in their final container. Aseptic technique is also necessary in sterility testing.

The methods which are used to prevent the access of microorganism during the preparation of parenteral products and their testing are called "Aseptic Techniques".

Good aseptic techniques can only be applied if one knows the possible source of contamination. The various sources of contamination are:

1. Atmosphere, which is contaminated with dust, droplet and droplet nuclei becomes the breeding ground of microorganism.
2. The hands are a major means of transmitting infection.
3. Coughing, sneezing and spitting can cause contamination at a considerable distance.
4. The clothes which absorb dust particles are also a source of contamination. A handkerchief is the richest source of contamination.
5. The hair, which is constantly exposed to atmospheric dust is source of contamination. These dust particles are liberated from the hair during brushing and shaking of the head.
6. The unsterile equipment.
7. The working surface.

Design of an Aseptic Room

For performing various techniques, it is desirable to maintain sterile conditions in the place of working. So, the following points must be taken into consideration before designing an aseptic room :

1. Site : It is desirable that the site selected for an aseptic room in the building should be away from stairs, lift and corridors, because these provide a route by which the airborne microorganism can travel in the building. The best site is the one where the workers can work undisturbed. There should be one or two rooms alongwith the aseptic room for providing washing and changing facilities.

2. Size : The proper size of an aseptic room depends on the maximum number of people which are going to use it. The maintenance cost can be reduced if the aseptic room is a bit smaller in size. The walls and the ceiling of the room should be of reasonable size so that it can be cleaned in routine without any difficulty.

3. Windows : The windows in the room are a source of dust particles which may enter and contaminate the atmosphere. In order to provide good light in the aseptic room, glass panes should be used. Ventilation should be provided by laminar air flow system.

4. Doors : The entrance to the aseptic room should be through an air-lock with double doors about 1 meter apart. This is necessary to prevent a sudden in-rush of air when the door is opened. The outer door is opened only when it is confirmed that the inner door (which opens into the aseptic room) is closed. For this purpose a small window is needed in the outer door. The inner door is opened when the outer door is closed.

5. Surface materials : The floors, walls and the bench tops of an aseptic room must be smooth, resistant to chemicals and easily clean-able. The floor of the aseptic room needs frequent washing to prevent the accumulation of dirt. The floor should be build with Terrazzo (mixture of cement and crushed marble), Linoleum (heavy grade) and plastics.

The walls and ceiling should be provided with tiles or coated with hard glass paint or smooth plaster or covered with plastic laminated boards. The working table tops should be made of stainless steel or plastic laminates so as to avoid accumulation of dust.

6. Services : An aseptic area generally requires the following services:

(*a*) *Ventilation* : It includes the removal of microorganisms, control of humidity and temperature and provision of fresh air. The clean air free from microorganism can be produced by mechanical filtration or electrostatic precipitation.

(*b*) *Electricity* : The electric supply is needed for lighting and functioning of equipment and machinery. The switches and sockets should be flush fitting and have finger plates of plastic. As far as possible, most of controls should be outside the room.

(*c*) Gas supply is needed for the burning of burners. Gas cocks may be on the walls or at the back of the bench.

(*d*) Vacuum arrangements for clarification and bacterial filtration.

(*e*) *Disposal of waste* : In order to control the dust, such arrangement should be made that majority of the pipes and fittings get hidden in the walls of the room or these are properly covered.

7. Furniture : Furniture, such as, working benches, chairs, trolleys and screens are used in an aseptic room. The furniture should be such that there is the least number of undesirable dust retaining cavities. Aseptic technique is usually carried out under a screen which is available in two designs:

(*i*) *Shack type* : This is made of wood or of plastic material. Plastic screens are transparent and hence give a good visibility of the

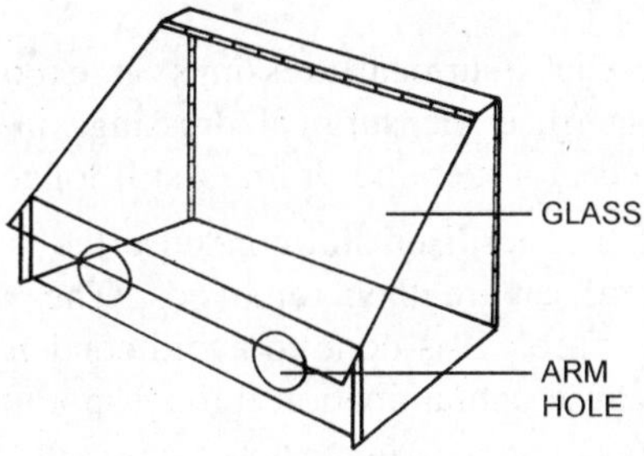

Fig. 13-5 Plastic folding shack-type screen

contents. Moreover, they are light in weight and can be moved from one place to another without any difficulty. The screen is a box like structure with a glass sloping front. This type of screen has two arm holes on the front side (as shown in Fig. 13.5) through which the worker can introduce his hands for doing various aseptic techniques. The U.V. tubes are fitted inside the screen in order to maintain the sterility inside the cabinet.

(*ii*) *Fume-cupboard type* : This type of screen is used in those cases where tall apparatus or equipment are needed in the aseptic work. These screens are generally made of wood. The design of the screen is just like a chemical fume cupboard used in a chemistry laboratory.

STERILISATION OF SURGICAL DRESSINGS

The materials like cotton-wool balls, gauze swabs, ribbon gauze, bandages *etc.* are used in surgery and in wards. These are commonly known as materials of surgical dressings. The following stages are involved in the sterilisation of surgical dressings:

1. Packing or wrapping of the unsterilised surgical dressings into a suitable container or packaging material. For this purpose, metal drums

are used. These drums are perforated in order to facilitate the free flow of steam during sterilisation. The surgical dressings can also be wrapped with fabrics like nylon film bags or muslin cloth or calico cloth.

2. The suitably packed dressings are correctly loaded into the steriliser. The packing should be done in such a way that it ensures satisfactory steam penetration and air removal. So, the pack should be kept as small as possible. The heavy materials should not be sterilised with soft material. The contents should be packed loosely and the spaces between the items and folds should be parallel.

3. The steriliser is closed and air inside the steriliser is replaced by steam.

4. The fabric pack (surgical dressings) is exposed for 30-45 minutes at 121°C to sterilise the surgical dressings in it. When surgical dressings are packed in a metallic drum, a still longer time is required.

5. Switch off the steriliser and condense the steam inside it. The contents of the steriliser are then removed. The warm packs are not placed on a cold surface. It is done to avoid condensation of steam into water which may cause contamination through porous wrappers.

6. The containers are labelled indicating the date of sterilisation so as to prevent overlong storage.

▪ STERILISATION OF TRANSFUSION FLUIDS ▪

It is easy to sterilise the transfusion fluids in bottles than the surgical dressing. The following steps are involved in the sterilisation of transfusion fluids:

1. The transfusion fluids or intravenous fluids are transferred into washed and dried bottles. These are then properly sealed to exclude any leakage.
2. The bottles are loaded into the steriliser and its door is closed.
3. The dry saturated steam is admitted into the steriliser. It will displace the air present in it.
4. The bottles are exposed to the desired temperature and pressure for the stated period.
5. The supply of steam is cut off.
6. The steam inside the steriliser is allowed to vent slowly to reduce the internal pressure to that of the atmospheric pressure. Then the load is left closed until the load in the steriliser has cooled down.

7. The sterilised bottles are taken out from the steriliser when these are cooled to less than 100°C.
8. The bottles are subjected to various quality control tests as required by the pharmacopœia.
9. The bottles of transfusion fluids are then labelled.

Precautions for Handling of Sterilisation Equipment

The main aim of aseptic technique is to prevent contamination of materials, instruments, containers, glass wares etc. during handling. The glass wares and containers should be thoroughly washed with detergent and water to remove the dirt and grease before sterilisation. They are stored under aseptic conditions immediately after their sterilisation.

As far as possible, the aseptic work should be done in a special room which is made for this purpose. The arrangement is made in such a way that there is positive pressure in the aseptic room so that the dust particles may not settle on the surface of the apparatus. The sterilised air is introduced in this room. The main sources of contamination are atmosphere, breath, the hands of the workers, clothes, hair and working surfaces. To maintain sterility it is desirable to minimise the contamination which can be done as under:

1. By wearing sterilised gowns, face masks and gloves before entering into aseptic room.
2. The hair should be properly covered with sterilised cap.
3. The hands should be thoroughly washed with soap and antiseptic solution before handling the sterilised equipment.
4. The working surface of the table or slab should be thoroughly cleaned with disinfectant before starting the aseptic work.
5. The sterilised equipment should be transferred from one place to another in a trolley or in a crate so that the aseptic room is not opened time and again.
6. The sterilised air should be introduced under pressure in the aseptic room to maintain sterility and positive pressure.

REVISION QUESTIONS

I. Very short answer type questions

Answer the following questions in brief.

1. Define the terms:

   Sterilisation, Antiseptic, Bactericide, Bacteriostatic, Disinfection, Germicide, Sterility

2. Explain the term "Thermal death time".
3. Name the different methods of sterilisation.
4. How are bacteria killed by dry heat method of sterilisation?
5. What is the temperature and time required to kill bacteria by dry heat method of sterilisation?
6. How fixed oils are sterilised?
7. What is the method used to sterilise the thermolabile powdered drugs?
8. How are bacteria killed by the moist heat method of sterilisation?
9. How is milk sterilised?
10. How is vaccine containing dead bacteria sterilised?
11. How will you sterilise the injections and transfusion fluids?
12. What is the temperation and time period at which bacteria get killed by pasteurisation?
13. Mention the wave length of ultra violet rays which has maximum antibacterial activity.
14. What is the source of gamma rays?
15. Give a list of chemicals which are used as bactericide.
16. How are bacteria killed by gamma rays?
17. How are bacteria killed by ethylene oxide gas?
18. What is the concentration of beta-propiolactone most effective as bactericide?
19. Why is sterility test necessary?
20. Name the factors which influence the efficiency of ethylene oxide.
21. Define the term "tyndallisation"
22. Explain the term "pasteurisation".

II. Short answer type questions

23. Classify the different methods of sterilisation.
24. Write the advantages and disadvantages of dry heat method of sterilisation.
25. What are the applications of dry heat sterilisation
26. What are precautions necessary to be taken while placing the material for sterilisation in a hot air oven?
27. What are the advantages and disadvantages of moist heat sterilisation?

28. Draw a labelled diagram of an autoclave.
29. Why is moist heat method of sterilisation more effective than dry heat method?
30. What is pasteurisation? How milk is pasteurised?
31. Write in brief about sterilisation by ultra violet light.
32. What are the applications of sterilisation by ultra violet rays?
33. What are the advantages and disadvantages of sterilisation by ionising radiations?
34. Write in brief about chemical methods of sterilisation.
35. How is formaldehyde inferior to ethylene oxide as sterilising agent?
36. Explain the factors which may influence the efficiency of ethylene-oxide.
37. Write the advantages and disadvantages of ethylene oxide used in gaseous sterilisation.
38. Write the applications of ethylene oxide when it is used in gaseous sterilisation.
39. What are the basic points to be followed in sterilisation by filtrations?
40. Write the advantages and disadvantages of sterilisation by filtration.
41. What is test for sterility? What are different methods to be used for performing this test?
42. What is the principle behind the tests for sterility?
43. What are aseptic techniques?
44. Describe the various sources of contamination.
45. How are surgical dressings sterilised?
46. Write the various steps involved in sterilisation of transfusion fluids.
47. What are the precautions to be observed for handling of sterilised equipment?

III. Long answer type questions

48. Enumerate the various methods of sterilisation. Discuss any two methods in detail.
49. Define the term "sterilisation". How it differs from disinfection? Describe dry heat method of sterilisation in detail.

50. Define the term "sterilisation". Why is moist heat method of sterilisation more effective than dry heat method? Write in detail about moist heat method of sterilisation.
51. What are the gases used in gaseous sterilisation? Explain in detail about ethylene oxide which is used in gaseous sterilisation. Write the various factors which may influence the efficiency of ethylene oxide.
52. Write the principle and methods used for test for sterility.
53. Explain the term "aseptic techniques". What are the various points to be considered while designing an aseptic room?
54. What do you know about sterilisation by mechanical methods? Explain in detail about various types of bacterial proof filters:—
55. Write in brief on any two of the following:
    (a) Sintered glass filter (b) Membrane filter
    (c) Seitz filter (d) Ethylene oxide
    (e) Pasteurisation (f) Tyndallisation
56. Write short notes on:-
    (a) Autoclave (b) Dry heat sterilisation
    (c) Moist heat sterilisation (d) Gaseous sterilisation
    (e) Radiation sterilisation (f) Sterilisation by filtration
57. How are the following sterilised?
    (a) Surgical dressings (b) Transfusion fluids

IV. Objective type questions

A. Completion type questions (Fill in the blanks with suitable word/words)

58. A substance which can kill pathogenic bacteria is called ____________.
59. A substance which can kill bacteria is called ____________
60. A preparation which is free from viable microorganism is called ____________.
61. Glass wares are sterilised by ____________ method.
62. Injections are generally sterilised by ____________ method.
63. In dry heat sterilisation method, bacteria are killed due to the ____________.
64. In moist heat method of sterilisation, the minimum holding time for sterilisation of injection at 121°C is ____________.

65. In moist heat method of sterilisation, bacteria are killed by ____________________.

66. U.V. light is used for sterilisation of air to prevent ____________________ in hospitals.

67. The solution to be sterilised is packed in final container and heated at 80°C for one hour on ________ in __________ method.

68. Ethylene oxide is very effective in concentration between _______ to ________/litre.

69. Beta-propiolactone is used in the concentration of _________ of space at __________ .

70. Asbestos pads may yield __________ and shed __________ into the filtrate and ___________ drugs from solution.

B. Matching type questions

71. Match the items of *Column I* with the appropriate items in *Column II*

Column I	*Column II*
A. Moist heat sterilisation is effective	(*i*) 160° for 2 hours
B. Tyndallisation method	(*ii*) The material is heated at 62.8°C for 30 mts.
C. U.V. light	(*iii*) used to sterilise the material after packing in final container.
D. Dry heat sterilisation	(*iv*) 115-116° for 30 mts.
E. Pasteurisation method	(*v*) The material is heated at 80°C for one hour on each of three successive days.
F. Gamma rays	(*vi*) used for sterilisation of air and to prevent cross infection in hospital.

KEY

5. 160°C for 2 hours
6. Dry heat method
7. Dry heat method
9. Pasteurisation
10. 55-60°C for one hour
11. Moist heat sterilisation
12. 62.8°C for 30mts or 71.6°C for 15 seconds
13. 265 nm
16. Cobalt 60 or Cesium-137

18. 2-4 mg/litre of space at 25°C
58. Germicide
59. Bactericide
60. Sterile product
61. Dry heat sterilisation
62. Moist heat sterilisation
63. Oxidation of essential cell constituents
64. 15 mts
65. Coagulation of protoplasm of bacterial cell
66. Cross infection
67. 3 successive days, tyndallisation method
68. 200 mg to 1g/litre
69. 2-4 mg per litre, 25°C
70. Alkali, fibres, asbestos
71. A(iv); B(v); c(vi); D(i); E(ii); F(iii)

14

Processing of Tablets

Tablets are the solid dosage form containing medicament or medicaments, usually circular in shape and may be flat or biconvex. Tablets are prepared by the compression method and are hence called the "Compressed Tablets".

Advantages of Tablets

1. The tablets are easy to be administered.
2. They are easy to be dispensed.
3. These are more stable dosage form.
4. They maintain the accuracy of dosage.
5. Bitter and nauseous substances can be given easily in tablet form after giving a suitable coating to the tablets.
6. They are the lightest and the most compact of all dosage forms.
7. Of all the dosage form, tablets are easiest and the cheapest as regard packing and transport.
8. They are better suited to a large scale production as compared with any other unit oral dosage form.
9. These are an economical dosage form.
10. They have longer expiry period due to lower moisture content
11. They are more temper proof in comparison to capsule.

Disadvantages of Tablets

1. Some drugs resist compression into tablet form due to their amorphous nature or low density character.
2. Bitter tasting drugs, drugs with objectionable odour or drugs that the sensitive to oxygen or atmospheric moisture may require encapsulation or a special type of coating which may increase the cost of the finished tablets.
3. Drugs with poor wetting and slow dissolution properties are difficult to convert into tablets which provide full drug

bioavailability.

4. The tablets cannot be used in case of emergency cases, because the rate at which active ingredient reaches the site to be treated slow.
5. Bioavailability of some drugs may be low due to poor absorption from the gastric tract.

TYPES OF TABLETS

Tablets are classified according to their route of administration or function. The following are the four main classification groups:—

(A) Tablets ingested orally

(*i*) Compressed tablets
(*ii*) Multiple compressed tablets or press coated tablets
(*iii*) Multilayered tablets
(*iv*) Sustained action tablets
(*v*) Enteric coated tablets
(*vi*) Sugar coated tablets
(*vii*) Film coated tablets
(*viii*) Chewable tablets

(B) Tablets used in the oral cavity

(*i*) Buccal tablets
(*ii*) Sublingual tablets
(*iii*) Lozenge tablets and traches
(*iv*) Dental cones

(C) Tablets administered by other routes

(*i*) Implantation tablets
(*ii*) Vaginal tablets

(D) Tablets used to prepare solutions

(*i*) Effervescent tablets
(*ii*) Dispensing tablets
(*iii*) Hypodermic tablets
(*iv*) Tablet triturates

Tablets Ingested Orally

A majority of the tablets manufactured are ingested orally. These tablets are designed to be swallowed as they are except the chewable tablets. The tablets covered in this category are:

Compressed tablets (C.T.) These tablets are uncoated and made by compression of granules. These tablets are usually intended to provide rapid disintegration and drug release. These tablets contain water soluble drugs which after swallowing get disintegrated in the stomach and its drug contents are absorbed in the gastrointestinal tract and distribute in the whole body.

Multiple compressed tablets (M.C.T.) These tablets are prepared to separate physically or chemically incompatible ingredients or to produce repeat-action or prolonged-action products. To avoid incompatibility, the ingredients of the formulation except the incompatible material are compressed into a core tablet and then incompatible substance alongwith necessary excipients are compressed over the previously compressed core tablet. A special type of tablet making machine is used which provides two compressions.

Multilayered tablets These tablets consist of two or more layers of materials compressed successively in the same tablets. The colour of each layer may be the same or different. The tablets having layers of different colours are known as "multicoloured tablets". These tablets are prepared to separate incompatible ingredients physically.

Sustained action tablets These tablets are used to get a sustained action of medicament. These tablets when taken orally release the medicament in a sufficient quantity as and when required to maintain the maximum effective concentration of the drug in the blood throughout the period of treatment. Controlled release of drug helps in getting the desired degree of action. These tablets are gaining popularity these days.

Enteric coated tablets These are compressed tablets meant for administration by swallowing and are designed to bypass the stomach and get disintegrated in the intestines only. These tablets are made to release the drug undiluted and in the highest concentration possible within the intestine. *e.g.* tablets containing anthelmentics and amoebicides.

Sugar coated tablets The compressed tablets having a sugar coating are called "sugar coated tablets". Sugar coating is done to mark the bitter and unpleasant odour and the taste of the medicament. The sugar coating makes the tablet elegant and it also safe guards the drug from atmospheric effects.

Film coated tablets The compresseu tablets having a film coating of some polymer substance, such as, hydroxypropyl cellulose, hydroxy propylmethyl cellulose and ethyl cellulose. The film coating protects the medicament from atmospheric effects. Film coated tablets are generally tasteless, having little increase in the tablet weight and have less elegance than that of sugar coated tablets.

Chewable tablets These tablets are chewed in the mouth and broken into smaller pieces. In this way, the disintegration time is reduced and the rate of absorption of the medicament is increased *e.g.* aluminium hydroxide tablets and phenolphthalein tablets.

(B) Tablets Used in Oral Cavity

The following types of tablets come under this category:

Buccal tablets These tablets are to be placed in the buccal pouch or between the gums and lips or cheek where they dissolve or disintegrate slowly and are absorbed directly without passing into the alimentary canal *e.g.* tablets of ethisterone.

Sublingual tablets These tablets are to be placed under the tongue where they dissolve or disintegrate quickly and are absorbed directly without passing into G.I.T. *e.g.* tablets of glyceryl trinitrite.

Lozenge tablets and troches These tablets are designed to exert a local effect in the mouth or throat. These tablets are commonly used to treat sore throat or to control coughing in common cold. They may contain local anaesthetics antiseptic, antibacterial agents, astringents and antitussives. These are prepared by compression at a high pressure or by the moulding process and generally contain a sweetening agent, a flavouring agent and a substance which produces a cooling effect alongwith medicaments.

Dental cones These are relatively minor compressed tablets meant for placing them in the empty sockets after tooth extraction. They prevent the multiplication of bacteria in the socket following such extraction by using slow-releasing antibacterial compounds or to reduce bleeding by containing the astringent. These tablets contain an excipient like lactose, sodium bicarbonate and sodium chloride etc. These cones generally get dissolved in 20 to 40 minutes time.

(C) Tablets Administered by other Routes

The tablets covered under this category are:

Implantation tablets These tablets are placed under the skin or inserted subcutaneously by means of minor surgical operation and are slowly absorbed. These may be made by heavy compression but are normally made by fusion. The implants must be sterile and should be packed individually in sterile condition. Implants are mainly used for administration of hormones such as testosterone and deoxycorticosterone etc.

Vaginal tablets These tablets are meant to dissolve slowly in the vaginal cavity. The tablets are typically ovoid or pear shaped to facilitate retention in the vagina. This tablet form is used to release steroids, antibacterial agents, antiseptics or astringents to treat vaginal infections. The tablets are often buffered to promote a pH favourable to the action of a specified antiseptic agent. They contain excipients, such as, lactose or sodium bicarbonate.

(D) Tablets used to Prepare Solutions

The following types of tablets come under this category:

Effervescent tablets These tablets when added in water produce effervescence. So they dissolved rapidly in water due to the chemical reaction which takes place between alkali bicarbonate and citric acid or tartaric acid or combination of both. These tablets are to be protected from atmospheric moisture during storage. So, these tablets should be stored in well-closed air tight containers.

Dispensing tablets This type of tablets are intended to be added to a given volume of water to produce a solution of a given concentration. The medicaments commonly incorporated in dispensing these tablets include mild silver proteinate, bichloride of mercury merbromin and quaternary ammonium compounds. These tablets contain excipient which gets dissolved quickly to form a clear solution. These tablets are highly toxic if taken orally by mistake. So, great care must be taken in the packaging and labelling of such tablets in order to prevent their misuse.

Hypodermic tablets These are compressed tablets which are composed of one or more drugs with readily water soluble ingredients. These tablets are dissolved in sterile water or water for injection and administered by parenteral route. So, special precautions are needed to be taken during their preparation. These tablets however are not preferred nowadays as there are chances that the solution prepared from hypodermic tablets may be a non-sterile.

Tablet triturates These are small tablets usually cylindrical, moulded or compressed, and contain a potent medicament with a diluent. On a small scale, tablet triturates are prepared by using hand-operated tablet triturates moulds but for bulk production, automatic tablet triturate machines are used.

MANUFACTURING OF COMPRESSED TABLETS

The following steps are involved during the manufacturing of compressed tablets:

I. Preparation of granules for compression : It includes—
   (*a*) Weighing the ingredients
   (*b*) Mixing the powdered ingredients and excipients
   (*c*) Converting the mixed ingredients into granules

II. Compression of granules into tablets.

III. Coating of tablets

IV. Quality control of tablets.

1. Preparation of Granules for Compression

The following steps are involved during the preparation of granules:

(*a*) Weighing of the ingredients : The ingredients should be weighed accurately using a balance of good quality. There should be a double check on the weighing in order to rule out any human error.

(*b*) Mixing the powdered ingredients and excipients : The main objective of mixing the medicaments and excipients is to prepare a homogeneous mass, so that uniform tablets can be manufactured. Mixing of ingredients should be done in an ascending order of their weight.

(*c*) Converting the mixed ingredients into granules : The crystalline medicament can be compressed to get good quality compressed tablets. In case the medicaments alongwith excipients are in powder from it cannot be compressed as such into tablets because:

TABLE 14-1

Fine powder	*Granules*
1. Fine powder does not flow evenly through the hopper of the tablet machine. Hence, the irregular supply of fine powder into the die of the tablet machine produces tablets of different weight.	1. Granules flow evenly through the hopper of the tablet machine. Hence tablets of uniform weight are produced.
2. In case of powder containing different ingredients the vibration of the tablet machine would help in its separation. The powder of high density forms an upper layer. So, it is not possible to get tablets of uniform composition.	2. The granules may be bigger or smaller but are uniform in composition. The ingredients are bound together and cannot separate. Therefore, separation of smaller granules at the bottom is not going to change the composition of the tablets.
3. Air is imprisoned during compression and may cause capping. Tablets are also broken down during transportation and handling.	3. Granules have more knitting power. Hence, on compression, the granules form a sound tablet.
4. Fine powder tends to blow out of the die and causes sticking of machine.	4. The granules being heavier, do not blow out of the die and therefore do not stick to the machine.

The granules can be prepared by the following methods:

1. Moist granulation method : This is the most widely used method of preparing granules. The powdered medicaments alongwith other excipients, such as, diluent, binding agent and a part of the disintegrating agent are moistened with a sufficient quantity of granulating agent in order to make a coherent mass. The coherent mass is then passed through sieve No. 8 or 10. If the mass sticks to the wire of the sieve it indicates over moistening. The wet granules are spread in trays and dried at 60°C in a hot air oven. The dried granules are passed through sieve number 20 to collect the granules of uniform size. The lubricating agent, any volatile substance and the remaining part of the disintegrating agent are mixed. These granules are then ready to be compressed.

2. Dry granulation : There are certain medicaments which are available in crystalline form or in the form of granules having its own binding property. Such medicaments are passed through sieve No. 20 or any other specified sieve and then mixed with any additional excipient. This method is used for making tablets of aspirin, sodium bromide, potassium chlorate and dried yeast etc.

3. Granules by preliminary compression : This method is also known as the "slugging method". The method is used in those cases where the medicament is unstable in presence of moisture.

In this process the dry powder is compressed into large tablets or "slugs". These slugs are broken into small pieces which are passed through a specified sieve to collect the granules of suitable size. A lubricating agent and a disintegrating agent are mixed with these granules before compression into the tablet machine.

Excipients used in formulation of tablets An excipient is an inert substance which is added along with medicaments to prepare the granules from the solid medicaments.

The following are some of the excipients which are generally required in the formulation of tablets:

1. Diluents
2. Granulating agents
3. Binding agents
4. Disintegrating agents
5. Lubricants
6. Adsorbents
7. Colouring agents, Flavouring agents and Sweetening agents.

1. Diluent : The diluent is needed in the formulation of a tablet, when the quantity of medicament in each tablet is very small and it is not possible to make a good tablet. The commonly used diluents are lactose, sucrose, sodium chloride, dextrose and starch, mannitol, sorbitol, dibasic calcium phosphate dihydrate and calcium sulphate dihydrate.

2. Granulating agents : These are used to convent the fine powder into granules. A granulating agent provided proper moisture to convert fine powder into damp mass, which after passing through a sieve of suitable number forms granules. The various granulating agents used are water, alcohol, mucilage of starch, mucilage of acacia, mucilage of tragacanth, gelatin solution, iso-propyl alcohol, acetone etc.

3. Binding agents : These are used in granulation to provide proper strength to the granules, in order to keep the tablet intact after compression. The various binding agents used are gum acacia powder, gum tragacanth, gelatin, sucrose, methyl cellulose etc. Binding agents are used along with granulating agents. The selection of proper binding agent and its concentration depends on the type of the tablets for which it is used. In lozenge tablets and implants the proportion of binding agent has to be very high, whereas in other cases where the tablets has to disintegrate quickly a binding agent with less binding property and in lower concentration is used.

4. Disintegrating agents : The substances which are added in the tablet formulation to ensure disintegrating of the tablets into smaller particles when swallowed are called Disintegrating Agents. These are added into the formulation of or oral tablets or sublingual tablets. When the medicament is insoluble in water a disintegrating agent is needed.

Disintegrating agents act in three ways:

(*i*) *By swelling* : Disintegrating agent gets swelled when it comes in contact with water or moisture *e.g.* potato starch, maize starch, wheat starch, methyl cellulose and bentonite. Potato starch is superior to other starches but maize starch is commonly used because it is very cheap.

(*ii*) *By producing effervescence* : They produce effervescence when they come in contact with moisture *e.g.* sodium bicarbonate, citric acid and tartaric acid.

(*iii*) They melt at body temperature *e.g.* cocabutter.

The disintegrating agent is generally divided into two parts. One part is mixed along with other excipients before the formation of granules. The other part is mixed with the dry granules before compression.

5: Lubricants : These are added to improve the appearance of tablets, flow properties of granules and to prevent the sticking of the materials to the dies and punches. On the basis of their function, the lubricants are divided into three groups.

(*i*) *Lubricants* : These are the substances that reduce interparticular friction during compression and friction between tablet and die wall during the ejection of tablet *e.g.* talc, magnesium stearate and calcium stearate etc.

(*ii*) *Glidants* : They improve the flow properties of the granules from hopper to die of the tablet machine *e.g.* talc, sodium chloride, magnesium stearate, boric acid, starch and calcium stearate.

(*iii*) *Anti-adhesive agents* : These prevent the sticking of tablet surface to dies and punches during compression *e.g.* liquid paraffin, magnesium stearate and stearate acid etc.

6. Adsorbing agents : These substances are used to adsorb volatile oil, liquid extract and tincture etc. which are included in the formulation of tablets. The commonly used adsorbents are magnesium carbonate, kaolin and starch.

7. Colours, flavours and sweetening agents : Colours of approved, certified F.D. and C dyes are used. The colours are used to improve the elegance of the tablet. The colours are added to the solution of the granulating agent or these are mixed with other ingredients before granulation.

Flavours are included in lozenges, effervescent tablets and chewable tablets. Flavours are volatile oils and hence they are added into the granules just before compression of tablets. Flavouring agent is dissolved in organic solvent and the solution is sprayed on the granules.

Sweetening agents are used to improve the taste of tablets. These are used in lozenges and chewable tablets. Artificial sweetening agents like saccharin and cyclamates, are not used nowadays. Sucrose, lactose and mannitol are some of the commonly used sweetening agents.

II. Compression of Granules into Tablets

The dried granules are compressed into tablets in a machine known as a tablet making machine. The various type of machines used for this purpose, are:

1. Single punch tablet machine which may be hand-operated or electrically operated
2. Multipunch tablet machine
3. Rotary tablet machine
4. Dry cota tablet machine

In all these tablet machines the compression is achieved by filling the required quantity of granules into the dies and then compressing them in between the lower punch and the upper punch. The single punch machine is used for small scale manufacturing, whereas the other machines are used for a large scale manufacturing. Rotary machines, having about 70 sets of dies produce about 1200 tablets in one minute.

1. Single punch tablet machine : The single punch tablet machine has the following major parts as shown in Fig. 14-1.

(*a*) *Hopper shoe* : To supply the granules to the die and remove the tablet after its compression.

(*b*) *Lower punch*

(*c*) *Upper punch*

(*d*) *Capacity regulator* : To adjust the position of the lower punch to accommodate the required quantity of granule by the die.

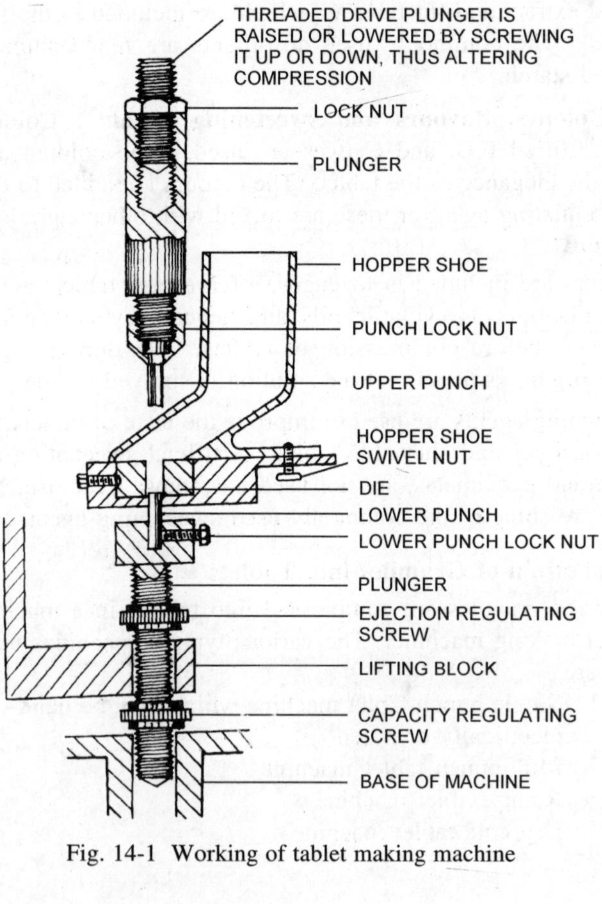

Fig. 14-1 Working of tablet making machine

(*e*) *Ejection regulator* : To adjust the position of the lower punch, so that its highest position is at par with the surface of the die.

(*f*) *Die* : It allows the lower punch and the upper punch to come close together to compress the granules.

(*g*) *Driving wheel* : It helps in the movements of the lower punch, the upper punch and the hopper shoe and also check their movements.

Working of a tablet making machine Several movements take place at a time to form a tablet in a tablet making machine. The cycle of movements is shown in Fig. 14-2.

1. The upper punch rises to allow the hopper shoe to move over the die.
2. The lower punch drops and the granules feed from the shoe into the die. The shaking movement of shoe helps in the flow of granules.
3. The shoe moves aside and the upper punch drops, thus compressing the granules into a tablet.
4. The upper punch rises upward and the lower punch rises upto the surface of the dies to eject the tablet.

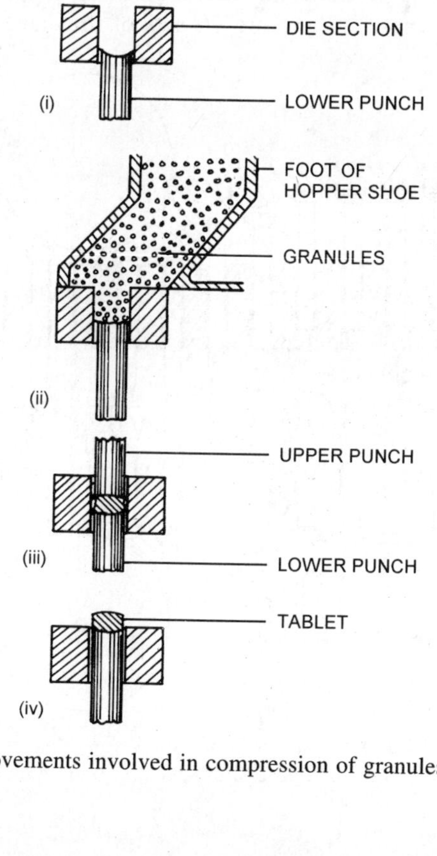

Fig. 14-2 Movements involved in compression of granules into tablets.

5. The hopper shoe again moves forward over the dies, pushing aside the newly formed tablet.
6. The lower punch drops and the cycle is restarted.

The tablet making machine is adjusted for ejection of tablets, capacity and compression. When these adjustments are done, the adjusting screws are locked in position. The machine is then ready for compression of the granules into tablets. It is necessary to check at regular intervals the setting of the tablet making machine during the course of the compression of granules into tablets on a large scale manufacturing.

2. Multi-punch tablet machine : In a multi-punch tablet machine, there are 2 to 12 dies on a big platform. The number of punches depends upon the number of dies fixed to the platform. The working of this machine is similar to that of a single punch machine but in this machine in one stroke as many tablets are compressed as the number of dies instead of just one tablet as in a single punch machine.

3. Rotary tablet machine : A rotary tablet machine is used for large scale economic production. In this machine about 1200 tablets are prepared in one minute. There are 70 sets of dies and punches, in this type of machine.

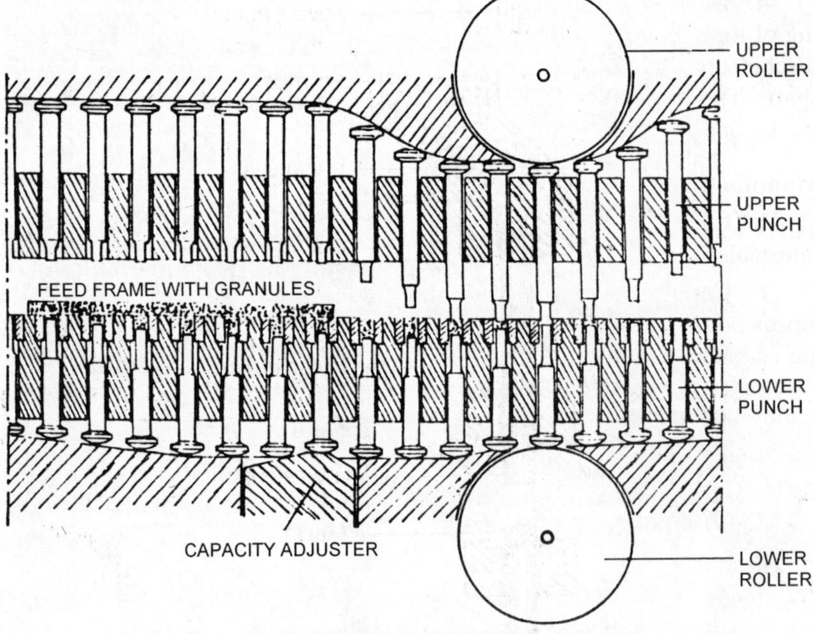

Fig. 14-3 Diagram of punch tracks of rotary tablet machine opened out to show cycle of one revolution

A rotary tablet machine has a circular rotating head, carrying a number of punch and dies assembles. The head revolves continuously while the tablet granulation runs from the hopper through a feed frame and into the dies placed in a large steel plate revolving under it. There is a uniform filling of the die due to this arrangement and therefore the tablets formed in rotary tablet machines have an accurate uniform weight. The compression of granules takes place as the upper and the lower punches pass between a pair of rollers. The tablet comes out when the lower punch lifts up.

Working Fix the upper punches and lower punches and dies in the rotary tablet machine. The feed frame is attached to the machine along with the feed hopper and the machine is adjusted for tablet weight and hardness. Fill the hopper with the granules. When the machine starts, the hopper delivers the granules to the feed frame placed over the central part containing the dies. The object of the feed frame is to confine the granules in position immediately over the die track. As the head revolves, the dies come under the feed frame in succession and are filled. These granules get compressed when the upper and the lower punch come close together. The cycle of events in one revolution of the rotary head is shown in Fig. 14-3.

4. Drycota tablet machine : The machine is used for manufacturing of multi-compressed, multi-coloured and press-coated tablets. In this machine two rotary machines work simultaneously by a single driven shaft. The core tablet is prepared in one machine which is transferred to the second machine for compress coating.

Manufacturing Defects in Tablets

The following defects may occur during the compression of granules into tablets.

1. Capping : In this case there is partial or complete removal of top or bottom portion of the tablet. The reasons for this defect usually are as under:

(*i*) Excessive fines in granules which entrap air in a tablet
(*ii*) Defective punches and dies
(*iii*) High speed of the tablet machine
(*iv*) The granules are too dry
(*v*) There is an usually high degree of compression

These defects can be removed by:

(*i*) Setting the dies and punches properly.
(*ii*) To reduce the percentage of fines.

(*iii*) Punches should be either buffed or polished before its use. Defective punches should be replaced.

(*iv*) Maintain the desired moisture content level in granules.

(*v*) Regulate the speed of tablet machine.

(*vi*) Regulate the pressure on the punches so as to maintain a proper degree of compression.

2. Picking and sticking : In picking the material is removed or picked up by the upper punch from the upper surface of the tablet. In case of sticking, the material sticks to the wall of the die. These defects appear due to the following reasons:

(*i*) Use of worn out dies and punches

(*ii*) Use of small quantity of lubricants

(*iii*) Presence of moisture in the granules

(*iv*) Excess of powder in the granules

(*v*) Scratches on the surface of the face of the punch

(*vi*) Defects in the formulation

These defects can be removed by using:

(*i*) A new set of die and punches

(*ii*) A proper quantity of lubricants in the granules

(*iii*) Dry granules

3. Mottling : Mottling means an unequal distribution of colour on the surface of a coloured tablets. This defect occurs due to the following reasons:

(*i*) Migration of dye in the granules during the process of drying

(*ii*) Use of different coloration of medicament and excipients

These defects can be avoided by:

(*i*) Drying the granules at a low temperature

(*ii*) Using the dye which can mask the colour of all the ingredients of tablet formulation

4. Weight variation : During the compression of granules in a tablet machine, the tablets do not have a uniform weight. Generally, following are the reasons for this defect:

(*i*) Granules are not uniform in size

(*i*) Presence of excess amount of powder in the granules

(*iii*) No proper mixing of lubricants

(*iv*) No uniform flow of granules from the hopper to the die

(*v*) During the course of compression of granules there is a change in the capacity of the die (*vi*) Variation in the speed of the tablet machine

These defects can be avoided by correcting and checking the above-mentioned points.

5. Hardness variation : Hardness variation is a problem having the same causes as weight variation. In this case, the tablets do not have a uniform hardness. Hardness depends on the weight of the material and the space between the upper and the lower punches during the stage of compression. If the volume of the material varies or the distance between punches varies, the hardness will also vary.

6. Double impression : This defect occurs when the lower punch has a monogram or some other engraving on it. During compression, the tablet receives an imprint of the punch. Due to some defect in the machine, the lower punch moves slightly upward before ejection of a tablet and gives a second, though light, imprint on the tablet. This defect can be removed by controlling the undesirable movement of the lower punch.

III. Coating of Tablets ▩

Tablets are coated for the following purposes:

1. To mask the unpleasant taste and odour.
2. To improve the appearance of tablets.
3. To prevent the medicament from atmospheric effects.
4. To control the site of action of drugs (Enteric coating).
5. To produce the sustained released product.

The tablet coating is generally done by using any of the following processes:

1. Pan coating
2. Press coating

1. Pan coating : In this technique the coating is done in a pan made up of copper or stainless steel. The pan is rotated with the help of an electric motor. The tablets to be coated are placed in the pan. Hot air is blown in. The speed of the pan is adjusted in such a way that the tablet remain separated from each other in the pan. After coating, polishing is done in a polishing pan. Pan coating technique is used for sugar coating, film coating and enteric coating.

2. Press coating : In this technique the granules of coating material are prepared and a layer of coating material is placed on the preformed tablet (below and above the tablet to be coated) in a Drycota Rotary Tablet Machine. The whole operation is carried out automatically in a number of steps.

Sugar Coating

Sugar coating is done by the pan coating method. It is one of the oldest arts to mask the unpleasant flavours and tastes of medicaments, but nowadays sugar coating of tablets is done for improving its aesthetic value. The various stages in the sugar coating process are:

1. Sieving
2. Sealing
3. Subcoating
4. Syrup coating
5. Finishing
6. Polishing.

Sieving The tablets to be coated are shaken in a suitable sieve to remove the fine powder or broken pieces of tablets.

Sealing Sealing is done to ensure that a thin layer of water proof materials, such as, shellac or cellulose acid phthalate is deposited on the surface of the tablets. The shellac or cellulose acid phthalate is dissolved in alcohol or acetone and its several coats are given in a coating pan. A coating pan is made of copper or stainless steel. The pan is rotated with the help of an electric motor. There is an arrangement of hot air to be supplied inside the coating pan. The coating pans are available in different sizes. The speed of the pan is adjusted in such a way that the tablets remain separated from each in the pan.

Nowadays it is possible to do the sealing of tablets by fluidised bed coating or by spraying techniques.

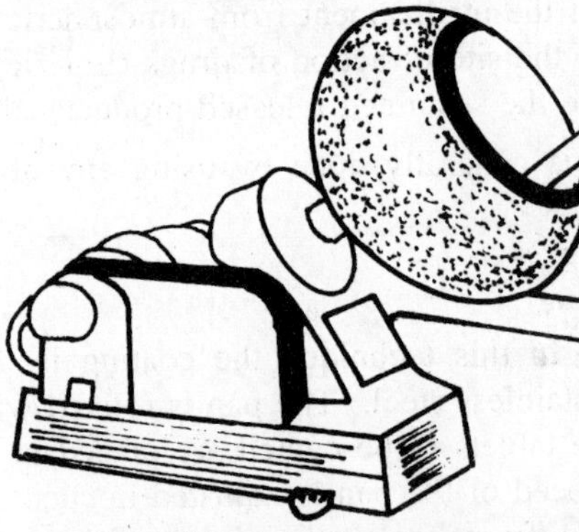

Fig.14-4 Tablet coating pan

Subcoating In subcoating several coats of sugar and other materials, such as, gelatin, acacia etc. are given to round off tablets and to help in building up the tablet size. Several coats of concentrated syrup containing acacia or gelatin are given. After each addition of the syrup, dusting powder is sprinkled. The dusting powder is a mixture of starch, talc and powdered acacia. The dusting powder does not allow the tablets to stick together. The hot air is blown inside the coating pan which is rotated at a suitable speed. This ensures proper drying of the syrup coat and thus prevents the tablets from getting stuck up with each other. The alternative addition of syrup and dusting powder is repeated until a coating of the required thickness is produced. Towards the end of the process, warm syrup without dusting powder is used to obtain a smooth surface.

Syrup coating This is done to give sugar coats, opacity and colour to the tablets. Several coats of the syrup are applied. Colouring materials and opacifying agents are also added to the syrup. The process of coating is repeated until uniform coloured tablets are obtained.

Finishing Three to four coats of syrup are applied in rapid succession without dusting powder and cold air is circulated to dry each coat. This forms a hard smooth coat.

Polishing Beeswax is dissolved in volatile organic solvent and a few coats of it are given. The finished tablets are transferred to a polishing pan which is made of canvas cloth. The polishing pan is rotated at a suitable speed so that the wax coated tablets are rubbed on the canvas cloth. This gives a proper shining to the tablets.

Sugar coating is an art. Only a skilled operator can judge the correct addition of syrup and dusting powder to give uniform coating to the tablets.

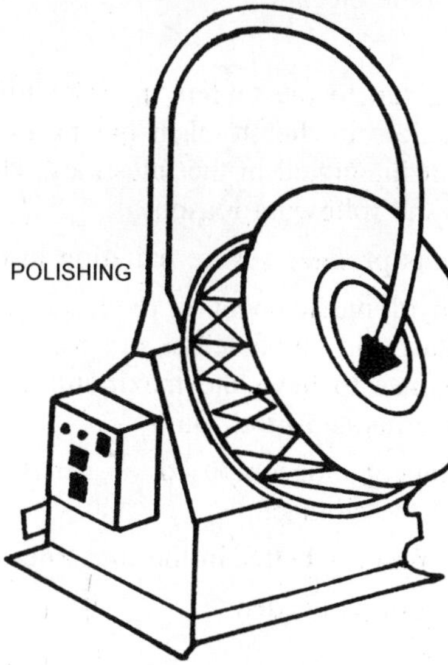

Fig. 14-5 Polishing pan

Film Coating

In this case the tablets are coated by a single or mixture of film forming polymers, such as, hydroxypropyl methylcellulose, hydroxyethyl methyl cellulose, carbowax, polyethylene glycol 400 etc. The polymer is dissolved in some volatile organic solvent and is sprayed over the tablets in a rotating pan. The process is continued till a uniform good film is formed over the tablets.

Film coating is also used to make the tablets water proof before the sugar coating. Film coating can be enteric or non-enteric.

Advantages of Film Coating

1. It is a less time-consuming technique.
2. Not much labour is required.
3. It has no adverse affect on disintegration of tablets.
4. The product cost is low because the material used for coating is quite cheap.
5. It protects the drug from atmospheric changes, such as, light, air and moisture.
6. Coating is resistant to cracking and chipping.
7. Film coating of tablet does not increase the weight of the tablet.
8. No water proof coating is required before the actual film coating.
9. The tablets become elegant.

Enteric Coating

Enteric coating is given to the tablets in order to ensure that these tablets will not disintegrate in the stomach but pass through it as they are. Such tablets get disintegrated in the intestines. This type of special coating is done-due to the following reasons:

1. Medicaments produce severe irritation in the stomach
2. The action of medicament is required in the intestine *e.g.* anthelmintics and amoebicides are required to be absorbed from intestines to have the maximum effect at the site of parasitic worms and protozoa
3. Medicaments get decomposed or destroyed by the acidic medium of the stomach
4. Drug absorption is better in the intestines
5. Delayed action is needed

An ideal enteric coating material has the following properties:

1. Resistance to gastric fluids
2. Non-toxic in the required quantity
3. Economical
4. Ease of application without specialized equipment
5. Compatible with the drug on which coating is done
6. Formation of a continuous film
7. The film of the coating material should not change on aging
8. Ready susceptibility to intestinal fluids

On a large scale, the enteric coating of tablets is done in a rotating pan. Solution of enteric coating material, such as, salol, cellulose acetate phthalate, shellac and its derivatives are prepared in a volatile organic solvent. The solution is sprayed over the tablets which are rotated in the coating pan. The hot air is blown into the pan which helps in the evaporation of organic solvent. Hence, a fine film of enteric coated material is made over the tablets. The process is repeated a number of times till the required number of coatings are done.

Microencapsulation

Microencapsulation is a process or technique by which thin coating can be applied to small particles of solids, droplets of liquids or dispersion, thus forming microcapsules. The microcapsules may consist of a single particle or clusters of particles. It differs from other coating methods because microencapsulation process is used to coat the particles having a particle size range from several tenths of a micro to 5000 μ.

Microencapsulation Techniques

There are a number of methods of microencapsulation which are reported in the literature. These are based on:

(*a*) Chemical processes in which there is a chemical or phase change.

(*b*) Mechanical processes in which there is a physical change in the system by using special equipment.

The following techniques are commonly used for microencapsulation:

1. Pan coating
2. Fluidised bed coating
3. Coacervation
4. Electrostatic deposition
5. Vacuum deposition
6. Polymerisation
7. Multiorific centrifugal process.

Pan coating This technique is suitable in those cases where the particle size is larger than 600 μ. The medicaments are charged on to spherical pellets of sugar which are then coated with a coating material in a coating pan. The coating material is dissolved in a suitable volatile organic solvent and sprayed in the pan. Hot air is circulated in the pan simultaneously in order to speed up the drying process. The process can be repeated if a subsequent coat is needed.

Fluidised bed coating In this method the particles of the solid core material are suspended in the turbulent current of air in a chamber. The solution of coating material is prepared in the volatile solvent and atomised in the chamber through nozzles. The temperature of the air inside the chamber is regulated in such a way that the volatile solvent gets vaporised. After coating, the solid particles become quite heavy and fall on the screen near the outlet from where these can be removed after suitable intervals. The thickness of the coat depends on particle size of core material, concentration and velocity of air and its temperature.

Coacervation Coacervation means the separation of a liquid or phase when solution of two hydrophilic colloids are mixed under suitable conditions. In this method, the three immiscible phases of core material, solvent and coating material are formed followed by deposition of coating material on the core. The coating material is dissolved in a suitable solvent and the core material is uniformly dispersed in the solution of the coating material. Then the coating material is phased out of its solution which starts getting deposited on the particles of the core material.

Electrostatic deposition The method is useful both for solid particles and liquid droplets. In this process, the core and coating materials are electrically charged by means of high voltage such as 10,000 volts etc. The core is charged and placed in the coating chamber. The coating material is also charged before it is sprayed as a mist. Because the charges are of opposite kind, the coating material gets deposited on the core due to electrostatic attraction.

Vacuum deposition In this method the coating material is vaporised in a chamber under vacuum of the order of 10^{-2} to 10^{-5} mm, in which the core material is present. The coating material gets deposited on the core particles.

Polymerisation This is a relatively new technique and is becoming popular with the drug manufacturers. In this technique the core material is dispersed in a liquid or a gas in which monomeric units of the coating material are present. These monomers get polymerised at the interface between the core particles and the liquid gas phase which form coats over the core.

Multi-orifice centrifugal process This is a mechanical process for producing microcapsules. The method is capable of microencapsulating liquids and solids. The particles of the core materials are forced through an envelope of coating material in solution by using centrifugal force. This results in a mechanical microencapsulation of the core particles.

Applications of Microencapsulation Process

1. It is used for masking the taste of bitter drugs.
2. It is used for preparing prolonged action dosage form.
3. It is used in modifying the physical characters of a material required in certain formulations.
4. The technique is used to separate an incompatible material.
5. It is used to protect chemicals against moisture and oxidation.

IV. Evaluation of Tablets

The following tests should be carried to maintain the quality control of tablets:

1. Shape of tablets
2. Appearance
3. Content of active ingredient in tablets
4. Uniformity of weight
5. Disintegration test for tablets
6. Dissolution test for tablets
7. Mechanical strength
8. Friability test

1. Shape of tablets : In the pharmacopoeia the shape of a tablet is defined as circular with flat or convex faces.

2. Appearance : When a broken section of an uncoated tablet is examined under a lens, either a relatively uniform texture (single-layer tablets) or a stratified structure (multi-layer tablets) is seen. There should be no signs of coating.

Coated tablets have a smooth and often coloured surface.

3. Content of active ingredient in tablets : The amount of active ingredient in tablet is determined by doing the assay as stated in the monograph. Generally 20 tablets or such other number as may be indicated in the monograph are used in the assay. The result lies within the range for the content of active ingredient stated in the monograph. Where 20 tablets cannot be obtained, a smaller number, which must not be less than 5, may be used. In such cases, the limits specified in the

TABLE 14.2

Weight of medicament in each tablet	*Subtract from the lower limit for sample of*			*Add to the upper limit for sample of*		
	15	10	5	15	10	5
0.12 g or less	0.2	0.7	1.6	0.3	0.8	1.8
More than 0.12 g and less than 0.3 g	0.2	0.5	1.2	0.3	0.6	1.5
0.3 g or more	0.1	0.2	0.8	0.2	0.4	1.0

monograph may be relaxed to the extent indicated in Table 14-2. The requirements of this Table apply when the stated limits are between 90 and 110 per cent. For limits less than 90 or greater than 110 per cent proportionately a larger allowance is to be made.

4. Uniformity of weight : It is desirable that every individual tablet in a batch should be uniform in weight, but a small variation in the weight of the individual tablet is liable to occur. Therefore a litter variation is allowed in the weight of a tablet by the pharmacopœia. The following percentage deviation in weight variation is allowed.

Weigh 20 tablets selected at random and determine their average weight. Not more than 2 of the individual weights may deviate from the average weight by more than the percentage deviation given in the Table 14-3 and none should deviate by more than twice that percentage.

TABLE 14-3

S.No.	*Average weight of a tablet deviation*	*Percentage*
1.	80 mg or less	10
2.	More than 80 mg and less than 250 mg	7.5
3.	250 mg or more	5

5. Uniformity of content : Tablets must comply with the requirements for uniformity of content specified in the individual monograph. Percentage of medicament is calculated by doing assay for a particular drug, the method of which is given in the pharmacopoeia against its monograph. The variation in percentage of medicament per tablet is due to the following reasons:

1. Weighing of materials before granulation
2. During the process of granulation
3. Variation in the weight of an individual tablet

4. Error of random sampling
5. Analysis error
6. Purity of medicament

As per the pharmacopœia, 20 tablets are taken, powdered and assayed. The average weight of medicament present in each tablet is calculated which is then compared with the desired weight. The pharmacopœia has prescribed the limit in percentage of medicament per tablet in the monograph.

6. Disintegration test for tablet : Disintegration of a tablet means to break the tablet into smaller particles after swallowing. The time required to disintegrate the tablet is called "Disintegration Time". The rate of disintegration depends upon the type of the tablet. The tablets which are dissolved by slow solution in the mouth or chewed or are to be dissolved in water before administration, do not need a disintegration test. The test of disintegration is required in tablets which are swallowed. The rate of disintegration differs from tablet to tablet because the nature of the drug. In some cases the disintegration time is as short as one minute and in other cases it may be as long as 30 mts. In general, Pharmacopœia prescribed a limited of 15 mts. for most of the tablets, unless otherwise indicated in the monograph.

The official disintegration test is as follows:—

The disintegration test apparatus as per I.P. specification is used for performing the test (Fig. 14-6). The apparatus consists of:

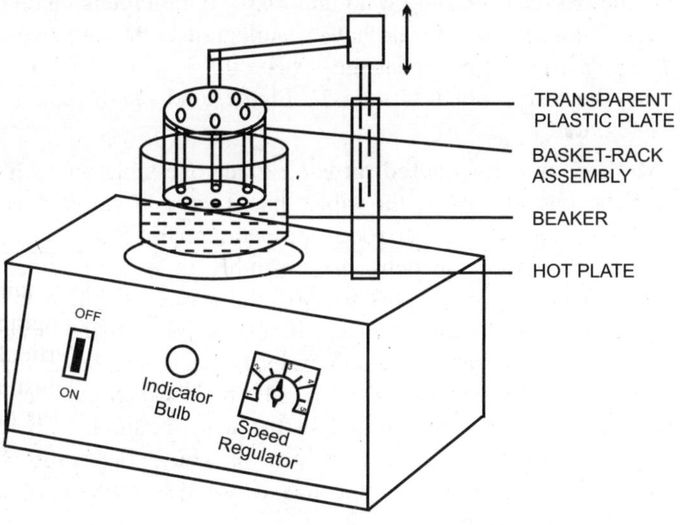

Fig 14-6 The disintegration test apparatus I.P. '85

A rigid basket-rack assembly supporting six cylindrical glass tubes. These tubes are held vertically by two superimposed transparent plastic plates with six holes having the same diameter as the tubes. These holes are at an equal distance from the centre of the plate and are equally spaced from one another. Woven wire gauze made from stainless steel is attached to the underside of the lower plate. The upper and lower plates are held in position by vertical metal rods at the periphery and a metal rod in the centre of the upper plate for attachment to a mechanical device. The assembly should be raised and lowered between 28 to 32 times per minute in the liquid at 37°C.

The tablets are kept immersed in the liquid within the tubes by means of cylindrical guides discs. A cylindrical disc is made of transparent plastic having thickness of 9.5 mm and a diameter of 20.7 mm

The assembly is suspended in the liquid medium in a 1000 ml beaker. The beaker may be filled in such a way that the wire mesh at the highest point is at least 25 mm below the surface of the liquid and its lowest point is at least 25 mm above the bottom of the beaker.

A separate method is used for each type of tablet, the detail of which is given below:

(*1*) Method used for uncoated tablets : Place one tablet in each of the 6 tubes of the basket. Add a disc to each tube and operate the apparatus, using water maintained at 37°±2° as the immersion liquid. At the end of 15 mts or after the time specified in the individual monograph, lift the basket from the liquid and observe the tablets. The tablets pass the test if all the size tablets have disintegrated. In case one or two tablets fail to disintegrate, repeat the test on 12 additional tablets. The tablets pass the test if not less than 16 of the total of 18 tablets tested have disintegrated.

(*2*) Method used for coated tablets : Place one tablet in each of the 6 tubes of the basket, and if the tablet has a soluble external coating, immerse the basket in water at room temperature for 5 minutes. Then add a disc to each tube, suspend the assembly in water maintained at 37°±2° and operate the apparatus for 60 minutes or as indicated in the monograph. The tablets pass the test if all six have disintegrated. In case any of the tablets has not disintegrated, repeat the test on further 6 tablets replacing water with 0.1 *N* HCl. The tablets then pass the test if all the six tablets have disintegrated in the acid medium. The test is repeated on 12 additional tablets if one or two tablets still fail to disintegrate. The sample passes the test if not less than 16 of the 18 tablets tested get disintegrated.

***(3)* Method used for enteric-coated tablets :** Place one table in a each of the six tubes of the basket. Immerse the basket in water for 5 minutes at room temperature in case the tablet has a soluble external coating. Operate the apparatus without using disc for two hours. The basket is immersed in 0.1 *N* HCl maintained at 37°±2°. If no tablet shows signs of disintegration or cracks, then add a disc to each tube and operate the apparatus using mixed phosphate buffer having pH 6.8 as the immersion liquid maintained at 37°±2°. After 60 minutes, remove the assembly from the liquid and observe the tablets. The tablets pass the test if all the six tablets have disintegrated. The test is repeated on 12 additional tablets in case one or two tablets fail to disintegrate. The tablets pass the test if not less than 16 of the total 18 tablets tested get disintegrated.

7. Dissolution test for tablets : The test is done for measuring the amount of time required for a given percentage of the drug substance in a tablet to go into solution under specified condition in vitro. The apparatus used for the test is as per specification given in I.P.

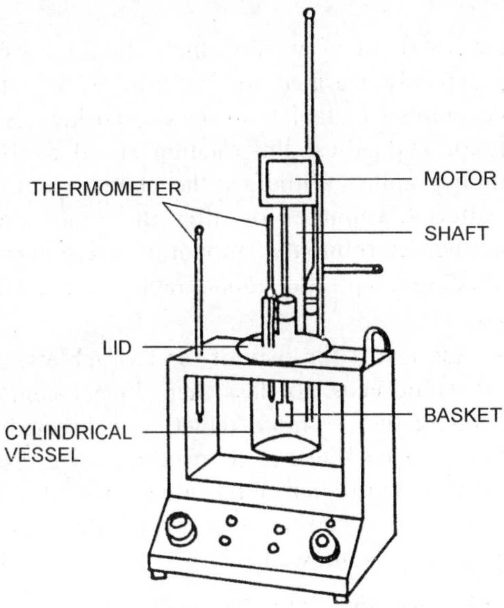

Fig. 14-7 Dissolution test apparatus

Apparatus It consists of the following parts:

1. A cylindrical covered vessel made of glass or other transparent material having 1000 ml capacity. The vessel is fitted with a lid having

four holes, one for having the shaft of the stirrer, second for placing the thermometer and remaining two for removing the sample.

2. An electric motor which is capable of rotating the basket in the vessel at varied speed between 25 and 150 revolutions per minute. The shaft is so adjusted that it enables the basket to revolve smoothly without much wobble.

3. A cylindrical stainless steel basket made of woven wire cloth having an aperture size of 425 µm. For use with dilute acid media, the basket may be coated with gold. The top of the basket is attached to the disc on the driving shafter.

4. The vessel is equipped with a suitable device for the withdrawal of the samples of the dissolution medium. The method of sampling should not interfere excessively with the normal pattern of flow of the dissolution medium in the apparatus.

5. The vessel should be securely clamped in a water bath maintained at 37°±0.5° having an arrangement for smooth motion of water during the test.

Method Place 1000 ml of water which should be free from dissolved air and previously warmed to 36.5° to 37.5° into the vessel. Place the specified number of tablets in the dry basket. Set the apparatus. Start the motor and adjust the rotation speed to 100 rpm or as directed in the monograph. Withdraw the stated volume of solution from the vessel after 45 minutes or after the time specified in the monograph. Filter and determine the amount of active ingredient present in it by the method given in the monograph. Repeat the complete operation 4 times.

The tablets pass the test if for each of the five tablets, the amount of active ingredient in solution is not less than 70 per cent of the stated amount. In case where two or more tablets are directed to be placed together in the basket for each test in the five replicate test, the amount of active ingredient in solution per tablet in each test should not be less than 70 per cent of the stated amount or of that specified in the monograph. No re-testing is allowed.

8. Mechanical strength : The Pharmacopœia has not fixed any standard for the mechanical strength or hardness of tablets. The manufacturers have employed their own tests to ensure that their tablets will withstand the normal risk of handling and transportation.

The following devices are commonly used by manufacturers to find out the mechanical strength of tablets:

(*1*) Monsanto hardness tester
(2) Pfizer tablet hardness tester

(*1*) Monsanto hardness tester : The Monsanto Chemical Co. Ltd had designed spring-pressure device to test the hardness of a tablet. It has a graduated scale which gives the reading in Kg/Sq cm. The tablet to be tested is placed between the spindle and the anvil. The desired pressure needed to hold the tablet in position is applied by moving the screw knob in clockwise direction. The scale is moved so that the indicator is fixed at zero. The pressure is then applied till the tablet breaks. The reading is noted, which indicates the pressure which is needed to break the tablet.

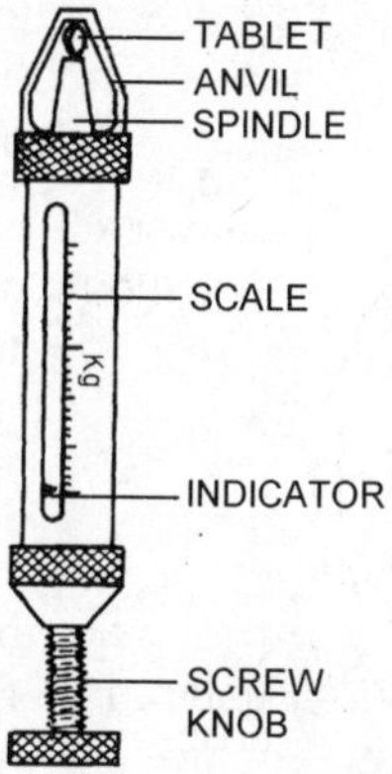

Fig. 14-8 Monsanto hardness tester

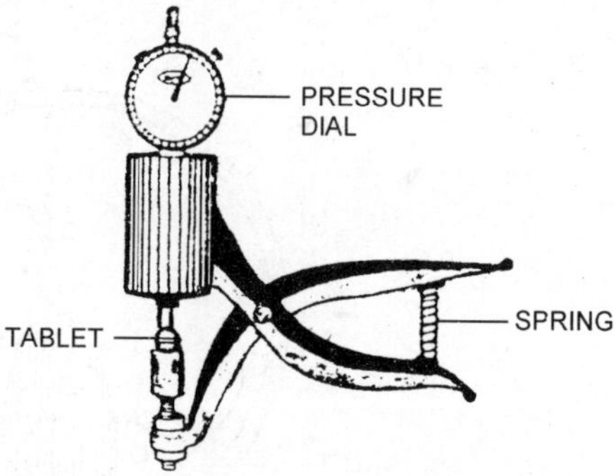

Fig. 14-9 Pfizer tablets hardness tester

(2) Pfizer tablet hardness tester : It is bases on the principle of an ordinary plier. Pfizer tablet hardness tester is a plier fitted with a pressure dial. The tablet is placed between the jaw of the plier and pressure is applied by pressing the handles with hand unit until the tablet breaks. The reading of the dial indicates the pressure needed to break the tablet.

9. Friability test : Normally during the course of compression of tablets a sufficient pressure is applied on the granules, so that the tablets can withstand the wear and tear during transportation and handling. But inspite of observing all the precautions, the tablets show considerable powdering after normal handling, giving an undesirable appearance. Friability test is performed to evaluate the ability of the tablet to withstand wear and tear in packing, handling and transporting. The apparatus used to perform this test is known as "Friabilator".

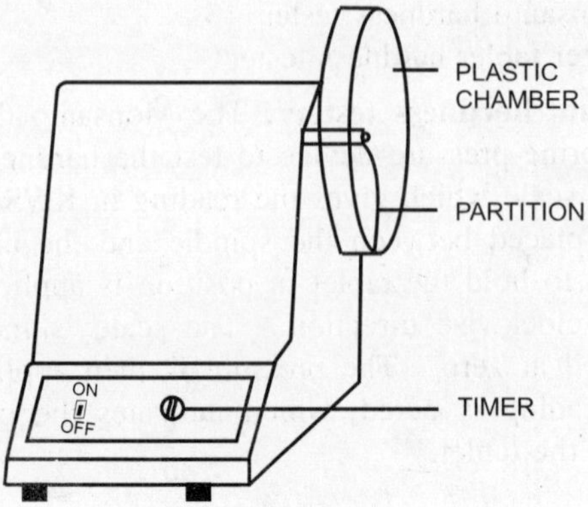

Friabilator

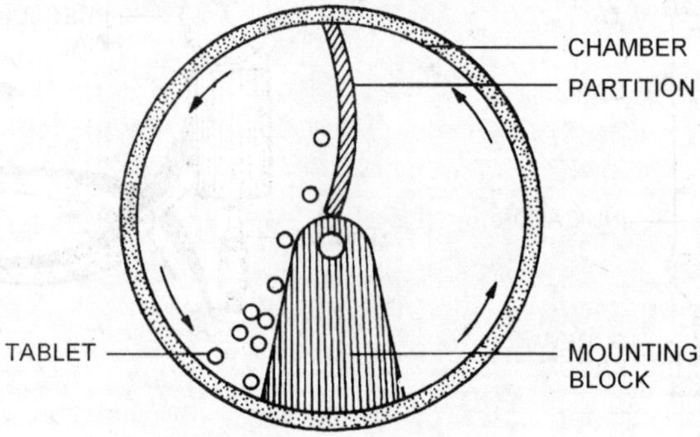

Plastic chamber of friabilator

Fig.14-10 Friabilator

The apparatus consists of a plastic chamber, which is divided into two parts and it revolves at a speed of 25 r.p.m. Twenty tablets are weighed and placed in the plastic chamber. The chamber is rotated for 4 minutes or 100 revolutions. During each revolution the tablet falls from a distance of 6 inch. The tablets are removed for the chamber after 100 revolutions and weighed. Loss in weight indicates the friability. The tablets are considered to be of good quality if the loss in weight is less than 0.8%.

▪ REVISION QUESTIONS ▪

I. Very short answer type questions ▪

Answer the following questions in brief.

1. Define a "Tablet".

2. Define the term "Excipient"
3. Name the different types of excipient used in formulation of tablets.
4. Why is diluent needed in certain tablet formulation?
5. Name the various diluent commonly used in tablet formation.
6. Give a list of granulating agents which are commonly used in moist granulation method.
7. Why is a binding agent required in certain types of tablets?
8. How is disintegrating agent helpful in disintegrating the tablets?
9. Why are lubricants needed as excipient in compressed tablets?
10. Name the various manufacturing defects in tablets.
11. Why is coating of tablets required?
12. What is the output of a rotary tablet machine?
13. Name the various tests which are carried to maintain the quality control of tablets.
14. What percentage deviation in weight is allowed in I.P. for tablets weighing 450 mg, 300 mg 200 mg, 60 mg and 250 mg?
15. Name the materials commonly used in enteric coating of tablets.
16. What are the materials used in film coating of tablets?
17. Define the term "Microencapsulation".
18. Name the various types of machines used for the compression of granules.

II. Short answer type questions

19. Write the advantages and disadvantages of tablets.
20. Classify the different types of tablets.
21. Write in brief about enteric coated tablets.
22. Why is the powdered drug not compressed as such into tablet form?
23. Give the advantages of film coating of tablets.
24. How does a disintegrating agent help to disintegrate a tablet in the stomach?
25. What are factors which cause variation in the percentage of medicament in each tablet?
26. Discuss in brief about moist granulation method.
27. Why are tablets still considered to be formulation of choice

among oral preparations?

28. What is "Capping"? How is this defect comes during preparation of tablets? How can this defect removed?
29. Why is coating of tablets done? What are the different methods of coating.
30. Mention the properties of an ideal enteric coated material.
31. What are the tests to be performed on the tablets to maintain its quality control. Write in brief about disintegration test for tablets.
32. Describe in brief about dissolution test for tablets.

III. Long answer type questions

33. Define a tablet. Classify the tablets. Write in brief about each type of tablet.
34. Discuss in detail the various steps involved in the manufacture of tablets.
35. Explain in brief the various types of excipients which are generally required in the formulation of tablets.
36. Write in brief about various defects which are commonly occurred during compression of granules into tablets.
37. Discuss in brief the various steps which are generally done to maintain the quality control of tablets.
38. Describe in brief on the following:—
    - (a) Friability test
    - (b) Disintegration test
    - (c) Dissolution test
    - (d) Enteric coating
    - (e) Film coating
39. Write short notes on the following:—
    - (a) Effervescent tablets
    - (b) Multicompressed tablets
    - (c) Lozenges
    - (d) Sustained action tablets
    - (e) Microencapsulation
40. Define the following terms:—
    - (a) Chewable tablets
    - (b) Sublingual tablets
    - (c) Capping
    - (d) Motting
    - (e) Picking and sticking

IV. Objective type questions

A. Completion type questions (Fill in the blanks with suitable word/words)

41. According to I.P., the shape of a tablet is defined as ________ ______________.

42. The film coating of tablets protects their medicaments from ________________.

43. The vaginal tablets are ______________ or ______________ shaped to facilite __________________ in the vagina.

44. The film coating of tablet is done to make them ____________ before sugar coating.

45. The dry cota tablet machine is used for the manufacturing of ______________, ______________ and ______________ tablets.

46. In capping, there is ______________ or ____________ removal of ______________ or ________________ portion of the tablet.

47. In picking the material is ____________ or ____________ by the upper punch from the ______________ surface of the tablet.

48. The disintegration time of uncoated compressed tablet is ______________.

49. The enteric coated tablets are disintegrated in the ____________.

50. Lozenges are made in such a way that it can exert a local effect in the __________ or ________________.

51. Buccal tablets are placed between the ______________ and ____________ or check so that they are dissolved and ______________ directly.

52. Pan coating technique is used for ________________ coating; ____________ coating and ______________ coating.

53. Press coating is done in ______________ tablet machine.

B. Matching type questions

54. Match the items of *Column I* with the appropriate items in *Column II*

Column I	*Column II*
A. Sugar coating of tablet	(*i*) is done to disintegrate it in the intestine.
B. The disintegration test is not required	(*ii*) for sugar coating, film coating and enteric coating.
C. Pan coating technique is used	(*iii*) in lozenge tablets and chewable tablets.
D. The enteric coating of tablet	(*iv*) is done to mask the unpleasant odour and taste of the medicament.
E. Lubricants	(*v*) improve the flow properties of the granules.
F. Glidants	(*vi*) reduces the interparticular friction.

KEY

12 1200 tablets/mt
14. 5, 5, 7.5, 10, 5
41. Circular with flat or convex faces
42. Atmospheric effect
43. Ovoid, pear, retention
44. Water proof
45. Multiple compressed, multicoloured press coated
46. Partial, complete, top, bottom
47. Removed, picked up, upper
48. 15 mts
49. Intestine
50. Mouth, throat
51. Gum, lips, absorbed
52. Sugar, film, enteric
53. Drycota rotary
54. A(iv); B(iii); C(ii); D(i); E(vi); F(v)

15

Processing of Capsules

Capsules are a solid dosage form in which the drug substance is enclosed in a water soluble shell or an envelope. A capsule shell is made from gelatin. The capsules are available both as hard capsule and soft capsule.

Advantages of capsules

A capsule is a very popular dosage form these days due to the following advantages:

1. The drugs having unpleasant odour and taste can be administered by enclosing them in a tasteless shell.
2. They are smooth, become very slippery when moist and can be easily swallowed.
3. They are economical.
4. They are easy to handle and carry.
5. The capsules release the medicament as and when desired in gastro-intestinal tract.
6. Capsules are made from gelatin and hence they are therapeutically inert.
7. They are attractive in appearance.
8. Capsules are available in various sizes and therefore suitable for all types of medicaments and for administering the desired quantity of medicament in a single dose.
9. Micro-capsulation provides the sustained released dosage form.

Disadvantages of capsules

1. The hygroscopic drugs cannot be filled in capsules. They absorb water present in the capsule shell and hence make it very brittle, which ultimately breaks into pieces.
2. The concentrated preparations which need previous dilution are unsuitable for capsules because it may lead to irritation in stomach if administered as such.

■ TYPES OF CAPSULES ■

Capsules are available in two types:

1. Hard gelatin capsules
2. Soft gelatin capsules.

1. Hard Gelatin Capsules ■

These are used for administration of solid medicaments. The capsule shell is prepared from gelatin, colour and titanium dioxide to make it opaque. It consists of two parts *i.e.* body and cap. The powdered material is filled into the cylindrical body of the capsule and then the cap is placed over it. The empty capsules are available in various sizes. They are numbered according to the capacity of the capsules. The number starts from 000 and goes up to 5. The approximate capacity of a capsule with respect to its number is given in the following Table:

TABLE 15-1

Capsule Number and its Approximate Capacity

Capsule number	*Approximate capacity in mg*
000	950
00	650
0	450
1	300
2	250
3	200
4	150
5	100

Excipients used in the filling of capsules While filling solid medicaments in a powder form into the body of a hard gelatin capsule, the following additives, too, are included in the formulation:

1. Diluents : The diluent is needed in certain cases where the quantity of the medicament is too small in bulk to get it filled in the smallest available capsule size. In such cases, diluent is added to bring the medicament upto the desired bulk. The commonly used diluents are lactose, mannitol, sorbitol, starch etc. The quantities of the diluent to be incorporated depends on the dose of the medicament and the capsule size.

2. Absorbents : Sometimes the medicaments are physically incompatible with each other *e.g.* eutectic substances or hygroscopic substances. In such cases, absorbents, such as oxides and carbonates of magnesium and calcium and kaolin are added to the powdered drug. These inert materials act as a protective sorbent.

3. Glidants : To ensure a regular flow of powder into the automatic capsule machine glidants are mixed with the medicaments. The various glidants used for this purpose are talc, magnesium stearate and calcium stearate.

4. Antidusting compounds : During the filling of capsules by an automatic filling machine, a lot of dust comes out of the machine. The dust is inhaled by the operator of the machine. It can pose a serious health hazard if allowed to be unchecked, especially, when the dust of the potent drugs is inhaled by the workers. To avoid this, some antidusting components, like inert edible oils, are added to the formulation.

Methods of filling the hard gelatin capsules

The capsules can be filled either by hand or by a semi-automatic device or by an automatic filling machine.

Capsule filling machine (Hand operated) It consists of:—

1. A bed having 200-300 holes
2. A loading tray having 200-300 holes
3. A powder tray
4. A pin plate having 200-300 pins
5. A sealing plate having a rubber top
6. A lever
7. A cam handle

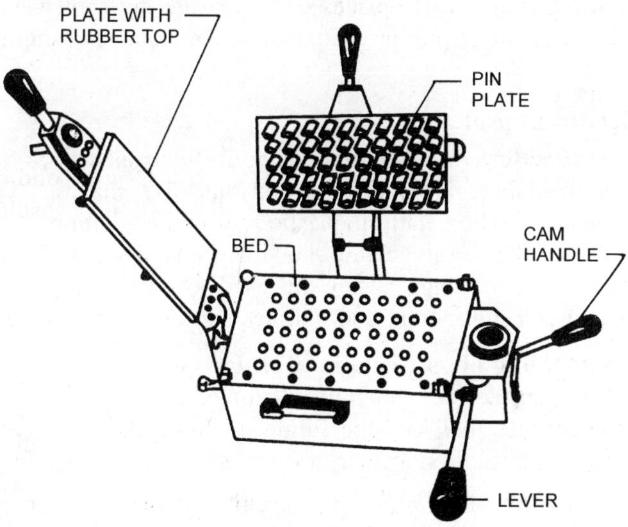

Fig. 15-1 Capsules filling machine (Hand operated)

The empty capsules are filled in the loading tray and it is placed over the bed. The cam handle is operated to separate the capsule caps from their bodies. The powder tray is placed in a proper position and filled with an accurate quantity of powder with scraper. The excess of powder is collected on the platform of the powder tray. The pin plate is lowered and the filled powder is pressed by moving the pin downwards. After pressing, the pin plate is raised and the remaining powder is filled into the bodies of the capsules. The powdered tray is removed after its complete filling. The cap holding tray is again placed in position. The plate with the rubber top is lowered and the lever is operated to lock the caps and bodies. The loading tray is then removed and the filled capsules are collected.

With a 200 hole machine, about 5000 capsules can be filled in one hour, whereas in a machine having 300 holes, about 7500 capsules can be filled in one hour.

Cleaning of capsules All capsules, whether they have been filled by hand or machine, will require cleaning. Small quantities of capsules can be wiped individually with soft cloth. But in case of large quantities, capsules are rotated or shaken with crystalline sodium chloride. The capsules are then rolled on cloth covered surfaces.

Sealing of capsules The capsules are then sealed, to ensure that the medicaments may not come out of the capsule due to rough handling. This can be done by banding them with molten gelatin, laid around the joint in a strip and dried. Capsules can be sealed by spot welding, by means of a heated metal pin, pressed against the cap and fusing it to the body.

2. Soft Gelatin Capsules

These are used for administration of liquid medicaments. Soft gelatin capsules are available in round, oval and tube like shapes. They are made from gelatin. The gelatin is plasticized by the addition of glycerin and sorbitol etc. The soft gelatin shell may contain a preservative to prevent the growth of fungi. They are used to enclose liquid medicaments—oils, suspensions, food concentrates and ophthalmic products.

Method of filling of soft gelatin capsules

Soft gelatin capsules are generally filled mechanically. The manufacturing of the capsule shell and the filling of the medicament take place simultaneously. Nowadays, a rotary machine is used for this purpose.

Rotary machine In a rotary die machine, the soft gelatin capsules are prepared and then filled immediately with the liquid medicaments.

The machine consists of two hoppers. Liquid gelatin mixture is placed in one hopper and the liquid medicament in the other hopper. There are two rotating dies which rotate in opposite directions (Fig. 15-2). When fluid gelatin mixture enters into the machine from the hopper, it produces two continuous ribbons. These ribbons come over

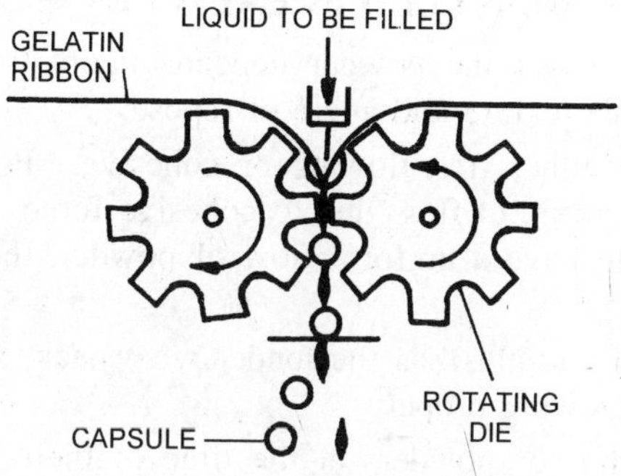

Fig.15-2 Rotary machine

the rotating dies from opposite directions and enter in between the dies. Thus, half shell of the capsule is formed. At this stage the measured quantity of the medicament is filled into it with the stroke of a pump. With the subsequent movement of the dies, the other half of the capsule is formed. The two halves of the capsules are sealed together by the

Differentiation between Hard Gelatin Capsules & Soft Gelatin Capsules

Hard gelatin capsules	*Soft gelatin capsules*
1. The hard gelatin capsule shell consists of two parts: (*a*) Body ; (*b*) Cap	1. The soft gelatin capsule shell becomes a single unit after sealing the two halves of the capsules.
2. They are cylindrical in shape.	2. They are available in round, oval and tube like shapes.
3. The contents of a hard gelatin capsule usually consist of the medicament or mixture of medicaments in the form of powder, beads or granules.	3. The contents of soft gelatin capsules usually consist of liquids or solids dissolved or dispersed in suitable excipients to give a paste-like consistency.
4. These are prepared from gelatin, titanium dioxide, colouring agent and plasticizer.	4. These are prepared from gelatin, plasticizer (Glycerin or Sorbitol) and a preservative.
5. Capsules are sealed after they are filled to ensure that the medicaments may not come out of the capsule due to rough handling.	5. Filling and sealing of soft gelatin capsules are done in a combined operation on machines.

heat and pressure of the rotating dies. The capsules formed are washed thoroughly and dried. These rotary machines are capable of producing between 25000 and 30000 capsules in an hour.

PROPERTIES OF THE POWDER TO BE FILLED IN CAPSULES

The flow properties of the powder depends upon its particle size, shape, density, surface texture and angle of repose.

Powders may be either free flowing or cohesive. Powders having very small particles, resist to flow due to cohesive forces between their particles. In order to have a uniform flow of powder, the fine powder should be removed.

Flat or elongated particles has the tendency to pack, whereas dense particles has a free flowing property.

The flow properties of powders at the time of their filling in capsules, can be increased by adding glidants like talc, stearic acid and magnesium stearate.

An inert edible oil is added to the material, which is to be filled in the capsules. This is necessary, because during the filling of the powder in the capsules on a large scale operation, the dust will come out of the automatic capsule filling machine. This may cause a serious health hazard for the workers.

Angle of Repose

The frictional forces in case of loose powder are measured by the angle of repose. The maximum angle which is formed between the surface of a pile of powder and horizontal surface is called the "angle of repose".

An angle of repose is defined by the equation:

$$\text{Tan } \varphi = \frac{2h}{D}$$

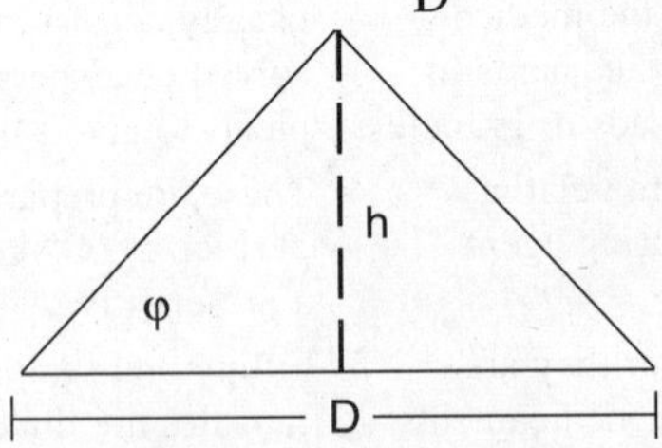

Fig. 15-3 Angle of repose

The angle of repose is not effected by the charge on the particles, but it depends on the shape of the particles. The angle of repose is quite high in case of the particles of a powder which are rough and have an irregular surface. Lubricants decrease the angle of repose to a certain extent but the excess quantity of the lubricant increases the angle of repose. The angle of repose depends upon the cohesive forces of the particles. The powder flows smoothly, if the angle of repose is 25°. The powder does not flow properly, if the angle of repose is more than 50°.

EVALUATION OF CAPSULES

The following tests should be carried out for evaluation of the capsules:

1. Uniformity of weight
2. Content of the active ingredients in the capsules
3. Disintegration test
4. Dissolution test.

1. Uniformity of weight : The 20 intact hard gelatin capsules are weighed individually and the average weight per capsule is determined. The capsule passes the test, if each of the individual weight is within 90-110% of the average weight. If the capsule does not come in this range, then the weight of the content of each individual capsule is determined and compared it with the average weight of the contents. As per the I.P., not more than two of the individual weights may deviate from the average by more than the percentage deviation shown in the following Table and none may deviate by more than twice that percentage.

TABLE 15-2

Average weight of capsule contents	*Percentage of deviation*
Less than 300 mg	10
300 mg or more	7.5

If the average net weight of two to six capsules deviates by the percentage deviation shown in the table and twice that percentage, determine the weight of the contents of additional 40 capsules and the average content of the 60 capsules. In a total of 60 capsules, not more than six of the capsules should deviate from average by more than the percentage deviation shown in the table and none by more than twice that percentage.

A similar method is followed for soft gelation capsules. After finding the individual gross weight of the capsules, the shells are carefully opened by cutting and the contents are removed by washing with a suitable solvent. After the shells have dried, they are weighed and the content weight of the individual capsule is calculated.

2. Content of active ingredients in capsules : It is applicable to all capsules which are used for oral administration. The assay is done as per the monograph of that drug in the pharmacopœia. An exception is made in those cases, where the assay method proves impracticable for the accurate determination of the drug contents of individual capsules. Generally, twenty capsules or such other number as is indicated in the monograph are used in the assay. The result lies within the range of the content of the active ingredients stated in the monograph. Where 20 capsules cannot be obtained, a smaller number, which must not be less than 5, may be used. In such cases, the limits specified in the monograph may be relaxed to the extent indicated in Table 15-3. The requirements of this table apply when the stated limits are between 90 and 110 per cent. For limits less than 90 or greater than 110 per cent a proportionately larger allowance should be made.

TABLE 15-3

Weight of medicament in each capsule	*Subtract from the lower limit for a sample of*			*Add to the upper limit for a sample of*		
	15	10	5	15	10	5
0.12 g or less	0.2	0.7	1.5	0.3	0.8	1.8
More than 0.12 g and less than 0.3 g	0.2	0.5	1.2	0.3	0.6	1.5
0.3 g or more	0.1	0.2	0.8	0.2	0.4	1.0

3. Disintegration test for capsules : The apparatus used for the disintegration test for capsules is the same as that used for the disintegration test for tablets.

Place one capsule in each of the six tubes of the basket and suspend the assembly in water maintained at 37° ± 2°. Do not use the discs for hard capsules except when the hard capsules float on the top of the water, the disc may be added. When testing soft capsules, discs may be used. Operate the apparatus for thirty minutes in the case of hard capsules and for sixty minutes in the case of soft capsules. The capsule passes the test if no residue is left on the screen of the apparatus or if a residue remains in the form of fragments of the shell.

If one or two capsules fail to disintegrate, repeat the test on twelve additional capsules so as not less than sixteen of the total number of eighteen capsules tested get disintegrated.

4. Dissolution test for capsules : The apparatus used for the dissolution test for capsules is the same as that used for dissolution test for tablets.

Place 1000 ml of water free from dissolved air having a temperature of 36.5° to 37.5° into the vessel. Place the specified number of capsules in the dry basket. Assemble the apparatus. Start the motor and adjust its speed to 100 rpm or such other speed as given in the monograph. Withdraw the required volume of the solution from the vessel after forty five minutes or after the period specified in the monograph. Filter and determine the amount of active ingredient present by the method given in the monograph. Repeat the complete operation four times.

The sample passes the test if the amount of active ingredients in the solution is not less than 70 per cent of the stated amount given in the monograph.

SPECIAL APPLICATIONS OF CAPSULES

1. Enteric-coated capsules : These capsules do not disintegrate in the stomach (acidic medium) but break-up in the intestine (alkaline medium). A special type of treatment or coating is given to the capsules so that these can pass unchanged through the stomach but get disintegrated in the intestine. On a commercial scale, a coating of cellacephate (cellulose acetate phthalate) and mixtures of waxes with fatty acids or their esters is given.

The following categories of drugs need enteric coatings.

(*i*) Drugs which cause irritation to the gastric mucosa and lead to nausea and vomiting.

(*ii*) Drugs which are destroyed by the gastric juices.

(*iii*) Drugs which are specially intended to act in the intestine *e.g.* amoebicides and anthelmintics.

(*iv*) Drugs which are required to produce a delayed action.

2. Sustained release capsules : In order to maintain a proper blood concentration of the medicament and reducing the number of doses per day, a capsule, containing numerous coated pellets, is administered that release the drug successively over a long period. The finely powdered drug is first converted into pellets. These pellets are treated with protective coatings that delay the release of the drug. The batches of pellets are mixed thoroughly and suitable doses are filled into capsules *e.g.*, a capsule may be filled with a mixture containing 30 per cent uncoated pellets for immediate release of the drug, 30 per cent each of the coated pellets, that release the drugs at 4-hour and 8-hour intervals and 10 per cent of the neutral pellets are used mainly to fill the capsule. In this way, there is a continuous release of the drug from a single capsule which maintains the concentration of the drug in the blood.

3. Rectal capsules : Soft gelatin capsules may be used as substitutes for rectal and vaginal suppositories. Various shapes and sizes are used for this purpose, but the pear-shaped form is commonly used. They are wider at one end which when inserted allows movement of the sphincter muscles to push forward the capsule into the rectum. Both liquid and solid medicaments can be filled into such capsules provided that the base used for incorporating the medicament is non-toxic, non-irritant and compatible with the capsule shell.

4. Capsules containing ophthalmic ointments : Nowadays ophthalmic ointments are packed in capsules. It is very important that the ophthalmic ointment is sterile. To keep such preparations sterile during their storage and later use, it is required to be filled in single-dose containers. The soft gelatin capsules are in common use for filling ophthalmic ointments. These capsules are intended for a single application to the eye. The capsule is punctured with a sterile needle and its contents are instilled into the eye and afterward the capsule shell is discarded.

■ PACKING AND STORAGE OF CAPSULES ■

Capsules should be packed in well-closed glass or plastic containers and stored at a temperature not exceeding 30°C. They should comply with such additional storage requirements as are specified in the individual monographs given in the pharmacopœia of India.

Capsules can be individually protected by enclosing them in a strip or blister packs. In strip packing, the capsule is hermetically sealed within the strips of an aluminium foil and/or plastic film. The contents are removed from the strip packs by tearing or cutting to separate the capsules. In case of blister packs, a press on the blister forces the capsule through the backing strip.

Generally, capsules have a longer shelf life in unopened glass bottles than in strip-packs but this is reversed, once a bottle has been opened.

■ REVISION QUESTIONS ■

I. Very short answer type questions ■

Answer the following questions in brief.

1. Define a "Capsule".

2. How are hard gelatin capsules made?
3. What are the excipients used in the filling of hard gelatin capsule?
4. Name the ingredients used in the preparation of soft gelatin capsule.
5. Write the approximate capacity in mg of a capsule having number 000, 00, 0, 1, 2, 3, 4, 5.
6. What is the output of hand-operated capsule filling machine, having 200 holes and 300 holes?
7. What is the output of rotary machine for filling soft gelatin capsule?
8. Define the term "Angle of repose".
9. What is the angle of repose for smooth flow of powder?
10. Write the equation of angle of repose.
11. Name the tests which are necessary for the evaluation of capsules.
12. How are enteric coated capsules made?
13. What are rectal capsules?
14. Why ophthalmic ointments are now-a- days packed in capsules?
15. What is the percentage deviation in weight allowed in the pharmacopoeia for a capsule weighing 420 mg?

II. Short answer type questions

16. What are the advantages and disadvantages of capsules?
17. Write in brief about hard gelatin capsule.
18. Describe in brief about soft gelatin capsule.
19. How will you differentiate between a hard gelatin capsule and soft gelatin capsule?
20. What are the excipients used in the filling of hard gelatin capsules?
21. What should be the properties of a powder to be filled in hard gelatin capsules?
22. What are sustained release capsules?
23. Write in brief about enteric coated capsules.
24. How are the capsules packed and stored?
25. Write in brief about dissolution test for capsules.

III. Long answer type questions

26. What are hard gelatin capsules? What are various numbers of capsules available in the market? Explain the construction and working of a capsule filling machine (hand operated).
27. Define the term "Capsule". Write the advantages and disadvantages of capsules. Differentiate between hard gelatin capsule and soft gelatin capsule.
28. Write in brief about a soft gelatin capsule. Describe the construction and working of a rotary machine with the help of labelled diagram.
29. What are various tests recommended by I.P. for the evaluation of capsules?
30. Write short notes on the following:
    (a) Angle of repose
    (b) Sustained release capsule
    (c) Enteric coated capsule
    (d) Capsule containing ophthalmic ointments
    (e) Hard gelatin capsule
    (f) Soft gelatin capsule

IV. Objective type questions

A. Completion type questions (Fill in the blanks with suitable word/words)

31. Capsules are available both as ________________ capsule and __________ capsule.
32. The ____________ drugs cannot be filled in hard gelatin capsule.
33. The hygroscopic/eutectic substances can be filled into hard gelatin capsule by mixing _________________ as absorbents.
34. The lubricants________ the angle of repose but excess quantities of lubricants ______________ the angle of repose.
35. In general the disintegration time of hard gelatin capsules is ____________ minutes and that of soft gelatin capsules is ____________ minutes.
36. The glidants such as __________ are used to ensure a __________ of powder into the automatic capsule machine.
37. The rectal capsules are ___________ shaped and are used as a substitute for _____________ and __________ suppositories.

B. Matching type questions

38. Match the items of *Column I* with the appropriate items in *Column II.*

Column I	*Column II*
A. Glidant	(*i*) required when quantity of medicament is small.
B. Protective coating on drug particles	(*ii*) used in enteric-coated capsule
C. Soft capsules	(*iii*) used to fill medicament in the form of powder, beads or granules.
D. Diluent	(*iv*) required to ensure a regular flow of powder into an automatic capsule machine.
E. Cellacephate	(*v*) used in a sustained release capsule.
F. Hard capsule	(*vi*) needed to fill liquid or paste.

KEY

5. 950, 650, 450, 300, 250, 200, 150, 100
6. 5000, 7500
7. 25,000 to 30,000
9. 25°
10. Tan Q = 2h/d
15. 7.5
31. Hard gelatin, soft gelatin
32. Hygroscopic
33. Oxides and carbonates of magnesium and calcium and kaolin.
34. Decreases, increases
35. 30 mts, 60 mts
36. Talc, magnesium stearate and calcium stearate, regular flow
37. Pear, rectal, vaginal
38. A(iv); B(v); C(vi); D(i); E(ii); F(iii)

16

Immunity and Immunological Products

The basic cause of disease in human beings is the invasion of pathogenic microorganisms (both bacteria and virus). The power of the body to resist the effects of the invasion of microorganisms is called *immunity*. The lack of such ability to resist infection caused by pathogenic microorganisms is called *susceptibility*.

FACTORS RESPONSIBLE FOR IMMUNITY

The following factors are responsible for producing immunity in human beings:

1. Phagocytosis
2. Antibody formation.

1. Phagocytosis : Phagocytosis means the ingestion of bacteria by certain cells of the body, which make them harmless. Phagocytosis is caused by two types of body cells:

(*i*) Cells of reticulo-endothelial system
(*ii*) White blood corpuscles (W.B.C.)

Cells of reticulo-endothelial system The cells of reticulo-endothelial system are present in the liver and spleen. These cells ingest the bacteria and make them harmless. From the blood circulation such harmless microorganisms enter lungs and disintegrate there.

White blood corpuscles (W.B.C.) W.B.C. help in the destruction of bacteria. When pathogenic bacteria enter the body, most of the leucocytes are carried to the infected area. They remain at the site of infection, ingest the bacteria and make them harmless. Leucocytes with their enclosed harmless microorganisms help in the formation of pus.

2. Antibody formation : The nature has given further protection from microorganisms by forming substances known as antibodies. Antibodies may be defined as substances formed in the body in response to the presence of foreign proteins and certain other materials in the tissues. The production of antibodies in the body is stimulated by the invasion of pathogenic microorganisms.

The nature of the antibodies depends upon the manner in which pathogenic microorganisms produce their harmful effects. For this purpose, pathogenic microorganisms may be divided into following two groups:

(*i*) Bacteria producing exotoxin
(*ii*) Bacteria producing endotoxin

Bacteria producing exotoxin During their growth, some pathogenic bacteria form poisonous substances which diffuse through the bacterial cell wall into the medium in which they are growing; hence called exotoxin. These toxins are carried to all parts, thus producing harmful effects. In response to these exotoxins, the human body produces antibodies to neutralise its effects. The antibodies which are capable of neutralising the exotoxin are called antitoxin.

Bacteria producing endotoxin The toxin produced by some pathogenic microorganism does not diffuse through the bacterial cell wall, but it remains in the cell of the bacteria and is therefore called endotoxins. Endotoxins are liberated only when the bacteria are disintegrated. In such cases, the antibodies produced should be very effective against such bacteria. They should reduce disintegration to the minimum, so that minimum amount of endotoxin will be liberated. These antibodies are named according to their mode of action. For example.

(*a*) *Opsonins* : Antibodies which make the bacteria more susceptible to phagocytosis are called opsonins.

(*b*) *Agglutinins* : Antibodies which cause agglutination of the bacteria are called agglutinins.

(*c*) *Precipitin* : Antibodies which precipitate the endotoxins are called precipitin.

(*d*) *Bacteriolysin*: Antibodies which prepare bacteria for lysis.

The blood and body fluids contain a substance known as complement. The complement is a complex of several components and is non-specific. It is responsible for the lysis. But it cannot act until the organisms have combined with their specific bacteriolysins (the effect is complementary) *i.e.*

Bacteria + specific bacteriolysin → No lysis
Bacteria + complement → No lysis
Bacteria + specific bacteriolysin + complement → Lysis of the bacteria

The antibodies which are antagonistic to viruses and rickettsia can be produced by the body but often with modes of action different from antibacterial antibodies.

TYPES OF IMMUNITY

IMMUNITY

- NATURAL IMMUNITY
  - * Age
  - * Race
  - * Species
  - * Individual
- ACQUIRED IMMUNITY
  - ACTIVE IMMUNITY
    - * Natural
    - * Artificial
  - PASSIVE IMMUNITY
    - * Natural
    - * Artificial

There are two types of immunities—*natural* and *acquired*

Natural Immunity

The resistance to disease is possessed by an individual due to the following factors.

1. Age : Majority of children in the age group between 2-5 years are susceptible to diphtheria disease, whereas adults are immune to it.

2. Race : While the Negroes have a high resistance to yellow fever, the white races are very susceptible to it.

3. Species : Men are susceptible to typhoid fever, whereas mice are immune to it. Fowls are immune to plague, whereas men are susceptible to it.

4. Individuals : Some persons have more resistance against cold and skin diseases than others.

Acquired Immunity

The immunity is acquired by an individual during his life time by producing antibodies in the body. It is of two types—*active* and *passive.*

1. Active immunity : The body takes an active part in the formation of antibodies to develop resistance against disease. It is of two types:

(*i*) *Naturally acquired active immunity* : The immunity is acquired as a result of infection by the causative organisms. The pathogenic microorganism may be virulent or attenuated. In the first case, the virulent bacteria may overpower the normal defensive measures and clinically the disease may occur. In the second case, the body resists the infection and clinically the disease may not occur. In both these cases, the infection stimulates the body to produce antibodies, which remain in the body to immune the person. This immunity may last for a life time *e.g.* smallpox, polio etc., or may be for a short duration *e.g.* pneumonia, influenza and gonorrhoea.

(*ii*) *Artificial acquired active immunity* : When the antigenic substances such as vaccines are introduced into the body, it stimulates the body to produce antibodies. Hence, immunity is produced in the body. The artificial active immunity is produced by injecting attenuated living microorganisms, dead bacteria and bacterial derivatives. The process is also called immunisation.

2. Passive immunity : The body does not play an active role in having immunity against a disease. Instead of this, it receives ready-made antibodies to produce immunity. This is of two types, namely—

(*i*) *Naturally acquired passive immunity* : Children aged less than a month, are generally immune to certain infectious diseases. This is because they have received the antibodies from the mother. These antibodies then gradually disappear and the children become susceptible to infectious diseases until they acquire active immunity either by natural or by artificial method. The antibodies of diphtheria, measles and chickenpox are transmitted in this way.

(*ii*) *Artificial acquired passive immunity* : The immunity is produced by injecting ready-made antibodies containing preparation (antiserum, sera) into the body. The passive immunity lasts for a short time only. Antiserum is injected for prophylaxis usually in the case of persons, who have been in contact with the infection, but have not yet shown the symptoms. In such cases immunisation is indicated.

IMMUNOLOGICAL PRODUCTS

Immunological products are the preparations which are meant for the prevention of diseases, such as, vaccines or for the treatment of diseases, such as, antitoxin and antiserum or for the diagnostic purposes *e.g.* bacterial toxin. These are biological products and are proteinous in nature except poliomyelitis vaccine.

Almost all immunological preparations are administered by parenteral routes except poliomyelitis vaccine which is administered by oral route. This is due to the fact that the immunological preparations become inactive when administered by oral route.

Storage of Immunological Products

Immunological products lose their potency on storage. The preservation of the potency of immunological products involves maintaining the viability of living cells or preventing the denaturation of protein *i.e.* antigens or antibodies. The reduction in potency is due to chemical changes which are directly proportional to the temperature of storage.

All immunological products are required to be stored below the room temperature. It is desirable that all immunological products should be stored in a refrigerator to ensure a reasonable life. The majority of immunological products (bacterial vaccines, bacterial toxoids and anti-toxin) should be stored in dark at temperatures between 2° and 8°C. The viral vaccines, such as, smallpox and oral poliomyelitis are more stable at or below their freezing point. The bacterial vaccines and antitoxins get deteriorated if they are allowed to freeze.

The required storage conditions are always mentioned on the label fixed on the container of the immunological products. To maintain the potency of these products, these instructions must be followed.

Light usually accelerates the decomposition of immunological products. So, they must be protected from it. The light resistant glass containers are not recommended for storage of immunological products because in that case it becomes difficult to detect the changes in the product.

Classification of Immunological Products

The immunological products can be classified into three categories on the basis of their use.

1. Immunological products for active immunisation : These include:—

(*a*) Bacterial vaccines
(*b*) Viral and rickettsial vaccines
(*c*) Toxoids.

2. Immunological products for passive immunisation : It includes preparations containing antitoxins and antiserum to produce passive immunity in human beings.

3. Immunological products as diagnostic agents : These are preparations containing toxins or preparations used for tuberculin and shick test.

IMMUNOLOGICAL PRODUCTS FOR ACTIVE IMMUNISATION

Bacterial Vaccines

Vaccines are preparations containing antigens which stimulate the body to produce antibodies. These antibodies make the person or animal immune to that disease for which the vaccine is given.

Bacterial vaccines are either sterile suspension of live or killed bacteria or sterile extracts of derivatives of bacteria. They may be simple vaccines prepared from one species or may be mixed vaccines prepared by mixing two or more simple vaccines from different species or varieties.

Bacterial vaccines may be prepared from cultures grown on suitable solid or liquid media. The bacteria are then suspended in normal saline solution or freeze dried.

Vaccines containing living bacteria may be prepared from strains which are avirulent for man but which can stimulate the production of antibodies active against pathogenic strains of the same species. The bacterial vaccines must be free from any substance known to cause toxic, allergic or other undesirable immunological reactions in man. *e.g.* B.C.G. vaccine.

Vaccines containing killed organisms may be prepared by killing the organism by chemical or physical means provided the antigenic potency of the vaccine is preserved *e.g.* cholera vaccine, pertussis vaccine and typhoid vaccine.

BCG Vaccine (Freeze-Dried)

BCG vaccine is in the form of white pellet which when reconstituted yields an opalescent suspension.

It is a freeze dried preparation containing live culture of the bacillus of calmette and guerin strain of *Mycobacterium tuberculosis*.

Preparation The bacilli are grown on a suitable culture media until 1 mg when plated out on suitable solid culture media, shows not less than 20 million colonies. The growth period should not be more than 14 days in any case.

After a suitable growth, they are separated by filtration in the form of a cake. The cake is homogenised in a grinding flask and suspended in a suitable sterile liquid medium designed to preserve the antigenicity and the viability of the vaccine. The suspension is transferred into the final sterile containers and freeze dried. Then containers are sealed so as to prevent contamination or deterioration of the vaccine. The vaccine contains no antimicrobial agent.

Storage Store in hermetically sealed light resistant glass containers at a temperature between 2° and 8°C. The reconstituted vaccine should be used immediately after its preparation.

Uses B.C.G. vaccine is used as an immunising agent which provides protection against tuberculosis.

Dose Prophylactic, 0.1 ml as a single dose by intracutaneous injection.

Cholera Vaccine

Cholera vaccine is a colourless, whitish or slightly coloured opalescent liquid.

IMMUNOLOGICAL PRODUCTS

- **FOR ACTIVE IMMUNISATION**
  - **BACTERIAL VACCINES**
    - BCG vaccine
    - Cholera vaccine
    - Pertussis vaccine
    - Typhoid vaccine
  - **VIRAL AND RICKETTSIAL VACCINES**
    - Smallpox vaccine
    - Yellow fever vaccine
    - Measles vaccine (live)
    - Poliomyelitis vaccine (oral)
    - Rabies vaccine
    - Typhus vaccine
  - **PREPARATIONS CONTAINING TOXOIDS**
    - Diphtheria toxoids
    - Tetanus toxoids
    - Diphtheria and tetanus vaccine (adsorbed)
    - Diphtheria, tetanus and pertussis vaccine (adsorbed)
- **FOR PASSIVE IMMUNISATION**
  - **ANTITOXINS**
    - Diphtheria antitoxin
    - Tetanus antitoxin
    - Gas-gangrene antitoxin
  - **ANTIVIRAL SERUM**
    - Rabies antiserum
  - **ANTIBACTERIAL SERUM**
  - **IMMUNE BLOOD DERIVATIVES**
    - Human normal immunoglobulin
    - Dried human normal immunoglobulin
- **AS DIAGNOSTIC AGENTS**
  - Schick test toxin
  - Old tuberculin
  - Tuberculin PPB

It is a sterile suspension of killed cholera vibrios (*Vibrio cholerae*) of a strains selected for high antigenic property and purity.

Preparation It is prepared from equal portions of suspensions of *cholera vibrios* of *Vibrio cholerae* Inaba and Ogawa strains selected for high antigenic efficiency. Either a single strain or several strains of each type may be used.

Each strain of cholera vibrios is grown separately on a solid medium for 24 to 48 hours. Bacteria are then washed with normal saline solution. The suspension of bacteria thus obtained is killed either by heating at 56°C for one hour or adding alcohol or other bactericide, such as, phenol or formaldehyde. All precautions must be taken to ensure that the antigenic property of the preparation is not destroyed. The preparation is then standardised so that 1 ml of vaccine contains not less than 12,000 millions bacteria. After adding a suitable preservative, it is transferred into final containers and then sealed.

The vaccine must comply with the tests for sterility and also the test for undue toxicity of vaccine.

Storage Store at a temperature between 2° to 8°C.

Uses It is used for immunisation against cholera. But it has a limited use as it has only about 50 % effectiveness for a period of 3 to 6 months. The vaccine does not prevent transmission of the disease.

Dose Prophylactic, initial dose 0.5 ml; second dose, 1 ml after an interval of 4 to 6 weeks.

Pertussis Vaccine (Whooping Cough Vaccine)

It is available as more or less turbid, whitish liquid nearly odourless or having faint odour due to antimicrobial agent.

Pertussis vaccine is a sterile bacterial suspension of killed pertussis bacilli (*Bordetella pertussis*) of a strain or strains selected for high antigenic efficiency.

Preparation It is prepared by culturing *Bordetella pertussis* in a suitable culture media. It is separated, washed and suspended in normal saline solution. The bacteria are killed either by heating or by adding some chemicals. The suspension is standardised. The vaccine may show abnormal toxicity in animal tests and this is removed by cold storage for upto three months.

Storage Store at a temperature between 2° to 8°C.

Uses For active immunisation of children against whooping cough especially when diphtheria and tetanus toxoids and pertussis vaccine (DPT) causes untoward reaction or is contraindicated.

Dose It is administered by subcutaneous injection in three doses of 0.5 ml, 1.0 ml and 1.5 ml at least 4 weeks apart.

Typhoid Vaccine

Typhoid vaccine is white or creamy white turbid liquid free from clumps.

It is a sterile suspension prepared from one or more strains of *Salmonella typhi* that are smooth and have the full components of O, H and VI antigens.

Preparation *Salmonella typhi* organisms are grown on a suitable culture media. The bacteria are killed by heat or by a bactericide such as phenol, formaldehyde or by a chemical such as acetone. It is then standardised, so that 1.0 ml of the typhoid vaccine contains not less than 1000 million bacteria (*S. typhi*). The vaccine must comply with tests for sterility and the test for undue toxicity for vaccine.

Storage Store at a temperature between 2° and 8°C. The vaccine must not be frozen.

Uses It is used for immunisation against infections caused by typhoid bacilli.

Dose Prophylactic, Initial dose 0.5 ml followed by second dose of 1.0 ml by subcutaneous injection after an interval of 4 to 6 weeks.

Viral and Rickettsial Vaccines

Viral and rickettsial vaccines are suspensions of viruses or rickettsial. They are prepared from infected tissue of blood obtained from artificially infected animals, from cultures in fertile eggs or from cell of tissue cultures. Viral vaccines may be live or killed. Live vaccines are usually prepared using attenuated strains of specific organism. Killed vaccine may be inactivated by suitable chemical or physical means. These vaccines may be freeze dried.

The following are some of the official viral and rickettsial vaccines—

Smallpox Vaccine (Freeze-Dried)

Smallpox vaccine (freeze dried) is almost white powder which reconstitutes to yield a viscid, straw coloured liquid. Smallpox vaccine contains living attenuated vaccinia virus. The vaccine is prepared by two methods:

1. By using animals
2. By using eggs

1. Preparation of smallpox vaccine using animals : Smallpox vaccine is prepared by using calves or sheep. The method of preparation can be divided into the following steps.

1. *Selection of animal free from disease* : Healthy calves or sheep are used for the production of vaccine. The animals are kept for 10-14 days in an isolated area under observation. They are given thorough examination to exclude communicable diseases.

2. *Preparation of animal for scarification* : The abdomen and flanks (the side of the body between ribs and ilium) are thoroughly scrubbed, washed and disinfected. The animal is taken to a special room where abdomen and flanks are shaved, scrubbed and then thoroughly disinfected.

3. *Inoculation* : Light incisions are made in the cleared skin without drawing blood with the help of scarifier. The scarified area is then rubbed with some of seed vaccine of known potency.

4. *Incubation* : During next 7-9 days pustules or vesicles form along the line of scarification. During the incubation period, every precaution is taken to keep the animal as clean and aseptic as possible. Any animal showing any sign of disease is rejected.

5. *Collection of viruses* : The animal is taken to the operation table and killed. A post mortem on the animal is made to check the absence of disease not detected otherwise. The abdomen and flanks are then washed with sterile water. The material in the pustules is withdrawn with the help of a sharp edged spoon under aseptic conditions.

6. *Purification* : The contents of pustules are mixed with equal volume of glycerin, cooled and then finely ground to form homogeneous mixtures. It is then stored for a long time at –10°C to remove impurities. This is an old method of purification.

Nowadays more efficient methods are used for purification such as—

(*i*) By using brilliant green.

(*ii*) By using trichlorofluro ethane.

(*iii*) By adding 0.4% phenol and then incubated at 22°C for 2 days.

(*iv*) By treating with a mixture of glycerin and peptone and then storing it at –10°C.

7. *Filling, sealing and storage* : It is filled into the final container under aseptic conditions and freeze dried. The containers are sealed to exclude the possibility of any contamination.

2. *Preparation of small pox vaccine by using eggs* : The eggs of hen are examined and selected for fertility. These eggs are incubated for 12 days. On the following day a small portion of the shell of the egg is removed and the chorio-allantoic membrane is inoculated with seed vaccine of known potency. The portion of the shell is replaced and sealed in position with a little melted paraffin wax. The eggs are incubated for 72 hours.

Using aseptic precautions the shell is removed and chorio-allantoic membrane is separated. It is placed in sterile saline solution at 0°C. Maintaining a low temperature, 50% glycerine is added. The material is ground to produce a homogeneous suspension. It is then transferred into final containers, freeze dried and sealed.

Storage Store at a temperature between 2° and 8°. The reconstituted vaccine may be expected to retain its potency for 7 days when kept at temperature between 2° and 8°C.

Uses Smallpox disease has been eradicated from India. The vaccine is indicated for a small number of laboratory workers who are likely to have contact with vaccinia virus and for travellers to those countries which require vaccination as a condition for entry.

Dose For prophylaxis of smallpox, about 0.02 ml is applied to the skin and inoculated by scarification or pressure.

Yellow Fever Vaccine ■

It is white, slightly yellow or light brown scale or powder. The vaccine is prepared before use by reconstitution of the dried vaccine with normal saline solution.

Yellow fever vaccine is an aqueous suspension of chick embryo tissue infected with the strains of yellow fever virus which is virulent for mice, but, although avirulent for man, still retains its immunising efficiency.

Preparation The virus is injected into the embryo of fertile eggs which have been incubated for 7-8 days. After incubation for further 3 to 4 days, the embryos are removed, pooled in batches, ground and then extracted with purified water. The suspension is then centrifuged. The supernatant liquid is separated, to which a suitable preservative may be added. It is then distributed into sterile glass ampoules and freeze dried. The air is removed from the ampoules or replaced by oxygen-free nitrogen before these are sealed.

Storage Yellow fever vaccine is stored in the dark at a temperature of approximately 0°C. The vaccine loses its potency within a few days if it is stored at a high temperature.

Uses It stimulates production of antibodies against yellow fever. Immunity develops within 7 days after vaccination and lasts for several years. Use of vaccine is recommended in the age group of 6 months or older, travelling or living in areas where yellow fever infection exists.

Dose Prophylactic, by subcutaneous injection not less than 1000 LD50 doses.

Measles Vaccine Live

The vaccine is white or nearly white friable mass.

Measle vaccine live is a bacterially sterile aqueous suspension of a suitable live, attenuated strain of measles virus grown on cultures of chick embryo cells.

Preparation The strain of attenuated measles virus used in the manufacture of live vaccine is tested on the monkeys for freedom from neuro virulence. The strain is grown with aseptic precautions in cultures of chick embryo cells. The chick embryos are derived from healthy and pathogens free flocks. Only primary cell cultures are used in the manufacture of the vaccine. The growth of virus is done within 14 days of inoculation. The virus suspension is tested for identity, sterility and for being free from adventitious viral agents.

The cultures which pass these tests are pooled and clarified to remove intact tissue cells. A suitable stabiliser is added and it is distributed into sterile containers, freeze dried and sealed. The vaccine must comply with the test for sterility and also the test for undue toxicity.

Storage The vaccine is stored in single dose in light resistant containers at a temperature between 2° and 8°C.

The reconstituted vaccine should be used immediately after preparation.

Uses It produces active immunity against measles in approximately 99% of recipients of a single dose. The immunity lasts for many years after vaccination.

Dose Paediatric, by subcutaneous injection, 0.5 ml of reconstituted vaccine.

Poliomyelitis Vaccine (Oral)

It is clear liquid which may have a reddish colour if phenol red has been used in its preparation.

Poliomyelitis vaccine (oral) is an aqueous suspension of one or a combination of 2 or 3 types of live attenuated strains of poliomyelitis virus tested for neuro-virulence on monkeys. It is a polyvalent vaccine.

Preparation It is prepared by using three strains of poliomyelitis virus type I, II and III. The virus of each type is grown separately in cultures of suitable tissue, with aseptic precautions. The tissue should be free from extraneous microorganisms and adventitious agents. Suitable antibiotic other than penicillin and streptomycin may be used in small concentration. The medium is maintained at a temperature not exceeding 35°C during the growth of the virus.

The growth of the virus is done within four days of inoculation and the virus suspension is tested for identity, sterility and freedom from adventitious viral agents. The final vaccine is prepared by combining the appropriate dilutions of three virus types and by the addition of approved bactericide.

The vaccine must comply with the tests for sterility and the test for undue toxicity for vaccine.

Storage The vaccine is stored in single dose or multidose containers in the frozen state at –28°C or below. When it gets melted, it should be kept at a temperature of 0°C to 40°C and used within three months. If stored at a temperature between 18°C and 20°C, it should be used within a few hours.

Uses It is used to produce active immunisation against poliomyelitis.

Dose The dose of each type of monovalent vaccine, 6 to 8 weeks apart and a fourth reinforcing dose of the trivalent vaccine, 8 to 12 months later.

Rabies Vaccine ▪

The vaccine is white, flocculent suspension in a clear liquid or white to brownish white turbid liquid.

Rabies vaccine is a sterile suspension in saline or other appropriate solution, isotonic with blood , of a suitable killed rabies virus in uncontaminated brain tissues from animals previously injected intracerebrally with rabies virus.

Preparation It is prepared by injecting sheep, rabbit, suckling rats, mice or other animals intracerebrally with rabies virus. The animals which show typical paralysis are killed. The brains are harvested under aseptic condition, tested for absence of bacteria and then finally suspended in sodium chloride injection or any other suitable liquid. The suspension is inactivated by using phenol or beta propiolactone or any other means until the virus will no longer infect mice. It is diluted to produce a vaccine of required strength. The vaccine is preserved by adding 0.01% *w/v* thiomersal. The pH is adjusted between 7.0 and 7.2. It is then transferred into sterilised containers and sealed. The vaccine must comply with the tests for sterility and the test for undue toxicity of vaccines.

Storage The vaccine should be stored in containers protected from light and at a temperature between 2°C to 8°C. It should not be used until the absence of live virus has been established.

Uses It is used as prophylactic against rabies, either for post exposure immunisation of person bitten by rabid animals or pre-exposure immunisation of high risk individuals.

Dose By subcutaneous injection 1 to 5 ml daily for 7 to 14 days according to the site and severity of the bite and the risk of exposure to infection.

Typhus Vaccine

Typhus vaccine is a sterile suspension of the killed rickettsia organisms of a strain or strains of epidemic typhus rickettsia (*Rickettsia prowazeki*) selected for antigenic efficiency.

Preparation It is prepared by injecting virulent rickettsia into the yolk sacs of fertile eggs which have been incubated for 7 days, within a period of 9-13 days after injection, the yolk sacs are collected under aseptic conditions. It is subjected to suitable treatment to liberate the maximum number of rickettsia. The material is suspended in normal saline solution. Formaldehyde solution is added, so that its concentration is between 0.2 to 0.5 %. The suspension containing 10 to 15 % *w/w* of yolk sac tissue is purified with solvent ether. The aqueous middle layer is collected and distributed into sterile containers under aseptic precautions. The vaccine must comply with tests for sterility and the test for undue toxicity for vaccines and sera. The vaccine can also be prepared from the lungs of small rodents in which rickettsial pneumonias have been caused by inhalation of large doses of virulent rickettsia or by giving intraperitoneal injections of rickettsia

Storage Store at a temperature between 2°C and 8°C.

Uses Typhus vaccine is used as a prophylactic agent to protect against epidemic typhus. It is not effective against endemic typhus.

Dose Prophylactic, by subcutaneous injection, 0.25 to 1.0 ml.

Toxoids

The pathogenic bacteria during their growth in a liquid media release a toxic substance known as "toxins". These toxins are disease producing and are antigenic in nature. These toxins cannot be used for immunisation purposes because of their toxicity. When these toxins are treated with chemicals, such as, formaldehyde, their toxic properties are destroyed without causing any significant loss of antigenic properties. These are called "toxoids". The following are some of the immunological products containing toxoids, which are official in Pharmacopœia of India (1966):—

Diphtheria Toxoid

It is a modified form of exotoxin of Corynbacterium diphtheriae.

Preparation A suitable strain of Corynbacterium diphtheriae is grown on a liquid medium at 37°C for 7-10 days or until the required toxin concentration is obtained. Phenol is added to kill the microorganisms and filtered through bacteria proof filters. The filtrate is a crude toxin. It is antigenic but highly toxic. So, the toxin is converted into toxoid which is less toxic in nature and has an equal number of antigenic properties as the parent toxin.

Four types of diphtheria toxoids are official, which are—

1. Formol Toxoid (*F.T.*) : It is prepared by adding about 1% formaldehyde into toxin and incubated at 37°C for 2-3 weeks. Due to undesirable reactions produced with this vaccine, it is not commonly used these days.

2. Toxoid Antitoxin Floccules (*T.A.F.*) : It is prepared hy adding Diphtheria antitoxin to formol toxoid and the floccules or precipitates thus obtained are suspended in normal saline solution. It has weaker antigenic properties but is free from harmful allergic reactions. Due to this reason it is useful for sensitive persons.

3. Alum Precipitated Toxoid (*APT*) : It is prepared by treating formal toxoid with an adequate quantity of potash alum which precipitates the diphtheria toxoid. The precipitates are separated, washed and suspended in normal saline solution containing some preservative.

4. Purified Toxoid Aluminium Phosphate (*PTAP*) : It is prepared by treating formol toxoid with hydrated aluminium phosphate.

Tetanus Toxoid

This is prepared from the exotoxin of *Clostridium tetani*, the specific toxicity of which has been completely removed by the action of chemical substances in such a way that it retains its antigenic properties.

Tetanus toxoid is available in the following forms—

1 Formol Toxoid (*F.T.*) : It is prepared by treating the sterile culture filtrate of *Clostridium tetani* with formaldehyde solution.

2. Alum Precipitated Tetanus Toxoid : It is prepared by adding alum to tetanus toxoid in simple solution in the proportion which is necessary to produce a suitable precipitate. The precipitates are separated, washed and suspended in normal saline solution.

Diphtheria and Tetanus Vaccine (adsorbed)

It is white turbid liquid, and is a sterile suspension of purified diphtheria vaccine and purified tetanus vaccine adsorbed on a mineral carrier, such as, aluminium hydroxide or aluminium phosphate.

Preparation The vaccine is prepared by mixing purified diphtheria toxoid containing not less than 1500 flocculation equivalents (1500 Lf) and purified tetanus toxoid containing not less than 1000 flocculation equivalents (1000 Lf) per mg of protein nitrogen with a suspension of aluminium hydroxide or aluminium phosphate in a normal saline solution. The vaccine contains a preservative other than any of the phenol or cresol groups. The vaccine must comply with tests for sterility and the test for undue toxicity for vaccines and sera.

Storage The vaccine is stored in single dose or multidose containers at a temperature between 2° and 8°. The vaccine should not be frozen.

Uses The vaccine is used to provide simultaneous active immunisation against both diphtheria and tetanus. The product should not be used after the age of 6 years since the diphtheria toxoid present in vaccine may cause undesirable reactions .

Dose The vaccine is administered in 3 doses by deep intramuscular injection. The first dose of 0.5 ml, followed by a second dose of 0.5 ml after 4 to 6 weeks, and a third dose of 0.5 ml 6 to 8 months later.

A dose of 0.5 ml of vaccine contains not less than 15 Lf of diptheria toxoid and not more than 5 Lf of tetanus toxoid.

Diphtheria, Tetanus and Pertussis Vaccine (adsorbed) ■

It is a white sterile suspension prepared by adsorbing formaldehyde treated diphtheria toxoid and tetanus toxoid on a mineral carrier, such as, aluminium hydroxide or aluminium phosphate and adding a suspension of killed *Bordetella pertussis*.

Preparation The diphtheria toxoid containing not less than 1500 flocculation equivalents (1500 Lf) and tetanus toxoid containing not less than 1000 flocculation equivalents (1000 Lf) per mg of protein nitrogen are added to a suspension of hydrated aluminium phosphate or aluminium hydroxide in a normal saline solution. It is then mixed with a quantity of suspension of killed *Bordetella pertussis* so that the final product contains not more than 20 x 10^9 bacilli in each dose. A suitable preservative other than of phenol or cresol group is added. The vaccine must comply with tests for sterility.

Storage It is stored in a single dose or multiple dose containers at a temperature between 2° and 8°C. The vaccine should not be frozen.

Uses The vaccine is used for simultaneous immunisation against diphtheria, tetanus and pertussis in infants and small children. The preparation is not generally used after the 6th year of age.

Dose The vaccine is administered in 3 doses by intramuscular injection. The first dose of 0.5 ml, followed by a second dose of 0.5 ml after 4 to 6 weeks and a third dose of 0.5 ml 6 to 8 months later.

A single dose of 0.5 ml contains not less than 15 Lf of diphtheria toxoid, 5 Lf of tetanus toxoid and 20×10^9 Bordetella pertussis.

IMMUNOLOGICAL PRODUCTS FOR PASSIVE IMMUNISATION

These products contain antibodies which produce passive immunity. These preparations are mainly used for the treatment of diseases or for immediate prophylaxis.

When a person or animal has been actively immunised either by natural or artificial means, the blood contains a large number of antibodies. If blood is withdrawn and allowed to clot, the antibodies are found in the serum. The serum is called *antitoxin*, if the antibodies it contains are antitoxin. The serum is called *antiserum*, if the antibodies in it are antibacterial antibodies. Similarly, if the antibodies are antiviral, the serum is known as *antiviral serum.*

A majority of the serum preparations are made from the serum of animals (Horse). The parenteral administration of products of animal origin may lead to immediate or delayed hypersensitivity reactions, such as, anaphylaxis and serum sickness. The products of human origin are preferred to those of animal origin because they rarely cause allergic reactions.

Antitoxins

The following are some of the antitoxin preparations which are official in the pharmacopœia of India—

Diphtheria Antitoxin

It is almost colourless, very faintly yellow or a slightly opalescent liquid.

Preparation The method of preparation of diphtheria antitoxin is divided into the following stages:—

1. Preparation of toxin for active immunisation of the horse : A pure culture of *Corynebacterium diphtheriae* is grown in a suitable culture media at 37°C for 4-7 days. After incubation, 0.5% phenol is added and the culture media is filtered through bacteria proof filters. The filtrate is a crude toxin. It is converted into toxoid.

2. Selection of the horse : Horses are selected because—

(*a*) They are easy to handle.

(*b*) They readily produce antitoxins because a horse resembles man in having a natural immunity against diphtheria.

(*c*) R.B.C. of horse's blood settles quickly and packs tightly. This property helps in the separation of the serum.

(*d*) Considerable volume of blood can be taken without any ill effects.

The horses selected must be free from disease. So the horses are kept in an isolated place for 7 days and then carefully examined. They are immunised against tetanus by injecting tetanus toxoid.

3. Active immunisation of the horse : To the selected horses diphtheria toxoid is given for active immunisation. The toxoid is given by i/m route in the gradually increasing doses. The first dose is of about 5 ml. Further injections are given at the interval of 2-3 days, by doubling the volume of the injection each time. In this way the volume of the last dose is about 600 ml.

4. Separation of serum from the horse : After a period of about 10 days from the final dose, the blood is collected under aseptic conditions to see if the adequate antitoxin has been obtained. Eight litres of blood is collected three times during a period of 8 days. After a rest of about 2 weeks, further injections of diphtheria toxoids are given as per the past schedule to stimulate the production of antibodies. Again 24 litres of blood is collected in three batches of 8 litres each. The process is again repeated, but it should not be more than 4 or 5 times.

After the collection of the blood, it is allowed to clot to separate the serum. The serum contains antitoxin along with other proteins, such as, beta-globulins, gamma-globulins and albumins. Antitoxins are largely associated with beta-globulin.

5. Concentration and refinement : Horse serum contains a high concentration of several other proteins which may cause undesirable reactions, such as, anaphylatic shock or serum sickness. So these undesirable proteins are separated by the following methods:—

Concentration by fractional precipitation The serum is mixed with sufficient ammonium sulphate to produce 25-33% saturation. The gamma globulin is precipitated, which is separated and discarded. More ammonium sulphate is added to produce 50% saturation. The beta globulin along with antitoxin is precipitated. The serum is filtered to remove liquid portion containing albumin. The filtrate is rejected. The precipitates are subjected to dialysis against sterile water to separate ammonium sulphate. The precipitates are passed into solution containing 0.3% tricresol or any other suitable preservative or the preparation is freezed dried without any preservative. The antitoxin activity of the original serum is increased only about 4 times.

Concentration by fractional proteolytic digestion The serum is diluted three times its own volume with normal saline solution. Pepsin is added and pH is adjusted to 4. It is incubated for about 2 days at 37°C. Gamma globulin is precipitated which is separated by filtration. The filtrate is subjected to special ultra filter. The transparent liquid is obtained which contains purified concentrated antitoxin together with beta globulin. In this way the antitoxin activity of the original serum is increased about eight times.

Diphtheria antitoxin has a potency of not less than 1000 international units per ml in the case of antitoxins obtained from horse serum and not less than 500 international units per ml for antitoxins obtained from other animals.

Storage It is stored in containers protected from light at a temperature between 2° and 8°C. It should not be allowed to freeze.

Dose It is administered by s/c or i/m injection in the following dose schedule:

(*i*) *Prophylactic* : 500 to 2000 international units
(*ii*) *Therapeutic* : not less than 10,000 international units

Tetanus Antitoxin ■

It is almost colourless or a very faintly yellow liquid.

Preparation It is prepared in the same way as diphtheria antitoxin. The toxin is obtained from *Clostridium tetani* which is used for active immunisation of the horse.

Tetanus antitoxin has a potency not less than 1000 international units per ml when intended for prophylactic use and not less than 3000 international units per ml when intended for therapeutic use.

Storage Same as diphtheria antitoxin.

Dose It is administered by s/c or i/m injection in the following dose schedule.

(*i*) *Prophylactic* : not less than 1500 international units.
(*ii*) *Therapeutic* : not less than 50,000 international units.

Gas-gangrene Antitoxin ■

It is almost colourless or a very faintly yellow liquid, free from turbidity. It is a preparation containing the specific antitoxic globulins obtained by purification from native serum and having the specific power of neutralising the a toxin formed by *Clostridium oedematiens* or *Clostridium perfringens*.

It has a potency of not less than 3750 international units per ml.

Storage Same as that of diphtheria antitoxin.

Dose It is administered by intravenous or intramuscular injection.

(*i*) *Prophylactic* : 10,000 international units

(*ii*) *Therapeutic* : not less than 30,000 international units.

Antiviral Serum

These preparations are antiviral and produce passive immunity *e.g.* rabies antiserum.

Rabies Antiserum

It is almost colourless or faintly yellow, slightly opalescent liquid free from suspended particles.

Preparation The suspension of dead rabies viruses are injected into healthy horses. After a specified time period, the blood is collected and by a suitable method, the gamma globulin is separated which contains antiviral antibodies (same as diphtheria antitoxin).

It contains the specific neutralising power equivalent to not less than 80 international units per ml.

Storage It is stored in single dose or multidose containers at a temperature between 2° and 8°. It is protected from light. It is not allowed to freeze.

Uses It is used along with vaccine for preventing rabies when a person is bitten in an area, such as, the head or neck by a rabid dog or any other rabid animal.

Dose By i/m or s/c injection, 40 international units per kg of body weight.

Antibacterial Serum

This type of serum is used to provide passive immunity to diseases caused by endotoxin producing bacteria, *e.g.* pneumonia, meningitis and typhoid. The serum contains antibacterial antibodies. The antibacterial serum or antiserum were used in the past but have now been replaced by chemotherapy.

These are prepared in the same way as antitoxins except that—

(*i*) The horse is injected with a dead or living suspension of the organism. The intravenous route is used because reactions often follow the injection of a large number of bacterial cells by i/m.

(*ii*) There are different methods of refining the sera.

Immune Blood Derivatives

These preparations produce passive immunity. The following are some of the preparations which are official in the Pharmacopœia of India:—

Human Normal Immunoglobulin ■

It is a transparent or slightly opalescent liquid, colourless or brownish in colour which on storage may show a slight granular deposits.

It is a sterile solution containing antibodies derived from human blood. It contains gamma-G globulins together with smaller amounts of other plasma proteins obtained from blood, blood plasma or blood serum of healthy donors.

Preparation It is prepared from the pooled material of a minimum quantity of 25 litres which is collected from about 1500 donors. The globulins are separated and are dissolved in a vehicle having a suitable preservative or a stabilising agent. It is sterilised by filtration through bacteria proof filter and distributed to the final containers which are then sealed.

Storage The preparation is stored in colourless, glass containers protected from light at a temperature between 2° and 10°C.

Uses The preparation is used for the prevention of measles in small children, infective hepatitis and rubella in a pregnant women.

Dose By intramuscular injection, a volume equivalent to the following amounts of protein is administered—

(*i*) For the prevention of measles : 250 mg for infants under one year of age, 750 mg for children aged three years and for attenuation of measles 250 mg.

(*ii*) For the prevention of rubella in pregnant women 750 mg.

(*iii*) For the prevention of infective hepatitis, 250 mg upto 10 years of age and 750 mg over 10 years.

Dried Human Normal Immunoglobulin ■

It is a white or slightly yellowish powder or a solid which is completely soluble in water for injection.

Preparation It is prepared from a pool of human normal immunoglobulin by freeze drying. The final solution of human normal immunoglobulin is distributed into its final sterile containers, freeze dried and the containers are sealed to prevent air, moisture and bacterial contamination.

Storage It is stored in a cool place, protected from light.

Dose Same as that of human normal immunoglobulin.

IMMUNOLOGICAL PRODUCTS AS DIAGNOSTIC AGENTS

These preparations which contain bacterial toxins, are used to test for:—

(*i*) Immunity or susceptibility to a particular infection
(*ii*) The presence of a particular disease
(*iii*) A proper degree of protection after immunisation.

The following preparations are official in the Pharmacopœia of India:

Shick Test Toxin

It is a clear, colourless liquid or very pale straw coloured liquid, which is used in the shick test to determine susceptibility to diphtheria.

Preparation It is a sterile filtrate, prepared from a culture of *Corynebacterium diphtheriae* grown on a sterile liquid medium. The filtrate contains diphtheria exotoxin. It is then diluted so that the test dose is contained in 0.1 ml or 0.2 ml with a diluent isotonic with blood and containing suitable bactericides and stabilisers. It is then distributed into sterile containers which are sealed in order to exclude the microorganisms.

Storage It is stored at a temperature between 2° and 10°C.

Dose 0.1 ml by intradermal injection.

Schick control or schick test control

It is a transparent liquid. Schick control is in fact a schick test toxin, the toxin of it is destroyed by heating at a temperature between 70° and 85°C for 5 minutes. The schick control must be prepared from the same batch of schick test toxin as that with which it is to be used.

Storage It is stored at a temperature between 2° and 10°C.

Dose 0.1 ml by interadermal injection.

SCHICK TEST

The schick test is performed to test the degree of immunity of an individual against diphtheria. Schick test toxin is injected intradermally into the left forearm and at the same time an equal volume of the Schick control is given into the right forearm. The arms are examined after 48 hours. The possible observations are given in Table 16-1.

From the above observations, it is concluded that a true positive persists longer than a pseudo reaction and therefore, the results at S. No. 3 and 4 below are re-examined after a week when the false results would have faded.

TABLE 16-1

S.No.	*Left arm (Schick test toxin)*	*Right arm (Schick control)*	*Explanation*	*Result*
1.	Large flushed area	No reaction	Toxin is not neutralised	Not immune
2.	No reaction	No reaction	Toxin is neutralised	Immune
3.	Large flushed area	Smaller flushed area	Not neutralised sensitivity to broth constituents	Not immune
4.	Small flushed area	Small flushed area	Neutralised, sensitivity to broth constituents	Immune and a pseudo-reactor

Old Tuberculin

It is transparent, yellow to brown viscous liquid, produced by the concentration of a fluid medium on which *Mycobacterium tuberculosis* has been grown.

Preparation The pure culture of Mycobacterium tuberculosis is grown on a liquid medium containing 5% *w/v* of glycerin or any other suitable medium at about 37°C for 6 weeks or more. The growth should be rapid and abundant. The culture is heated in steam for one hour and then filtered. The filtrate is concentrated to about 1/10th of original volume by evaporation under reduced pressure. A suitable preservative such as 0.5 per cent *w/v* of phenol is added and assayed. It is then diluted to produce a product of the required strength. The product is then distributed in sterile glass containers and sealed. The final product is free from live tubercle bacilli.

Old tuberculin contains not less than 100,000 international units per ml.

Storage The old tuberculin is stored at a temperature between 2° and 10°, protected from light.

Dose 0.1 ml by intradermal injection.

Tuberculin Purified Protein Derivative or Tuberculin (PPD)

It is colourless or pale, straw coloured liquid or cream coloured powder or pellet made from the heat treated products of growth and lysis of the *Tubercle bacillus* (*Mycobacterium tuberculosis* or *Mycobacterium bovis*).

Preparation *Mycobacterium tuberculosis* is grown in a suitable medium which is used in the preparation of old tuberculin. The culture is filtered through paper pulp to remove the bacteria and then subjected to ultra filtration to remove the glycerin and mineral salts. The protein precipitant, such as, ammonium sulphate or trichloro acetic acid is added to precipitate the protein which is purified and converted into freeze dried powder, hypodermic solution, tablets or a concentrated solution. The final sterile product is distributed into sterile glass containers and then sealed.

The liquid preparation contains 100,000 international units per ml and the freeze dried preparation contain 30,000 international units per mg.

Storage It should be stored at a temperature between 2° and 10°C, protected from light.

Dose 0.1 ml containing 10 or 100 international units by intradermal injection.

TUBERCULIN TESTS

The following tests are performed to detect the immunity or susceptibility to tuberculosis:—

1. Mantous test : A dose of 5 tuberculin units of old tuberculin or an equivalent dose of PPD is injected intradermally. After 48 to 72 hours the reaction of the test is observed at the site of the injection. A positive reaction consists of a raised indurated area. Induration measuring 10 mm or more is interpreted as positive for past or present infection with *Mycobacterium tuberculosis.* Induration of 5 to 9 mm is regarded as of doubtful significance. The induration of less than 5 mm is interpreted as a negative. The presence of erythema without induration is not significant.

2. Tine test : In this test, a stainless steel disc with four tines (teeth) 2 mm long is attached to a plastic handle. The tines are dipped into the solution of old tuberculin containing acacia and lactose as stabilisers. These are then dried and sterilised using ethylene oxide gas.

The uncovered disc is placed over the volar surface of the upper 1/3rd of the patient's forearm, over a muscle belly and a sufficient pressure is exerted on the plastic handle so that the four puncture site of the tines and a circular depression of the skin from the plastic base are visible. The criteria for evaluating the reactions are same as used in the Mantous test.

REVISION QUESTIONS

I. Very short answer type questions

Answer the following questions in breif.

1. Define the term "Immunity"
2. Explain the term "Phagocytosis"
3. Define the term "Opsonins".
4. What do you mean by "Immunisation"?
5. What do you mean by "Immuniological products"?
6. What is "Active Immunity"?
7. What is "Passive Immunity"?
8. Define the term "Vaccine".
9. Give some examples of bacterial vaccine.
10. Name the vaccines prepared from virus.
11. What are immunological products used as diagnostic agent?
12. How are immunological products classified?
13. Define the term "Toxoids".
14. What do you know about antitoxin and antiserum?
15. What are the diseases which produce life long immunity after its occurence?

II. Short answer type questions

16. What is the mechanism of producing immunity by cells of reticulo-endothelial system?
17. Explain how W.B.C. helps in fighting against a disease.
18. Write in brief about storage of Immunological products.
19. Discuss natural immunity in brief.
20. How are Immunological products classified? Give suitable examples of each class.
21. Write in brief about Phagocytosis.
22. Discuss in brief about B.C.G vaccine.
23. Give in brief the method of preparation of smallpox vaccine.
24. Write in brief about tetanus toxoid.
25. What is the storage condition of oral poliomyelitis vaccine?
26. Why are horses preferred in preparing diphtheria antitoxin?
27. How is the "Schick test" done?

28. Write in brief about "Mantous test".
29. Discuss old tuberculin in brief.
30. Write in brief about human normal immunoglobulin.

III. Long answer type questions

31. Define the term "Immunity". What are the factors responsible for producing immunity in human beings?
32. Define the term "Vaccine". What are different types of vaccines? Write the method of preparation of smallpox vaccine.
33. Explain the term "Immunological products". Discuss any two vaccines in brief.
34. How are antitoxin differs from antiseurm? Write in brief about diphtheria antitoxin.
35. What are the preparation which produce active immunisation? Explain different types of vaccines with suitable example. Write in brief about rabies vaccine.
36. Describe briefly:
    (*a*) B.C.G. vaccine
    (*b*) Smallpox vaccine
    (*c*) Measles vaccine (oral)
    (d) Diphteria antitotxin
    (e) Rabies vaccine
    (f) Human normal immunoglobulin
37. Differentiate between the following:
    (*a*) Antitoxin and antiserum
    (*b*) Toxin and toxoid
    (*c*) Exotoxin and endotoxin
    (*d*) Active immunity and passive immunity
    (*e*) Natural immunity and artificial immunity
38. Write short notes on the following:
    (*a*) Phagocytosis
    (*b*) Bacterial vaccine
    (*c*) Artificial immunity
    (*d*) Schick test toxin
    (*e*) Old tuberculin
    (*f*) Active immunity
    (*g*) Passive immunity

IV. Objective type questions

A. Completion type questions. Fill in the blanks with suitable word/words.

39. Antibiotics which make the bacteria more susceptible to phagocytosis are called ___________ .

40. Antibiotics which are capable of neutralising the exotoxin are called ___________ .

41. The children in the age group between 2-5 years are susceptible to ___________ disease.

42. Negroes have a high resistance to ___________ disease.

43. The serum containing antibacterial antibodies is called ________ .

44. A person who has already suffered from smallpox becomes immune to the disease because of ___________ .

45. The immunity produced by injecting a preparation containing ready-made antibodies is called ___________ .

46. The immunity which is produced by injecting a vaccine in the body is termed as___________ .

47. B.C.G. vaccine contains living culture of the ___________ strain of ___________ .

48. Pertussis vaccine is a sterile bacterial suspension of killed ___________ .

49. The majority of bacterial vaccines are stored at a temperature between ___________ to ___________ .

50. The cholera vaccine contains not less than ___________ bacteria per millilitre.

51. The human normal immunoglobulin is used for the prevention of ________ in small children and ___________ in pregnant women.

52. The schick test is done to detect the immunity or susceptibility to ___________ .

53. The mantous test is done to detect the immunity or susceptibility to ___________ .

B. Matching type questions.

54. Match the items of *Column I* with appropriate items in *Column II*.

Column I		*Column II*
A. Phagocytosis	(*i*)	produced by artificial acquired active immunity
B. Active immunity	(*ii*)	produced by injecting antiserum and antitoxin
C. Vaccine	(*iii*)	preparation containing ready-made antibodies
D. Bacterial vaccine	(*iv*)	produces immunity in human beings
E. Passive immunity	(*v*)	produced by injecting vaccine
F. Antiserum	(*vi*)	preparation containing antigens which stimulate the body to produce antibodies
G. Measle vaccine	(*vii*)	is bacterial vaccine and bacteria are grown on artificial media
H. B.C.G. vaccine	(*viii*)	is viral vaccine and virus are grown on chick embryo cells

KEY

15. Smallpox and Polio
39. opsonins
40. Antitoxin
41. Diptheria
42. Yellow fever
42. Diphtheria
43. Antiserum
44. Naturally acquired active immunity
45. Artificial acquired passive immunity
46. Artificial acquired active immunity
47. Bacillus calmette guerin, Mycobacterium tuberculosis
48. Bordetella pertussis bacilli
49. 2° to 8°C
50. 12000 millions
51. Measles, hepatitis
52. Diphtheria
53. Tuberculosis
54. *A*(*iv*); *B*(*v*); *C*(*vi*); *D*(*i*); *E*(*ii*); F(*iii*); *G*(*viii*); H(*vii*).

APPENDIX-I

Selected Technical and Medical Terms

Abortion is also called miscarriage. It means a separation and expulsion of the contents of the pregnant uterus before seven months of pregnancy.

Abrasive an agent that rubs off an external layer, such as dental plaque *e.g.* pumice.

Abscess a localised collection of pus.

Absorbent a drug that takes up chemicals into the drug substance, useful in reducing the free availability of toxic chemicals *e.g.* gastrointestinal absorbent.

Acne a chronic skin disease affecting the sebaceous glands of the nose, prehead, chin and chest.

Addiction a severe degree of drug dependence wherein the individual is compelled to take the drug.

Adsorbent a drug that binds chemicals to the drug surface, useful in reducing the free availability of toxic chemicals *e.g.* kaolin.

AIDS acquired immuno-deficiency syndrome *i.e.* a set of sign and symptoms which result from the destruction of the body defence by HIV.

Anaemia a condition in which there is decrease of haemoglobin and consequently of the oxygen carrying capacity of the blood.

Anaesthesia a condition, induced by drugs, in which there is complete loss of sensations.

Analgesic a drug that selectively suppresses pain perception without inducing unconsciousness *e.g.* aspirin, paracetamol, morphine sulphate.

Anaesthesia a condition, induced by drugs, in which there is complete loss of sensations.

Anaesthetic, General a drug that eliminates pain perception by inducing unconsciousness *e.g.* thiopental sodium.

Anaesthetic, Local a drug that eliminates pain perception in a limited body area by local action on sensory nerves *e.g.* procaine hydrochloride.

Androgen a hormone that stimulates and maintains male reproductive function and sex characteristics *e.g.* testosterone propionate.

Anginapectoris a condition in which there is pain in the chest and left arm.

Anorexic a drug that suppresses appetite usually by central stimulation of mood.

Antacid a drug that neutralizes excess acid in the stomach locally *e.g.* aluminium hydroxide gel.

Antagonist an agent or a drug which exerts an action opposite to that of another.

Anthelmintic a drug that kills or inhibits the intestinal worm *e.g.* piperazine citrate.

Antibacterial an agent that checks the growth of bacteria.

Antidote an agent that counteracts a poison.

Anticonvulsant a drug that arrests convulsions by inducing general anaesthesia.

Antidepressant a drug that selectively induces mood elevation, useful in treating mental depression.

Antiemetic a drug that prevents vomiting.

Antifungal a drug that kills or inhibits pathogenic fungi that causes infection.

Antigen a protein which is not normally present in the body but when introduced into the blood stream stimulates production of antibodies which reacts specifically with it.

Antihistaminic a drug that prevents response to histamine.

Anti-inflammatory a drug that inhibits the physiological response to cell damage (inflammation).

Anti-malarial a drug that kills or inhibits pathogenic protozoa that cause malaria.

Antipyretic a drug that lowers body temperature in the presence of fever.

Antiseptic a substance destructive to microorganism.

Antiserum a serum containing antibodies.

Antitussive a drug that suppresses coughing.

Anxiety a feeling of apprehension, uncertainty and fear.

Arteriosclerosis degenerative changes in arteries which is a part of the normal ageing process.

Arthritis an inflammation of the joint.

Artherosclerosis a condition in which cholesterol is deposited in the inner layer of the artery.

Astringent a mild protein precipitant suitable for topical application to toughen and shrink tissues.

Attenuated bacteria a bacteria which loses its virulence.

Bacteriostatic an agent which inhibits or retards the growth of a bacteria.

Bactericidal an agent which destroys the bacteria.

Bronchiodilator a drug that expands bronchiolar airways, useful in treating asthma and related conditions.

Bronchitis an inflammation of the bronchial tubes.

Carcinoma a malignant new growth made up of epithelial cells tending to infiltrate the surrounding tissues and give rise to metastases.

Carminative an agent that relieves flatulence.

Cathartic a drug that promotes defecation, or causes purgation.

Cirrhosis of the liver a liver disease in which there is destruction of the liver cells and over-growth of fibrous tissues.

Coitus a sexual connection per vaginum between the male and the female.

Colic an acute abnormal pain or pertaining to the colon.

Colitis an inflammation of the colon.

Coma a state of unconsciousness from which the patient cannot be aroused even by powerful stimulation.

Congenital means which exists at birth.

Congestion means excessive or abnormal accumulation of blood in a part.

Congestive heart failure a condition in which the output of the blood from the heart is inadequate for the requirements of body tissues.

Counter-irritant a drug which produces counter irritation.

Convulsion a series of contractions of the voluntary muscles.

Crystalluria the excretion of crystals in the urine producing renal irritation.

Cutaneous means pertaining to the skin.

Cyst any sac, normal or abnormal, especially one which contains a liquid or semi-solid material.

Decongestant an agent which relieves congestion or swelling.

Delirium a mental disturbance marked by illusions, hellucinations and cerebral excitement.

Dermatitis an inflammation of the skin.

Detergent a substance which combines the properties of wetting and emulsifying agents facilitating the removal of oil and dirt.

Diarrhoea an abnormally frequent discharge of more or less fluid faecal matter from the bowl.

Diuretic a drug that promotes renal excretion of electrolytes and water.

Dysentery a condition which is marked by the inflammation of the large intestines. There is pain in the abdomen with the passage of stools containing mucous and blood.

Eczema an inflammatory skin disease which is characterised by lesions.

Emetic a drug that induces vomiting, useful in removing unabsorbed, accidentally ingested poisons.

Emollient a topical drug used to soften the skin *e.g.* cold cream.

Encephalitis an inflammatory condition of the brain produced by an acute systemic infection.

Epilepsy a disorder of brain function usually associated with a disturbance of consciousness due to sudden and excessive discharge from the area of the brain.

Expectorant a drug that increases respiratory tract secretion, lowering its viscosity and promoting its removal.

Flatulence the presence of an excessive amount of gas in the stomach and intestine.

Gastroenteritis inflammation of the mucous membrane of stomach and intestine.

Glaucoma a condition of the eye, characterised by an increase in the intraocular pressure.

Glossitis an inflammation of the tongue.

Glycosuria the presence of an abnormally large amount of sugar in the urine.

Gonorrhoea a contagious inflammation of the genital mucous membrane transmitted chiefly by coitus.

Gout a disease in which there is recurrent attacks of acute pain and swelling of the joints.

Haemophilia a bleeding disorder in which there is tendency to excessive haemorrhage and prolonged coagulation time.

Hematopoiesis or Hemopoiesis the process of formation and development of various red blood cells

Hepatitis an inflammation of the liver due to an infection or toxic agent.

HIV Positive means the presence of antibodies against HIV (human immunodeficiency virus) in human body.

Hypertension a condition in which the blood pressure is above normal limits.

Hypnotic a central nervous system depressant that induces sleep.

Incubation development, especially of pathogenic microorganism within the body.

Insomnia an inability to sleep.

Instilled put in by drops.

Induration an abnormally hard spot at the site of injection.

Inoculation introduction of pathogenic microorganisms into the body to stimulate the production of antibodies and immunity *or* introduction of infectious material into culture medium in an effort to produce growth of the causative organism.

Jaundice a condition in which there is increase in bilirubin level above the normal range.

Lactation means the secretion of milk from the breast.

Lysis destruction of cells by a specific antibody.

Meningitis an inflammation of the meninges (surrounding membrane of the brain and spinal cord).

Migraine a recurring pulsating headache often unilateral associated with nausea or vomiting and visual disturbances.

Miosis a contraction of the pupil.

Mydriasis a dilation of the pupil.

Narcotic an agent that produces insensibility.

Narcotic a drug that induces sleep by reacting with central nervous system receptors.

Neuralgia means paroxysmal pain which extends one or more nerve.

Neuritis an inflammation of a nerve.

Obesity an increase in body weight beyond the limitation of skeletal and physical requirements as a result of excessive accumulation of fat in the body.

Oedema means the excessive presence of an abnormally large amounts of fluid inn the intracellular tissue spaces of the body.

Oestoarthritis a degeneration of the articular cartilages and formation of bony out-growths at the edges of the affected joints.

Oestomalacia means the weakness of bones due to decalcification (Vitamin D deficiency), there is pain in the skeleton.

Oestomyelitis an inflammation of the bones.

Peptic ulcer an ulcer which is found either in the lower end of the oesophagus, stomach, duodenum or the small intestine.

Pernicious donating a disease of severe character and usually fatal.

Pruitis means itching.

Prophylactic a drug tending to ward off disease for which it is given.

Pustule a pus-containing lesion of the skin, upto 5 mm in diameter.

Relaxant a drug that inhibits contraction of voluntary or involuntary muscles.

Rheumatism a disease marked by inflammation of the connective tissues structure of the body, especially the muscles and joints accompanied by pain in these parts.

Rubefacient a drug that induces mild irritation to produce reddening of skin.

Scarification the making of small superficial incisions on the skin with the help of scarifier.

Sedative a central nervous system depressant which, in suitable dosage, induces mild relaxation and reduces emotional tension.

Sinusitis an inflammation of a sinus.

Spasm means the contraction of involuntary muscles.

Spondylitis an inflammation of the vertebrae.

Suppressant a drug that inhibits the progress of a disease but does not cure it.

Systemically Acting Drug a drug administered for absorption into systemic circulation, from which the drug diffuses into all tissues including the site of therapeutic action.

Tachycardia an increase in the heart rate above 100 per minute.

Therapeutic pertaining to the treatment of disease.

Tonsilitis an inflammation of the tonsils.

Topically Acting Drug a drug applied to the body surface for local therapeutic action without drug absorption into systemic circulation.

Tranquillizer a drug used in treating varying degree of tension, anxiety and agitation without significant sedation.

Ulcer a lesion on the surface of the skin or mucous membrane.

Vasodilation means the dilation of blood vessels.

Virulence ability of an organism to produce infection in its host.

Vesicle a fluid-containing elevated lesion of the skin up to 5 mm in diameter.

APPENDIX-II

Recommended Readings

1. Ansel, H. C., *Introduction to Pharmaceutical Dosage Forms,* Lea and Febiger, Philadelphia.
2. Gennaro, A. R., *Remington's Pharmaceutical Sciences,* Mac Publishing Co., Easton, Pa.
3. Lachman, L., Lieberman, H. A., Kanig, J. L., *The Theory and Practice of Industrial Pharmacy,* Lea and Febiger, Philadelphia.
4. Staklosa, M. J., Ansel, A. C., *Pharmaceutical Calculations,* Lea and Febiger, Philadelphia.
5. Martin, A. N., Swarbrick, J. and Cammarata, A., *Physical Pharmacy,* Lea and Febiger, Philadelphia.
6. Denyer, S. P., Baird, R. M., *Guide to Microbial Control in Pharmaceuticals,* Ellis Horwood, New York.
7. Lawrence, C. A. and Block, S. S., *Disinfection, Sterilisation and Preservation,* Lea and Febiger, Philadelphia.
8. Banker, G. S. and Chalmers, R. K., *Pharmaceutics and Pharmacy Practice,* Lippincott.
9. Little, A., and Mitchell, K. A., *Tablet Making,* The Northern Publishing Co. Ltd., England.
10. Leon Shargel, et al, *Pharmacy Review,* A Wiley Medical Publication, John Wiley and Sons, Singapore.
11. Rawlins, E. A., *Bentley's Text Book of Pharmaceutics,* Bailliere, Tindall and Cox, London.
12. Cooper and Gunn's *Tutorial Pharmacy*, The Kothari Book Depot, Mumbai.
13. Carter, S. J., *Dispensing for Pharmaceutical Students,* Pitman Publishing Co. Ltd., London.
14. Mithal, B. M., *A Text Book of Pharmaceutical Formulation,* Vallabh Prakashan, New Delhi.
15. Jain, N. K., Sharma S. N., *A Text Book of Professional Pharmacy,* Vallabh Prakashan, New Delhi.
16. Schroff's *Professional Pharmacy,* Part III, Volume III, National Book Centre, Kolkatta.
17. Pharmacopœia of India.
18. British Pharmacopœia.
19. British Pharmaceutical Codex.
20. National Formulary of India.
21. Extra Pharmacopœia.

INDEX